Infection Control in the Everyday Built Environment

Raja Singh • Nirupam Madaan
Anil Dewan

Infection Control in the Everyday Built Environment

Springer

Raja Singh
Founder/Researcher
The Built
New Delhi, Delhi, India

Former Post Doctoral Fellow, Department of Environmental and Occupational Health, Dornsife School of Public Health, Drexel University, Philadelphia, Pennsylvania, USA

Nirupam Madaan
Department of Hospital Administration
All India Institute of Medical Sciences
New Delhi, Delhi, India

Anil Dewan
Department of Architecture
School of Planning and Architecture
New Delhi, Delhi, India

ISBN 978-981-95-8623-3 ISBN 978-981-95-8624-0 (eBook)
https://doi.org/10.1007/978-981-95-8624-0

This Springer imprint is published by the registered company Springer Nature Singapore Pte Ltd.
The registered company address is: 152 Beach Road, #21-01/04 Gateway East, Singapore 189721, Singapore

This book is dedicated to the countless patients and the healthcare workers who fought against COVID-19, a disease that spreads through the airborne route, and one which changed the human experience of living, forever.

The book is further dedicated to all the people who created the vast amount of evidence-based research for dealing with infection control and other public health measures in the built environment.

Prologue

My mother developed tuberculosis when my father was posted in Mumbai, one of India's most densely populated cities. Tuberculosis (TB) is often imagined as a disease of poverty or one that belongs to the past, long eradicated. In reality, its burden remains substantial and difficult to quantify because it frequently exists in a latent form—present within the body without manifesting the symptoms commonly associated with active disease, such as persistent cough. In my mother's case, the infection involved her lymphatic system. She eventually recovered, but thousands continue to die from TB every year.

For an architect applying to pursue research within a department of architecture, one must also become a convincing storyteller. To link a personal experience of TB to a credible research agenda in architecture required more than technical reasoning—it demanded persistence. Multiple rounds of persuasion, including personal meetings with members of the research committee, were necessary to explain the legitimacy of interdisciplinary inquiry linking architectural design with disease prevention. The National Education Policy of 2020, which today actively encourages interdisciplinary research, was not yet in place. Matters became even more complex when I proposed to study ventilation design for reducing airborne infection transmission—an area situated at the intersection of architecture, engineering, and medicine/public health. After initial hesitation, I was admitted as a doctoral scholar, albeit with the expectation that I would refine and strengthen my research protocol. At the time, none of us could have anticipated that within 6 months the world would confront a global pandemic.

The arrival of COVID-19 transformed abstract research questions into urgent societal concerns. Cities changed visibly: circles were painted on pavements to enforce distancing, masks became ubiquitous, and thermal screening and hand sanitization became routine. Yet the most striking validation of my research focus came from a quieter behavioral shift—people began opening their windows and switching off air-conditioners. The metro system in Delhi disabled its cooling systems in the early morning hours and relied exclusively on fresh-air ventilation. International studies rapidly emerged linking infection clusters to poor ventilation in buildings. During online research review meetings, the same reviewers who had once expressed reservations now remarked that the work addressed one of the most critical public health needs of the time.

When I began this journey, however, COVID-19 was not on the horizon. My initial exploration took the form of a modest write-up titled *Reduction of*

Hospital-Acquired Infection Through Architectural Design of Hospitals, which I shared with our known physician in the neighborhood. He spoke at length about clinical practices used by healthcare workers to reduce infections and expressed caution about the difficulty of establishing a direct link between architectural design and infection outcomes. Yet he also pointed me towards one category where the physical environment plays a decisive role: airborne infections. That conversation became a turning point. As I began to read further, it became clear that tuberculosis—still endemic in India and targeted for national elimination—was fundamentally an airborne disease.

A review of Indian scientific literature revealed that much of the work on TB transmission came from a small number of institutions, many located in Delhi. One such institution, the Lala Ram Swarup Tuberculosis Hospital, appeared both accessible and academically active. With some hesitation, I approached a senior professor there and explained my interest in the relationship between architecture and airborne infection. He listened carefully and, after a pause, handed me a pen drive containing one of his published papers on ventilation in tuberculosis facilities. That moment marked the true beginning of my academic engagement with dilution ventilation and its role in infection prevention.

Prior to the COVID lockdowns, I consulted another senior tuberculosis researcher while exploring methods to directly measure airborne bacterial presence. I had imagined experiments involving microbial sampling and ventilation intervention. He cautioned me firmly that working with TB bacteria without advanced laboratory facilities and biosafety protocols would be dangerous. Conventional plate-count methods, he explained, were not applicable to tuberculosis. This forced me to reconsider my approach and return to foundational literature.

The answer lay in a landmark study in which air exhausted from a tuberculosis ward was directed into an enclosure housing laboratory animals. Higher ventilation rates were associated with lower rates of disease transmission. This empirical relationship along with future work was later formalized into the Wells–Riley equation, which estimates the probability of infection based on parameters such as room volume and air changes per hour—both of which fall directly within the domain of architectural design. This insight proved transformative.

I designed a simple but meaningful experiment in my own living space. Using a carbon dioxide cylinder purchased from personal savings and a CO_2 monitor gifted by a friend, I evaluated ventilation performance using carbon dioxide as a proxy for exhaled air. Faster decay of indoor CO_2 concentrations after release indicated higher ventilation rates. The results were clear: opening doors and windows fitted with wire mesh significantly improved air change rates and reduced calculated infection probability. This led to a further hypothesis—that occupants often do not open windows even when they are technically operable. A field survey in an affluent South Delhi neighborhood confirmed this: nearly half of the homes lacked wire mesh on windows, effectively discouraging regular window opening. While this also implied a vulnerability to mosquito entry, my primary concern at the time was the public health implication for ventilation and infection risk.

Applying the Wells–Riley equation to real-world spaces demonstrated the profound impact of ventilation. For example, doubling ventilation in a library reduced theoretical infection probability from 76% to 51% during a 15-minute exposure scenario involving one infectious occupant. Similar analyses across multiple building typologies consistently showed substantial risk reductions through improved ventilation or increased spatial volume.

We often assume that ventilation is inherently beneficial, yet contemporary building practices may frequently undermine it—through sealed façades, non-operable windows, and the absence of basic features such as wire mesh. The evidence suggests that access to adequate ventilation should not be treated as a luxury or a design preference, but as a fundamental public health right embedded within the built environment.

Raja Singh

First author of this book; doctoral work supervised by Prof. Dr. Anil Dewan (third author), with academic guidance from Prof. Dr. Nirupam Madaan (second author), in the interdisciplinary field of built environment and public health.

Preface

In the midst of a plethora of literature available on Hospital Infection Control, this book takes a leap forward to address infection control, which has transformed from a medical topic to everyday lingo. The interventions that were focused earlier only in hospitals, that too in certain areas, are now an everyday reality in most public and private spaces. This book aims to demystify infection for everyday users, designers, and facility administrators. As a small example, this book will provide the right answers to airborne infection control by appropriate ventilation to spaces that may be using physical distancing, but may lack adequate ventilation.

This book also takes a bold step in addressing the issue of vector control of diseases through the built environment. As most vectors require source control and screening, this book will be a handbook for people who design and use spaces.

This book is based on evidence-based design, which is backed on research and endorsed by practitioners. This book will be like a handbook, which will sit on the shelves of most architects, space planners, interior designers, hospital administrators, facility managers of public spaces, and even owners of small clinics. This will address the multidisciplinary nature of the issue which aims at shaping the well-being of the building occupants.

This book is all the more relevant after the COVID-19 pandemic, which has suddenly brought the spotlight on the infection control requirements for buildings that previously were not in the infection control radar. The buildings that now fall in the purview are every building that may be public in nature.

In this book, we will cover mainly airborne and vector borne spread of diseases and the measures of their control.

Who is the book for?

Primary:

1. Architects, planners, and interior designers
2. Doctors and hospital administrators
3. Facility managers of public buildings

Secondary:

1. Researchers working in the area of infection control
2. Policymakers preparing master plans and building byelaws
3. General public, who wants a demystified understanding of infection control

Overall, this book may help architects at the undergraduate level and hospital administration students at the MD level. This may serve as a handbook for the design of everyday spaces.

Salient Features of the Book

- Demystifies infection control for the design of everyday buildings
- Addresses the key concerns regarding spread of vector borne of diseases, which is least discussed by building designers
- Forms the basis of the post pandemic design of spaces

New Delhi, Delhi, India Raja Singh
New Delhi, Delhi, India Nirupam Madaan
New Delhi, Delhi, India Anil Dewan

Acknowledgments

The authors would start by thanking the publishers, especially Dr. Naren Agarwal, Dr. Jagjeet Kaur Saini, Sinchu Mohan, Badri Nath and Thilageshwari S for their kind support before, during, and after the work on this publication. The authors would like to thank their home institutions for the kind support provided. Special thanks to all the researchers who provided their support in enriching the manuscript by providing their valuable inputs or research work or any other support. The first author would also like to especially thank his wife Sandeep Kaur and family members for the kind support through the book development process. The authors would like to thank the Indian Judiciary for passing directions related to airborne infection control in the built environment, especially dilution ventilation. This is particularly directed toward the Hon'ble National Green Tribunal and the Hon'ble Delhi High Court at New Delhi. Without their action, the work on infection control during COVID-19 as a matter of public policy and public action would have been decelerated if not been absent. The first and third authors particularly want to thank Advocate K.C. Mittal, Yugansh Mittal, Amit Shahi, and Keshav P Singh for taking important matters to the Hon'ble Delhi High Court and the Hon'ble National Green Tribunal. The first author would also like to thank Rajshekhar Pullabhatla and Group Captain P Aanand Naidu (retd.) for their kind support. Many thanks to all the faculty and staff at the School of Planning and Architecture, New Delhi; Drexel University, USA; and the All India Institute of Medical Sciences, New Delhi, for their perpetual support. This is foremost to the Directors and Deans of the institutes, and other Professors. Special thanks to Dr. Milind Umre; Dr. Vohra of National Institute of Tuberculosis and Respiratory Diseases; Dr. Amit Pandey of Translational Health Science and Technology Institute, Faridabad, India; Dr. Anjali Joseph of Clemson University, South Carolina, USA; Dr. Dyson Misquitta of Tata Institute of Social Sciences; Dr. Yuguo Li of Hong Kong University; Dr. Arthur L Frank of Drexel University; Dr Ulla Haverinen Shaughnessy of University of Oulu; Dr. Jugal Kishore of the Department of Community Medicine at Vardhman Mahavir Medical College & Safdarjung Hospital, New Delhi, among others. Special thanks to the heads of the Department of Architecture at School of Planning and Architecture, New Delhi, and the heads of Department of Hospital Administration, All India Institute of Medical Sciences, New Delhi. This includes Dr. Ranjana Mital and Dr. Mandeep

Singh. Special thanks to Dr. Hina Zia, Dr. T Srinivas, Dr. G Subbaiyan, Dr Rohit Kumar, Dr Malhotra Ruchi Mishra and Dr. Vijay Yeldandi. Thanks to the All India Institute of Medical Sciences, New Delhi. Many thanks to Dr. Satish Kaipilyawar for his support and the exposure he provided in real-life tuberculosis facilities for airborne infection control. Many others have been thanked in the chapters as we move forward.

Contents

About the Authors

Raja Singh has been working in the area of Performance-based design of buildings. This ranges from work at the master's degree level on fire performance of naturally ventilated buildings to the extensive work on Infection Control by Dilution Ventilation at the doctoral level. He has led classrooms for architects teaching infection control in the everyday built environment at School of Planning and Architecture, New Delhi, as a visiting faculty in the past. He has been a post doctoral fellow at the Department of Environmental and Occupational Health, Dornsife School of Public Health, Drexel University, PA, USA, for work related to toxic indoor pollutants and mesothelioma-related work in India. He has been the Secretary of the Scientific and Technical Committee STC34 on IEQ Guidelines of ISIAQ, an international body working on indoor air quality. He has published in internationally reputed journals like *Environment International*, *Indoor and Built Environment*, *Tobacco Prevention & Cessation*, *Cities & Health*, *Cureus Journal of Medical Sciences*, *Public Health Action*, the *International Journal of Tuberculosis and Lung Diseases*, the *American Journal of Industrial Medicine*, and the *International Journal of Environmental Research and Public Health*. He also serves as a peer reviewer for *Cureus*, *Cities & Health*, and *Indoor and Built Environment*, among others. He has addressed national and international gatherings and conferences and works actively in spearheading policy in this area. In the advocacy role, he has been pushing for airborne infection control in the built environment through judicial action in the Delhi High Court. He has also been Built Environment and Public Health Research Fellow at Tathatara Foundation, Bobbili, India, and Advisor, ISAC Centre for Built Environment Policy, India. He currently works as a researcher at The Built apart from being an independent consultant. He is also a research observer at the Department of Pulmonary Medicine at Safdarjung Hospital/VMMC, New Delhi.

Nirupam Madaan is currently Medical Superintendent at All India Institute of Medical Sciences, New Delhi. She is also a Professor in the Department of Hospital Administration. She has also been the in charge of the AIIMS COVID hospital during the pandemic. She was responsible for the planning and execution of the new RAK OPD, the upcoming National Centre for Ageing, the CSSD at AIIMS, New OPD in Provincial Hospital Jammu, waste disposal projects at grassroots-level rural hospitals in Jammu, and more. She has worked in settings from primary level healthcare to the largest tertiary level care hospital in India. She has worked previously in the National Rural Health Mission. At the policy level, she was responsible for implementing Moily Commission Guidelines at AIIMS and was one of the first professionals to give a wakeup call for the provision of oxygen to small towns of India. She is also the recipient of the prestigious Chevening Gurukul Fellowship. She is an alumna of Sher-E-Kashmir Institute of Medical Sciences, Srinagar.

Anil Dewan was former Dean of Research at the School of Planning and Architecture, New Delhi, which is an institute of national importance created by an act of Parliament. He has decades of experience in the healthcare design and planning sector, where he has led studios and designed healthcare facilities nationally and internationally. He also led an online teachers training program for architecture faculty on hospital design under the SWAYAM ARPIT Platform of the Government of India. He has previously worked for World Bank and is currently member of committees at NCDC, Delhi. He is also the Convener of MHD 14: P02 of the Bureau of Indian Standards dealing with Hospital Planning. He is an active speaker and is currently leading research in the area of Hospital Resilience, Indoor Air Quality, and other topics related to infection control through the built environment. He has previously authored a book on Hospital Design and Planning published by Springer Nature. He has been working on hospital projects internationally.

Abbreviations

μ	Micro
AAI	Airports Authority of India
ACH	Air Changes per Hour
ASHRAE	The American Society for Heating, Ventilation and Air Conditioning Engineers
AHU	Air Handling Unit
AC	Alternate Current | Air Conditioner
AIIMS	All India Institute of Medical Sciences, New Delhi
AIDS	Acquired Immune Deficiency Syndrome
BC	Before Christ
BRI	Building Related Illnesses
BS	Bio Safety
COVID-19	Corona Virus Disease, 2019
CEPT	Centre for Environmental Planning and Technology, University
CO_2	Carbon Dioxide
CFM	Cubic Feet per Minute
CMH	Cubic Meter per Hour
CPCB	Central Pollution Control Board
CPU	Central Processing Unit
CPWD	Central Public Works Department
CSSD	Central Sterile Supply Department
DOTS	Directly Observed Treatment, Short Course
DC	Direct Current
GBCI	Green Building Certification Inc.
GRIHA	Green Rating for Integrated Habitat Assessment
HVAC	Heating, Ventilation and Air Conditioning
HKU	Hong Kong University
HCW	Health Care Workers
HEPA	High Efficiency Particulate Absorbing, Filter
HVLS	High Velocity Low Speed, fan
ICU	Intensive Care Unit
IAQ	Indoor Air Quality
IGBC	Indian Green Building Council
IICC	India International Convention and Expo Centre, New Delhi

ISSN	International Standard Serial Number
ISBN	International Standard Book Number
ISHRAE	The Indian Society of Heating, Refrigerating and Air Conditioning Engineers
LEED	Leadership in Energy and Environmental Design
LTBI	Latent Tuberculosis Infection
MNRE	Ministry of New and Renewable Energy
MERV	Minimum Efficiency Reporting Value
MERS	Middle Eastern Respiratory Syndrome
NITRD	National Institute of Tuberculosis and Respiratory Diseases
NACO	National AIDS Control Organisation
NTBI	No Tuberculosis Infection
NIST	National Institute of Standards
NDIR	Non Dispersive Infrared
NBC	National Building Code, 2016
NIT	National Institute of Technology, Tiruchirappalli
OEM	Original Equipment Manufacturer
OSHA	Occupational Safety and Health Administration
OT	Operation Theatre
PVC	Poly Vinyl Chloride
PIL	Public Interest Litigation
$PM_{2.5}$	Particulate Matter of aerodynamic diameter of 2.5 micron
ppm	Parts Per Million
PHFI	Public Health Foundation of India
R_0	R-Nought, the basic reproduction number of a virus
SARS	Severe Acute Respiratory Syndrome
SCIE	Science Citation Index Expanded
SARS-CoV-1	Severe Acute Respiratory Syndrome, Corona Virus, 1, 2003
SARS-CoV-2	Severe Acute Respiratory Syndrome, Corona Virus, 2, 2019
SBS	Sick Building Syndrome
SPA	School of Planning and Architecture, New Delhi
STEM	Science, Technology, Engineering and Mathematics
TVOC	Total Volatile Organic Compounds
TB	Tuberculosis Disease I *Mycobacterium tuberculosis* bacteria
THSTI	Translational Health and Technology Institute
TERI	The Energy and Resources Institute
USD	United States Dollar
USA	United States of America
UVGI	Ultra Violet Germicidal Irradiation
UV	Ultra Violet
USGBC	United States Green Building Council
VOCs	Volatile Organic Compounds
VRV	Variable Refrigerant Volume
VRF	Variable Refrigerant Flow
XDR	Extensively Drug Resistant; Tuberculosis

List of Figures

List of Tables

Introduction, Relationship Between Built Environment and Public Health, Sick Building Syndrome, and How Small Changes in the Built Environment Lead to Big Public Health Effects

1

Raja Singh, Nirupam Madaan, and Anil Dewan

1.1 Introduction

1.1.1 The Indoor Species

It is a profound biological paradox that humanity, a species that evolved on the savannas of Africa under the open sky, has transformed into an organism that exists almost exclusively within sealed containers. We are no longer truly outdoor creatures; we are an indoor species. Contemporary exposure science and environmental epidemiology have converged on a singular, staggering statistic: in industrialized nations, human beings spend approximately upto 90% of their lives indoors [3, 37]. We are born in hospitals, educated in schools, productive in offices, and recover in homes or healthcare facilities. Consequently, the air we breathe, the surfaces we touch, and the microbial ecosystems we interact with are not determined by nature, but by the mechanical systems, architectural designs, and maintenance protocols of the built environment.

For decades, the primary focus of building engineering and architecture was structural integrity, aesthetic expression, and, following the energy crises of the 1970s, energy efficiency. The building was viewed as a shelter from the elements—a static envelope designed to keep the rain out and the heat/cool in. However, this

R. Singh
Founder/Researcher, The Built, New Delhi, Delhi, India

Former Post Doctoral Fellow, Department of Environmental and Occupational Health, Dornsife School of Public Health, Drexel University, Philadelphia, Pennsylvania, USA

N. Madaan
Department of Hospital Administration, All India Institute of Medical Sciences, New Delhi, Delhi, India

A. Dewan
Department of Architecture, School of Planning and Architecture, New Delhi, Delhi, India

R. Singh et al., *Infection Control in the Everyday Built Environment*,
https://doi.org/10.1007/978-981-95-8624-0_1

perspective may be dangerously incomplete. As we sealed our buildings to conserve energy, we inadvertently created incubators for biological and chemical contaminants, fundamentally altering the relationship between the host (humans) and the pathogen (microorganisms) [40, 70]. The built environment is not merely a passive backdrop to human life; it is an active determinant of public health, functioning as either a formidable shield against infection or a highly efficient vector for transmission.

The outbreak of the COVID-19 pandemic, caused by the severe acute respiratory syndrome coronavirus 2 (SARS-CoV-2), acted as a violent catalyst, forcing a global re-evaluation of this relationship. It shattered the complacent assumption that modern buildings were inherently safe. Instead, it revealed that our offices, schools, and transport hubs were often engineered in ways that may have facilitated, rather than mitigated, the spread of airborne infectious diseases [60, 82]. The realization that a building's ventilation rate, filtration efficiency, and airflow patterns could help contribute to dictate the trajectory of a pandemic has elevated the role of the building professional—the architect, the engineer, the facility manager—to that of a frontline public health worker. This book serves as a comprehensive guide to this new reality, bridging the chasm between the biological sciences and the building sciences to define the principles of infection control in the everyday built environment.

1.1.2 The Evolution of "Safe" Air

To understand the current imperative for infection control, one must examine the historical trajectory of indoor environmental quality (IEQ). Prior to the mid-twentieth century, the prevailing medical theory of "miasma" (bad air) drove architectural decisions, prioritizing high ceilings and large windows to dissipate foul odours believed to carry disease [47, 80]. While the germ theory of disease eventually displaced "miasma" theory, the intuition regarding ventilation remained valid. However, the energy crisis of the 1970s introduced a conflicting priority: conservation. To reduce reliance on fossil fuels, buildings were tightened. Infiltration was minimized, windows were sealed, and mechanical ventilation rates were slashed for some cases to as low as 5 cubic feet per minute (cfm) per person in some codes [27, 40].

This hermetic sealing of the built environment gave rise to a new class of occupational hazards. By the 1980s, clinicians began observing clusters of nonspecific symptoms—headaches, lethargy, mucosal irritation—among office workers, a phenomenon that came to be known as "sick building syndrome" (SBS) [20, 70]. While SBS was often associated with chemical off-gassing and insufficient oxygen, it also signaled a failure to manage the biological load of the indoor environment. The same reduced ventilation that trapped volatile organic compounds (VOCs) also trapped bioaerosols—bacteria, fungi, and viruses [57, 75].

Today, we stand at a new inflection point. The challenge is no longer just about preventing the chronic malaise of SBS, but about preventing acute, life-threatening transmission of pathogens like SARS-CoV-2, influenza A, and mycobacterium tuberculosis. Contemporary aerosol science increasingly rejects rigid droplet-airborne dichotomies, instead emphasizing a continuum of respiratory particle behavior governed by physical and environmental processes. The scientific community now recognizes that the distinction between "droplet" and "airborne" transmission is largely artificial, a relic of antiquated experiments from the 1930s and 1940s [61, 82]. We now understand that human expiratory activities—speaking, coughing, breathing—generate a continuum of particle sizes. While large droplets fall quickly, smaller aerosols (often defined as <5 μm or even up to 100 μm depending on environmental conditions) can remain suspended for hours, traveling far beyond the conversational distance of 1–2 m [42, 49]. This establishes the air distribution system of a building as one of the primary "highway" for infection.

1.1.3 Scope and Objectives

This text, *Infection Control in the Everyday Built Environment*, aims to deconstruct the complex interactions between building physics and microbiology. It is designed for a dual audience: the technical professional who needs rigorous data on air exchange rates (ACH) and filtration efficiency (MERV/HEPA), the public health official or the building owner who requires a strategic framework for risk mitigation.

In this first chapter, we lay the foundation. We explore the intrinsic link between the built environment and public health, tracing the epidemiological evidence that connects building parameters to disease outcomes. We delve into the definitions of building-related illness (BRI) and sick building syndrome (SBS), distinguishing these historical concepts from the urgent, pathogen-specific focus of modern infection control. Finally, we establish the critical distinction between managing a "sick building" (often a chemical-like VOCs or psychological issue) and managing "infection control" (a biological and physical issue), setting the stage for the technical interventions detailed in later chapters.

1.2 Relationship Between Built Environment and Public Health

1.2.1 The Biological Enclosure

The relationship between the built environment and public health is foundational, reciprocal (complementing each other), and often overlooked until a failure occurs. Historically, public health advancements were largely civil engineering achievements: the separation of sewage from drinking water, the reduction of overcrowding in tenements, and the ventilation of factories [45]. Today, as urbanization intensifies, the "indoor environment" has become the dominant ecosystem for the human species. The built environment functions as an external immune system; when it functions correctly, it excludes pathogens and pollutants, but when it is compromised, it amplifies exposure [2, 52].

The health of building occupants is determined by a complex interplay of physical, chemical, and biological factors regulated by the building's envelope and mechanical systems [84]. Research has consistently demonstrated that specific building parameters—ventilation rates, humidity levels, filtration efficiency, and surface materials—directly influence the incidence of respiratory infections, allergies, and systemic inflammation [21, 80]. For instance, a seminal multidisciplinary review by Sundell et al. [80] established a strong association between lower ventilation rates and increased rates of respiratory inflammation, infections, and sick leave. Conversely, higher ventilation rates (up to 25 L/s per person) have been positively associated with a significant reduction in the prevalence of SBS symptoms and improved productivity [76, 89].

1.2.2 The Physics of Transmission: Airflow as a Vector

The most critical intersection of building science and public health lies in the physics of airflow. In the context of infectious disease, the air in a room is a "vehicle". When an individual speaks or coughs, they release a turbulent cloud of multiphase gas (exhaled jet or puff of air carrying droplets) containing mucosal droplets [9, 49]. In a still room with poor ventilation, this cloud remains concentrated. However, the building's HVAC (heating, ventilation, and air conditioning) system dictates the fate of this cloud.

Recent studies utilizing computational fluid dynamics (CFD) and epidemiological trace-backs have proven that airflow patterns can facilitate long-range transmission. For example, the outbreak of COVID-19 in a Guangzhou restaurant was traced to the air conditioning unit's strong airflow, which recirculated the virus-laden aerosols across specific tables, infecting patrons who were well outside the range of direct contact [43, 46]. Similarly, Li et al. [42] demonstrated through mechanistic modeling that poor ventilation exacerbates even short-range transmission. Traditionally, it was believed that ventilation only mitigated long-range (room-scale) risk. However, Li's work revealed that in poorly ventilated spaces (<10 L/s per person), the concentration of aerosols in the "short-range" cone (less than 2m) remains dangerously high because the background air is not being cleared, allowing the expiratory jet to penetrate further and linger longer [12, 42].

This redefines the relationship between the building and the user. The building is not just a container; it is a dynamic fluid environment where thermal plumes from human bodies, forced air from diffusers, and infiltration through cracks interact to determine whether a pathogen is removed or delivered to a susceptible host. Therefore, public health policy cannot be separated from building codes. The "People Source and Room Source" rule used in older standards like to determine ventilation rates may now be viewed through the lens of infection risk, not just odor control [7, 42].

1.2.3 The Microbiome of the Built Environment (MoBE)

Beyond the transient transmission of viral pathogens, the built environment hosts a resident ecology known as the microbiome of the built environment (MoBE). Just as the human gut has a microbiome essential for health, buildings have complex microbial communities on surfaces, in dust, and in the air. These communities consist of bacteria, fungi, and viruses derived from outdoor air, soil, and the occupants themselves [26, 33].

Research into the MoBE has revealed that building design influences the diversity and composition of these communities. For instance, Kembel et al. [34] showed that architectural choices, such as the source of ventilation (natural vs. mechanical), significantly alter indoor bacterial diversity. Mechanically ventilated rooms tend to contain bacterial communities more closely related to human skin and oral cavities, whereas naturally ventilated rooms show a higher abundance of outdoor, soil-associated microbes [34, 51].

This has profound public health implications. The "Old Friends" hypothesis or hygiene hypothesis suggests that reduced exposure to a diverse array of environmental microbes in sanitized, sealed indoor environments may contribute to the rise in atopic diseases, asthma, and immune dysregulation in developed countries [26, 71]. Further, this may also mean that our infection surveillance measures based only on counts may be relooked at and now the diversity may be a key factor. We have engineered our buildings to be biologically "tight," effectively severing the link between the human immune system and the natural microbial world it co-evolved with. This creates a dichotomy in infection control: while we must aggressively eliminate pathogens like SARS-CoV-2 or *Legionella pneumophila*, indiscriminate sterilization of the indoor environment may have unintended negative consequences for long-term immune health and mental well-being [26, 78].

1.2.4 Socioeconomic Determinants: Housing as Health

The relationship between the built environment and health is also a story of inequality. The quality of housing and infrastructure is a primary social determinant of health. Inadequate housing—characterized by overcrowding, poor ventilation, dampness, and insufficient sanitation—may be a major driver of infectious and other disease transmission [16, 36]. Systematic reviews assessing housing conditions have repeatedly linked overcrowding and poor ventilation to the incidence of tuberculosis (TB) and COVID-19. For example, a review by J.Y. Lee et al. [39] highlighted that residents of inadequate housing, particularly the homeless and those in dense urban slums, face significantly higher risks of TB due to shared airspaces and lack of isolation facilities.

During the COVID-19 pandemic, these disparities were magnified. Lockdowns forced populations to remain indoors, increasing the exposure time to indoor pollutants and pathogens. In low-income settings, where multi-generational families often share small, poorly ventilated dwellings, the secondary attack rate of SARS-CoV-2 was significantly higher [36, 39]. Furthermore, the lack of "sick bays" or isolation rooms in standard residential architecture may have meant that once the virus entered a household, transmission to all members was almost inevitable. This underscores that building standards may not be merely technical specifications; they are instruments of public health equity.

1.2.5 The Role of Stress and Psychosocial Factors

The built environment influences health not only through biological and chemical exposures but also through psychosocial pathways. The concept of "sick building syndrome" initially focused heavily on chemical pollutants, but subsequent research revealed that psychosocial work factors—such as high workload, lack of control, and poor social support—are strong predictors of symptom reporting [15, 73].

However, the physical environment itself acts as a stressor. Poor lighting, excessive noise, thermal discomfort, and the perception of "stale" air trigger physiological stress responses that may be linked to weakening of the immune system, making occupants more susceptible to infection [19, 26]. Conversely, "bioinformed" design that incorporates natural light, views of nature (biophilia), and adequate fresh air may reduce cortisol levels and enhance immune function [3, 26]. Thus, infection control in the built environment may not solely be about "killing bugs"; it may be extended to designing resilient spaces that support the physiological and psychological robustness of the occupants, allowing them to better resist infection at all levels.

1.2.6 The Shift from Reactive to Proactive Building Health

Historically, the approach to building health may have been reactive. Interventions may typically have been triggered only after occupants complained or an outbreak occurred—fixing a leak after mold appeared or cleaning cooling towers after a Legionnaires' disease cluster. The paradigm advocated in this book is proactive resilience. This aligns with the concept of "infection-resilient environments" proposed by the Royal Academy of Engineering [72]. This approach demands that infection control be integrated into the lifecycle of the building, from the strategic definition and design phase through to construction, handover, and daily operation.

This shift requires a fundamental change in how we value buildings. As a starting point, we may consider moving beyond the metric of energy efficiency (Money/kWh) to a metric of health performance. As highlighted by Allen and Macomber [2], the cost of salaries in an office building dwarfs the cost of energy by a factor of 100. Therefore, a building that saves energy but makes its occupants sick or facilitates infection spread during a pandemic spread may by one lens be economically disastrous. Investing in robust dilution-based ventilation, advanced filtration (e.g., MERV 13 and/or HEPA), and air disinfection technologies (e.g., UVGI) may not be a sunk cost but a high-yield investment in human capital and public health stability [21, 72].

In the following sections, we will dissect the specific pathologies of the built environment—building-related illness and sick building syndrome—to understand the baseline from which we must improve.

1.3 Describing Building-Related Illness and Sick Building Syndrome

1.3.1 The Taxonomy of Indoor Malaise

To navigate the complex landscape of infection control in the built environment, one must first distinguish between the historical classifications of building-associated health problems. For decades, environmental health and occupational medicine have utilized two primary categories to describe adverse health effects linked to indoor environments: *sick building syndrome (SBS)* and *building related illness (BRI)*. While these terms are often used interchangeably in lay discourse, they represent distinct clinical and environmental entities with vastly different implications for diagnosis, remediation, and building operation. Understanding these concepts is a prerequisite for appreciating the shift toward the modern paradigm of "infection resilience."

1.3.2 Sick Building Syndrome (SBS): The Syndrome of the Unknown Definition and Scope

Sick building syndrome (SBS) is used to describe a situation in which the occupants of a building experience acute health- or comfort-related effects that appear to be linked directly to the time spent in the building, yet no specific illness or cause can be identified. It is a diagnosis of exclusion and association; the complaints may be localized to a particular room or zone or widespread throughout the building, but the defining characteristic is the temporal relationship with occupancy: symptoms worsen while in the building and improve or disappear shortly after leaving [10].

The World Health Organization (WHO) formally recognized the syndrome in 1982, estimating that up to 30% of new and remodeled buildings worldwide might be subject to complaints related to indoor air quality (IAQ). Unlike specific diseases, SBS defines a constellation of nonspecific symptoms. These are generally grouped into five major categories:

1. *Mucous membrane irritation:* Eye, nose, and throat irritation, including dryness, stinging, or hoarseness.
2. *Neurotoxic effects:* Headaches, mental fatigue, reduced memory, lethargy, drowsiness, dizziness, and irritability.
3. *Asthma and asthma-like symptoms:* Chest tightness, wheezing, and dry cough.
4. *Skin irritation:* Dryness, itching, and rashes (often on the face, hands, or neck).
5. *Chemosensory changes:* Complaint of unpleasant odors or altered taste.

The Historical Context of the "Tight" Building The emergence of SBS is believed to be linked to the energy crises of the 1970s [31]. In response to rising fuel costs, building codes and construction practices shifted dramatically toward energy conservation. Architects and engineers designed "tight" buildings with sealed windows and heavily insulated envelopes to minimize thermal loss. Ventilation standards may have been lowered to reduce the energy load required to condition outdoor air. For instance, the American Society of Heating, Refrigerating and Air-Conditioning Engineers (ASHRAE) Standard 62-1981 reduced the minimum outdoor air requirement for some cases from 15 cubic feet per minute (cfm) per person to 5 cfm per person in non-smoking areas (Note: Historically, ASHRAE Standard 62-1981 lowered recommended minimum outdoor air ventilation rates—for example, introducing values near 5 cfm (≈2.5 L/s) per person in certain non-smoking areas—reflecting energy-conservation priorities of the time rather than a health-based rationale, whereas earlier practice had relied on higher rates (≈10–15 cfm per person) for odor control and air quality.) This reduction in air exchange created a "thermodynamic bottle" where internally generated pollutants—volatile organic compounds (VOCs) from furniture, bioeffluents from people, and ozone from copiers—accumulated to levels capable of triggering sensory irritation.

Etiology: A Multifactorial Puzzle The etiology of SBS is notoriously multifactorial, rarely attributable to a single toxic agent [25]. Instead, it is the cumulative result of multiple low-level stressors.

- *Chemical Contaminants:* Volatile organic compounds (VOCs) such as formaldehyde, benzene, and trichloroethylene are ubiquitous in modern interiors, emitted by adhesives, carpeting, upholstery, and manufactured wood products. While individual concentrations usually remain below occupational safety thresholds, the "cocktail effect" of hundreds of VOCs can produce additive or synergistic sensory irritation [5]. For example, 2-ethyl-1-hexanol (2EH), a degradation product of the plasticizer DEHP found in PVC flooring, has been specifically linked to mucosal irritation and SBS symptoms in damp buildings [88].
- *Bioaerosols:* The presence of mold, bacteria, and their metabolic byproducts (endotoxins, mycotoxins) contributes significantly to SBS. Fungi like *Cladosporium*, *Penicillium*, and *Stachybotrys chartarum* colonize damp building materials and HVAC components, releasing spores and microbial volatile organic compounds (MVOCs) that trigger immune responses and irritation. Research has shown that maintaining indoor relative humidity between 40% and 60% is critical; levels outside this range can promote microbial growth or cause mucous membrane drying, both exacerbating SBS.
- *Psychosocial Factors:* It is critical to acknowledge that the built environment impacts the occupant psychologically as well as physically. High workload, lack of control over environmental conditions (temperature, lighting), and poor management relations have been consistently associated with higher reporting rates of SBS symptoms. This does not imply the symptoms are psychosomatic; rather, stress may lower the physiological threshold for irritation or alter the perception

of the environment. This "neurogenic switching" hypothesis suggests that chemical irritants triggering sensory nerves at one site (e.g., the nose) can lead to inflammation at a distant site (e.g., the head or skin) via the central nervous system, a mechanism potentially amplified by stress.

1.3.3 Building-Related Illness (BRI): The Specific Pathology Defining the Distinction

In contrast to the vague and subjective nature of SBS, *building-related illness (BRI)* refers to discrete, well-defined medical conditions with identified etiologies that can be directly attributed to airborne building contaminants [6]. BRI is mainly characterized by objective clinical findings—fever, leukocytosis, antibodies, or specific tissue pathology—and unlike SBS mostly, the symptoms of BRI may persist long after the occupant leaves the building and may require medical treatment.

Categories of BRI BRI generally falls into three pathologic categories: infections, immunologic diseases, and toxic reactions.

1. *Infections:* The most notorious example is *Legionnaires' disease*, caused by the bacterium *Legionella pneumophila*. This organism thrives in warm, stagnant water systems like cooling towers, humidifiers, and showerheads, disseminating via aerosols to cause severe pneumonia. Other building-associated infections include Pontiac fever (a milder, non-pneumonic form of legionellosis) and viral infections such as influenza or measles spread via ventilation systems.
2. *Immunologic/Allergic Diseases:*
   - *Hypersensitivity Pneumonitis (HP):* Also known as extrinsic allergic alveolitis, HP is an inflammation of the lung parenchyma caused by an immune reaction to inhaled organic dusts, fungus spores, or bacterial antigens (e.g., thermophilic actinomycetes) often found in contaminated HVAC systems. It presents with fever, cough, and shortness of breath, and can lead to permanent lung fibrosis if exposure continues.
   - *Humidifier Fever:* A flu-like illness caused by inhalation of aerosols from contaminated humidifiers, distinct from HP as it typically does not cause long-term lung damage and resolves spontaneously after exposure ceases.
   - *Building-Associated Asthma:* Occupants may develop new-onset asthma or experience exacerbation of pre-existing asthma due to indoor allergens (dust mites, cockroaches, molds) or irritants.
3. *Toxic Reactions:* Exposure to high levels of specific toxins, such as carbon monoxide from faulty combustion appliances or pesticides applied indoors, can result in acute systemic toxicity. While less common in office settings, cases of "mass psychogenic illness" have also been documented, where symptoms spread rapidly through a workforce via social contagion triggered by a perceived environmental threat (e.g., a strange odor), although this diagnosis is controversial and should be one of exclusion.

Table 1.1 Comparison of sick building syndrome and building-related illness

Feature	Sick building syndrome (SBS)	Building-related illness (BRI)
Symptoms	Nonspecific: headache, fatigue, irritation	Specific: fever, cough, muscle aches, pneumonia
Etiology	Multifactorial; often unknown	Defined; usually identifying specific agent
Onset	Gradual; linked to occupancy.	Acute or gradual; linked to specific exposure
Recovery	Rapid relief after leaving building	Prolonged; may require medical treatment
Prevalence	High (can affect >20% of occupants)	Low (affects specific susceptible individuals)
Diagnostic signs	None; diagnosis by exclusion	Clinical signs (X-ray, labs, antibodies)

Comparison: The Diagnostic Divergence The distinction between SBS and BRI is clinically and operationally vital [90]. If a patient presents with vague headaches and fatigue that clear on weekends, the investigation focuses on ventilation rates, VOC sources, and general hygiene (SBS). However, if a patient presents with pneumonia . (Legionnaires') or interstitial lung disease (HP), the investigation becomes a forensic hunt for a specific microbial reservoir within the building's infrastructure (BRI). Table 1.1 summarizes these key differences.

1.4 Creating a Distinction: From "Sick Buildings" to Infection Control

1.4.1 The Paradigm Shift: Comfort vs. Survival

While the concepts of SBS and BRI provided the framework for indoor environmental quality (IEQ) for the last 40 years, the COVID-19 pandemic has forced a radical re-evaluation of our priorities. Traditionally, building codes and standards (like older versions of ASHRAE 62.1) may have been designed primarily to control body odors and manage SBS-type comfort issues. If a building provided enough fresh air to keep CO_2 levels below 1000 ppm and prevented mold growth, it was considered "healthy."

However, SARS-CoV-2 demonstrated that a building can be fully code-compliant, thermally comfortable, free of mold and VOCs—and thus not a "sick building" in the traditional sense—yet still be a lethal environment for the transmission of an airborne pathogen. This necessitates a conceptual separation between *general IEQ* (focused on chemical pollutants and comfort) and *infection control* (focused on pathogen viability and transmission).

1.4.2 The "Everyday" Building as a Vector

Historically, infection control was the domain of hospitals (nosocomial infections). Specialized ventilation systems, negative pressure rooms, and high-efficiency filtration were reserved for healthcare settings. The current crisis has revealed that infection control is a fundamental requirement for the *everyday built environment*—schools, offices, restaurants, and public transport.

- *The Vector is Human, the Medium is Building:* In SBS, the building itself (materials, systems) is often the source of the pollutant (e.g., formaldehyde from carpets). In general infection control, the source is usually the human occupant. The building acts as the medium that modulates the transmission. The ventilation system, airflow patterns, and humidity levels determine whether an infectious aerosol exhaled by one person reaches the respiratory tract of another.
- *The "Healthy" Super-Spreader:* A key distinction is that SBS typically arises from chronic exposure to low-level irritants affecting many people mildly. Airborne infection can result from a single acute exposure event (e.g., a choir practice or a business meeting) in a room that otherwise feels "fresh" and comfortable. The "quanta" of infection (infectious dose) behaves differently than a chemical concentration; it is probabilistic in nature.

1.4.3 Moving Toward Infection Resilience

This book focuses on the "infection-resilient environment." This concept transcends the avoidance of SBS. It acknowledges that while we must continue to prevent dampness and chemical toxicity (traditional IEQ), we must overlay a new set of performance criteria designed to break the chain of infection.

- *Dynamic Response:* Unlike SBS management, which aims for a steady state of low pollution, infection control requires dynamic responsiveness—the ability of a building to "surge" its ventilation or filtration in response to increased biological risk (e.g., flu season or a pandemic wave).
- *The Invisible Threat:* SBS often presents with sensory warnings (odors, stuffiness). Viral aerosols are odorless and invisible. Therefore, infection control requires reliance on proxies (like CO_2 monitoring) and engineered defenses (UVGI, HEPA) that operate beyond human sensory perception.

In summary, while SBS and BRI taught us that buildings can harm us through accumulated pollutants, the modern challenge of infection control teaches us that buildings must actively protect us from each other. The following chapters will explore the technical means to achieve this protection without sacrificing the energy efficiency and comfort hard-won over the last half-century.

1.5 The Transmission Dynamics in Indoor Spaces: A Physics-Biology Interface

1.5.1 The Intersection of Disciplines

To effectively manage infection control within the everyday built environment, we must first dismantle the traditional silos that have separated medicine from building engineering. For decades, the medical community may have defined transmission routes based on clinical observations of infection patterns, while building engineers may have focused on thermal comfort and air distribution based on fluid dynamics. The separation of these disciplines led to a critical gap in our understanding of how pathogens navigate the indoor environment. The "infection-resilient environment" requires a new synthesis: one where the building is understood not merely as a static container for human activity, but as a dynamic fluid medium that actively transports, dilutes, or concentrates biological agents [72].

The fundamental premise of this book is that the transmission of infectious disease in buildings is governed by the laws of physics—specifically fluid mechanics, thermodynamics, and particle physics—just as much as it is by virology or epidemiology. When an occupant exhales, coughs, or speaks, they are not just releasing a pathogen; they are injecting a multiphase turbulent gas cloud into the room air [49]. The trajectory of this cloud, its rate of evaporation, and the ultimate fate of the infectious cargo are determined by the building's design and operation. Therefore, the architect and the facilities manager are, de facto, key players in the chain of infection prevention.

1.5.2 The "Continuum" of Airborne Transmission

One of the most significant paradigm shifts necessitated by recent pandemics is the re-evaluation of "airborne" versus "droplet" transmission. Historically, medical dogma relied on a binary classification: "droplets" were defined as particles larger than 5 microns that fell rapidly to the ground within 1–2 m, while "aerosols" were smaller particles that remained suspended [41]. This dichotomy underpinned decades of building standards, leading to the assumption that if people stood 2 m apart (social distancing), the building's ventilation system was largely irrelevant to direct person-to-person transmission.

However, recent research has dismantled this binary view in favor of a "continuum model" of transmission [41]. Empirical evidence and advanced modelling have demonstrated that human expiratory events produce a spectrum of particle sizes. Crucially, the behavior of these particles is not governed solely by gravity but by the complex interaction between the exhaled jet and the ambient room air. Li et al. [41] demonstrated that the distinction between short-range and long-range transmission is fluid. In a poorly ventilated room, the "short-range" hazard is magnified because the exhaled jet of pathogen-laden air does not dissipate; instead, it penetrates further and lingers longer, effectively bridging the gap between occupants. This finding challenges the adequacy of the traditional "people source" and "area source" framework embedded in older ventilation standards estimate outdoor air requirements using occupant density and floor area but does not explicitly account for short-range aerosol exposure, interpersonal distance, or airflow structure relevant to infection risk [7, 41]

Furthermore, the physical transformation of droplets plays a critical role. Upon leaving the humid respiratory tract, droplets immediately encounter the drier indoor air and begin to evaporate. A particle that leaves the mouth as a heavy "droplet" can rapidly evaporate into a lighter "droplet nucleus" (aerosol) capable of remaining airborne for hours [49]. The rate of this evaporation is dictated by the building's relative humidity and temperature. Thus, the building's psychrometric setpoints are not just comfort parameters; they are biological control variables that determine whether a pathogen falls to the floor or floats across the room [49].

1.5.3 The Building as a Vector

If we accept that the air is a primary vehicle for pathogen transport, the building itself becomes a potential vector. A "vector" in epidemiology is typically an organism (like a mosquito) that transmits a disease. In the built environment, the HVAC (heating, ventilation, and air conditioning) system can function analogously. If an air handling unit recirculates air without adequate filtration (e.g., just utilizing MERV 8 filters that capture dust but pass viral aerosols), it actively distributes the pathogen from a source room to unaffected parts of the building.

Historical outbreaks serve as stark reminders of this mechanism. The SARS-CoV-1 outbreak at the Amoy Gardens housing estate in Hong Kong demonstrated how defective plumbing traps and exhaust fans could aerosolize fecal-borne viruses and transport them vertically through a building's light wells/plumbings [41]. Similarly, investigations into outbreaks of Legionnaires' disease have repeatedly shown how cooling towers and water systems can amplify bacteria and disseminate them through air intakes [27]. These are not failures of medicine; they are failures of building physics and maintenance.

Consequently, the definition of a "healthy building" must evolve. It is no longer sufficient for a building to be free of toxic materials (asbestos, lead) and obvious moisture damage (mold). A truly healthy building must be "infection resilient," possessing the surge capacity to increase ventilation rates, improve filtration efficiency, and potentially deploy active air disinfection technologies (like UVGI, among others as needed, without harming health of occupants) during periods of heightened risk [63, 72].

1.6 The Microbiome of the Built Environment

1.6.1 The Indoor Ecosystem

While pathogens like SARS-CoV-2 garner immediate attention, they exist within a much broader biological context known as the *microbiome of the built environment (MoBE)*. Every building hosts a complex community of bacteria, fungi, and viruses that populate our surfaces, air, and water systems [81]. Research indicates that we spend 90% of our lives indoors, interacting constantly with this invisible ecosystem [26].

The composition of the MoBE is heavily influenced by architectural design. Kembel et al. [34] found that the source of ventilation—natural versus mechanical—significantly alters the indoor bacterial diversity. Mechanically ventilated spaces tend to be dominated by human-associated microbes (skin and oral bacteria), whereas naturally ventilated spaces show a higher abundance of outdoor, soil-associated microbes. This suggests that sealing our buildings has effectively created a "human-centric" microbial monoculture, isolating us from the environmental biodiversity with which we co-evolved [26].

1.6.2 The "Old Friends" Hypothesis and Building Design

This isolation has profound implications for public health, encapsulated in the "Old Friends" or "Hygiene" hypothesis. This theory suggests that the rise in chronic inflammatory disorders, allergies, and asthma in the developed world is linked to reduced exposure to the diverse immunoregulatory microorganisms present in the natural environment [26, 71]. By engineering increasingly sealed and highly sanitized indoor environments, we may be reducing exposure to environmental microbial diversity which may help our immune systems with the training inputs required to distinguish between harmless environmental antigens and dangerous pathogens.

Thus, infection control in the everyday built environment faces a delicate paradox: we must design buildings that can rigorously exclude or remove specific acute pathogens (like Coronavirus or Legionella) while ideally maintaining a connection to the beneficial or commensal microbial world. This nuance is often lost in "deep cleaning" protocols that sterilize environments indiscriminately. Future building standards may need to consider "bio-informed design"—strategies that not only ventilate to remove toxins but also incorporate elements (like biophilic design, natural ventilation modes, or even emerging experimental approaches such as probiotic or bio-active surfaces) that support a healthy indoor microbiome [26].

1.6.3 Fungal Contamination: The Silent Occupant

Within the MoBE, fungi represent a specific challenge related to building failure [30]. Unlike viruses which require a host, or bacteria which often require specific water conditions, fungi are uniquely adapted to exploit the building envelope itself. Cellulose-rich materials like drywall paper, ceiling tiles, and wood serve as nutrients, requiring only a transient source of water to support growth.

Research by Straus [79] and others has highlighted the correlation between "damp buildings" and adverse health effects, ranging from sick building syndrome (SBS) symptoms to specific building-related illnesses (BRI) like hypersensitivity pneumonitis. *Stachybotrys chartarum*, often termed "toxic black mold," has been shown to produce macrocyclic trichothecene mycotoxins that can exist on spores and be dispersed into the air [79]. The presence of such organisms is a direct indicator of building envelope failure—specifically, the failure to manage moisture. Therefore, infection control extends to the building facade, roofing, and plumbing; an effective moisture control in the building envelope is a critical first line of defense against fungi-related respiratory risks [48].

1.7 Defining the "Everyday" Built Environment

1.7.1 Beyond the Hospital

Historically, rigorous infection control standards (like ASHRAE 170) were reserved for healthcare facilities—operating theatres, isolation rooms, and ICUs. The "everyday" built environment—schools, offices, homes, retail spaces, and transport hubs—was governed by standards focused primarily on comfort and odour control. The COVID-19 pandemic shattered this distinction. It revealed that certain everyday settings, such as classrooms or choir practice rooms can, under conditions of poor ventilation, reach transmission risks comparable to those observed in some healthcare environments [41, 59].

This book focuses specifically on these *everyday environments*. They present unique challenges compared to hospitals:.

1. *Occupant Density:* Classrooms and public transport often have far higher occupant densities than hospital wards, increasing the "people source" load of potential pathogens.
2. *Lack of Monitoring:* Unlike hospitals, everyday buildings rarely have real-time monitoring of pressure differentials or air change rates.
3. *Behavioral Variability:* Occupants in offices or homes are not trained in infection control protocols (PPE usage, hand hygiene) to the same degree as healthcare workers.

1.7.2 The Socioeconomic Dimension of Indoor Air

We must also recognize that the quality of the indoor environment is a major stratifier of public health. Low-income populations are disproportionately likely to live and work in buildings with poor ventilation, older filtration systems, and higher occupant densities. Studies have shown that housing characteristics, such as overcrowding and poor ventilation, are significant risk factors for the transmission of respiratory infections like tuberculosis and COVID-19 [36, 39]. In this context, upgrading building infrastructure is not just an engineering task; it is a public health equity intervention. Providing "clean air" in public housing and schools is arguably as vital as providing clean water.

1.7.3 Moving Forward

In summary, the built environment is a complex, biologically active interface. It is the medium through which respiratory pathogens travel, influenced by the physics of airflow and thermodynamics. It is also a habitat for a vast microbiome that interacts with our immune systems. As we move to the next section of this chapter, we will delve deeper into the specific distinctions between "Sick Building Syndrome"—a condition of non-specific malaise—and the specific, quantifiable risks of infectious disease transmission, paving the way for targeted engineering solutions.

1.8 The Pathogen "Palette": Specific Agents in the Built Environment

1.8.1 The Biological Complexity of Indoor Air

While the physics of airflow provides the mechanism for transport, the biological nature of the particle determines the consequence of exposure. The "everyday built environment" is not a sterile void; it is a complex ecosystem teeming with microscopic life. To design infection-resilient environments, architects and engineers must understand the specific biological behaviors of the pathogens they are trying to exclude or contain. The "pathogen palette" of the indoor environment is broadly categorized into viruses, bacteria, and fungi, each interacting with building physics in distinct ways.

1.8.2 Viral Dynamics: Enveloped vs. Non-enveloped

Viruses are the primary drivers of modern pandemics and seasonal respiratory morbidity. From a building science perspective, the most critical structural classification of a virus is the presence or absence of a lipid envelope.

- *Enveloped Viruses (e.g., Influenza, SARS-CoV-2, RSV):* These pathogens possess a lipid bilayer derived from the host cell membrane. While this envelope contains the spike proteins necessary for infection, it is also the virus's "Achilles' heel." The lipid layer is susceptible to desiccation and disruption by detergents and environmental stressors. Research indicates that the stability of enveloped viruses in the air is highly dependent on relative humidity (RH). At intermediate humidity (40–60%), the evaporation of droplets concentrates salts and solutes that can disrupt this lipid envelope, reducing viability [83]. However, in dry air (<40% RH)—common in heated buildings during winter—the rapid desiccation can preserve viral infectivity by rapidly desiccating droplets into stable aerosol residues [49].

- *Non-Enveloped Viruses (e.g., Norovirus, Adenovirus, Rhinovirus):* These viruses lack a lipid envelope and consist of a robust protein capsid. They are notoriously resilient in the built environment, capable of persisting on dry surfaces for prolonged periods under favorable environmental conditions and resisting common disinfectants like alcohol and quaternary ammonium compounds [69, 86]. In the context of building design, non-enveloped viruses drive the need for rigorous surface hygiene and plumbing design, as they are frequently transmitted via the fecal-oral route and aerosolized during toilet flushing [86].

1.8.3 Bacterial Persistence: The Biofilm Reservoir

Unlike viruses, which are obligate parasites requiring a host to replicate, many bacteria can colonize the built environment itself. They find niches in cooling towers, showerheads, and humidifiers, forming *biofilms*—complex, slime-encased communities that protect them from desiccation and chemical disinfection [62].

- *Legionella pneumophila:* This bacterium is the causative agent of Legionnaires' disease and Pontiac fever. It thrives in warm, stagnant water systems within buildings. Its transmission is predominantly airborne but originates from the building's infrastructure (showers, cooling towers) rather than human occupants [27]. This distinguishes it as a classic "Building Related Illness" (BRI) where the building is the source.
- *Mycobacterium tuberculosis* (TB)*:* TB remains the archetype of airborne bacterial infection. Unlike *Legionella*, it is obligate human-to-human transmission(as Legionella comes from environmental sources unlike TB). The bacteria are carried in droplet nuclei that can remain suspended in room air for prolonged periods. Historical studies in hospitals and office buildings have demonstrated that standard ventilation rates are often insufficient to prevent TB transmission, necessitating the use of enhanced ventilation rates, administrative controls-outdoor waiting halls, ultraviolet germicidal irradiation (UVGI) or high-efficiency filtration in high-risk settings [63].

1.8.4 Fungal Contamination: The Toxic Home

Fungi represent a unique intersection between structural failure and human health. Fungal growth in buildings is almost always a symptom of moisture control failure—leaking roofs, condensation on thermal bridges, or rising damp.

- *Stachybotrys chartarum*: Often referred to in the media as "toxic black mold," *Stachybotrys* requires high water activity to grow on cellulose-rich building materials (drywall, ceiling tiles). It produces macrocyclic trichothecene mycotoxins, which are potent inhibitors of protein synthesis [48]. While *Stachybotrys* spores are heavy and sticky, not easily aerosolized, they can become airborne attached to dust particles during renovation or disturbance. Inhalation of these mycotoxin-laden particles has been associated in some studies with severe respiratory outcomes, including pulmonary hemorrhage in infants, although causality may be debated [18, 48].
- *Aspergillus* and *Penicillium*: These genera are common aeroallergens but can also cause invasive disease in immunocompromised individuals. Research has shown that *Penicillium* spores can induce allergic inflammation in animal models, suggesting a direct pathway for "damp building" asthma [14, 79].

1.9 The Neurogenic Hypothesis: Bridging SBS and Chemical Sensitivity

1.9.1 Beyond Toxicity: The Nervous System as a Sensor

A persistent challenge in building science is explaining why some occupants develop severe symptoms in "sick buildings" while others remain unaffected, and why symptoms sometimes persist even after the building is remediated. Traditional toxicology, which relies on dose-response relationships of specific poisons, often fails to explain the sick building syndrome (SBS) or multiple chemical sensitivity (MCS). To understand these phenomena, we must look to *neurogenic inflammation*.

1.9.2 The Common Chemical Sense

Humans possess a "common chemical sense" mediated by the trigeminal nerve (Cranial Nerve V), distinct from the olfactory nerve (smell). This system detects irritants and protects the airway by triggering reflexes like coughing, sneezing, and breath-holding. However, research by Meggs [53] and others suggests that chronic exposure to low-level volatile organic compounds (VOCs) and irritants in indoor air can sensitize this neural pathway.

- *Neurogenic Switching:* Ideally, inflammation is a localized response. However, Meggs [54] proposed the hypothesis of "neurogenic switching," where a chemical stimulus at one site (e.g., the nasal mucosa irritated by formaldehyde) triggers an inflammatory response at a distant site (e.g., a headache or skin rash) via the central nervous system. This mechanism helps explain the protean nature of SBS symptoms, where occupants report diverse systemic issues ranging from fatigue to joint pain [8, 54].

- *C-Fiber Activation:* The sensory nerves involved are often slow-velocity C-fibers. Upon stimulation by indoor pollutants (tobacco smoke, solvents), these nerves release neuropeptides like substance P and calcitonin gene-related peptide (CGRP). These neuropeptides induce vasodilation, plasma protein extravasation (edema), and the recruitment of inflammatory cells [8, 53].

1.9.3 The "Remodeling" of the Airway

Crucially, biopsy studies of patients with chemical sensitivities have revealed objective pathological changes in the nasal mucosa, including defects in tight junctions between epithelial cells, glandular hyperplasia, and proliferation of sensory nerve fibers [55]. This suggests a positive feedback loop: an initial acute exposure (e.g., a chemical spill or a new building off-gassing) damages the epithelial barrier, allowing lower levels of irritants to penetrate and stimulate nerve endings, which in turn release more inflammatory neuropeptides, perpetuating the damage [55]. This biological reality refutes the dismissal of SBS as merely "psychogenic" or "mass hysteria." While psychosocial stress plays a role in symptom reporting, there is a tangible, physiological basis for the hypersensitivity observed in building occupants exposed to the "chemical soup" of modern interiors [15, 40].

1.10 The Fomite-Aerosol Continuum: A Re-evaluation

1.10.1 The Surface as a Storage Medium

For decades, infection control focused heavily on *fomites*—inanimate surfaces contaminated with pathogens. The logic was visual and intuitive: we touch surfaces, then our faces. Indeed, pathogens like *Staphylococcus aureus* (including MRSA) and Norovirus are readily transmitted via surfaces. However, the SARS-CoV-2 pandemic forced a re-evaluation of the hierarchy of transmission. While viral RNA is frequently found on hospital surfaces (bed rails, door handles), the recovery of *viable* (infectious) virus is significantly rarer [67]. This suggests that while surfaces are a reservoir, their role in the transmission of respiratory viruses may be secondary to the airborne route, particularly in non-hospital settings.

1.10.2 Re-aerosolization: The Hidden Vector

A critical and often overlooked mechanism is *re-aerosolization*. Pathogens that have settled on floors or surfaces do not necessarily stay there. Human activity—walking, vacuuming, or even the draft from a door opening—can resuspend settled dust and pathogens back into the breathing zone.

- *The "Pig Pen" Effect:* Humans generate a thermal plume and a wake of turbulence as they move. Research has shown that walking can resuspend settled particles, increasing the concentration of airborne bioaerosols in the immediate vicinity of the walker [44].
- *Fungal Spores:* This mechanism is a major route of exposure for heavy fungal spores like *Stachybotrys*. They accumulate in dust and are lofted into the air during disturbance. Therefore, "cleaning" that involves vigorous dry sweeping or high-velocity air can paradoxically increase inhalation risk [79].

1.10.3 Materiality and Persistence

The persistence of pathogens on surfaces is dictated by the material properties. Porous materials (fabrics) tend to trap pathogens but transmit them less efficiently to hands, while non-porous surfaces (steel, plastic) allow for higher transfer efficiency but may not support survival as long as previously thought for enveloped viruses.

- *Antimicrobial Surfaces:* Copper and its alloys have intrinsic antimicrobial properties, rapidly inactivating viruses and bacteria via ion release that destroys genomic material [87].
- *Viral Half-life:* The half-life of SARS-CoV-2 on plastic and steel can range from hours to days, but this is heavily influenced by temperature and humidity [32]. Higher temperatures and humidity generally accelerate viral decay on surfaces [85, 87].

1.11 Vulnerable Typologies: Office and School

1.11.1 The Modern Office: A Density Problem

The open-plan office, designed for collaboration and density efficiency, presents a unique challenge for infection control.

- *The "Sealed" Box:* Since the 1970s energy crisis, offices have been designed as sealed envelopes dependent on mechanical ventilation. Inadequate fresh air supply leads to the accumulation of CO_2 and bioeffluents. Studies have consistently shown that lower ventilation rates are associated with higher rates of sick leave and respiratory symptoms [58, 76].
- *Presenteeism:* The culture of "presenteeism"—working while sick—turns the office into an amplification node. An infected worker in a poorly ventilated open-plan office can generate a viral aerosol plume that affects colleagues rows away, as demonstrated in the Guangzhou restaurant outbreak analysis [43].

1.11.2 The School: High Mixing, Low Ventilation

Schools represent perhaps the most critical intervention point for public health. They are characterized by high occupant density (often exceeding office standards), high mixing rates (children interact intensely), and frequently, aging infrastructure with poor ventilation.

- *The "Petri Dish" Effect:* Schools are known amplifiers of community influenza transmission. The close contact and poor hygiene etiquette of younger children facilitate both droplet and fomite transmission.
- *Ventilation Deficits:* Many schools rely on natural ventilation (opening windows) which is often compromised by weather conditions, noise, or security concerns. Research indicates that increasing ventilation rates in classrooms not only reduces infection risk but also significantly improves cognitive performance and student attendance [77, 80].

1.11.3 The Home: The Final Frontier

While workplace and public regulations exist, the home remains unregulated regarding infection control. Yet, household transmission is often the primary driver of sustained epidemics.

- *Isolation Difficulty:* In many homes, especially in lower socioeconomic demographics, effective isolation of a sick family member is impossible due to crowding and shared facilities (bathrooms, kitchens) [68].
- *Infiltration vs. Ventilation:* Most homes rely on infiltration (leakage) rather than controlled ventilation. This uncontrolled air exchange can be insufficient to dilute viral loads when a household member is infectious, leading to high secondary attack rates among families [41].

In summary, the transition from "sick building syndrome" to "infection resilience" requires us to treat the building as a medical device. We must understand the specific pathogens we are fighting, the physics of their transport, and the neurogenic mechanisms that make occupants sensitive to the chemical milieu. The next section will explore the specific engineering interventions—ventilation, filtration, and disinfection—that serve as the "immune system" of the built environment.

1.12 The Physics of Proximity: Rethinking the "Safe Distance"

1.12.1 The Continuum of Transmission

For much of the past century, infection control in the built environment has been governed by a binary paradigm: the distinction between "droplet" and "airborne" transmission [23]. This dichotomy, entrenched in public health dogma, dictated that heavy droplets (>5 microns) fall rapidly to the ground within a 1–2 m radius, while only specific "airborne" diseases (like measles or tuberculosis) generate droplet nuclei small enough to remain suspended. Consequently, architectural and engineering interventions were bifurcated; standard buildings relied on social distancing and surface cleaning to manage droplets, while specialized negative-pressure isolation rooms were reserved for airborne threats.

However, recent mechanistic modeling has dismantled this binary view, replacing it with a "continuum model" of transmission that fundamentally alters our understanding of spatial safety [42]. The human expiratory event—be it coughing, sneezing, or speaking—does not release discrete categories of particles, but rather a turbulent, multiphase gas cloud containing a spectrum of droplet sizes. The trajectory of these particles is not determined solely by gravity, but by the interaction between the momentum of the exhaled jet and the background airflows of the room [42].

1.12.2 Ventilation and Short-Range Transmission

A critical, counterintuitive finding emerging from recent building physics research is the impact of ventilation on *short-range* transmission. Traditionally, it was believed that general room ventilation (dilution) only mitigated long-range (room-scale) risks, while protection from close contact required physical distancing or masks. However, Li et al. [42] demonstrated that in poorly ventilated spaces, the exhaled jet plume does not dissipate; instead, it penetrates further and maintains a high concentration of pathogens for a longer duration [29].

Using a mechanistic model, researchers showed that when the background ventilation rate is low (e.g., <10 L/s per person), the concentration of exhaled aerosols in the "short-range" cone (less than 1.5 m) remains substantially elevated because the background air is saturated, preventing the dilution of the jet [42]. This implies that the "safe distance" is not a fixed static metric (e.g., 6 feet) but a dynamic variable dependent on the building's air change rate. In a stagnant room, the infectious plume from a speaker can bridge the physical distance between occupants more effectively than in a well-ventilated room where the jet is rapidly entrained and diluted. Thus, ventilation is not merely a background control; it is an active disruptor of close-contact transmission chains [42].

1.12.3 Evaporation and the "Droplet Nuclei" Transformation

The physical fate of an infectious particle is further complicated by thermodynamics. Upon exiting the warm, humid respiratory tract, droplets encounter the relatively drier indoor environment and immediately begin to evaporate. Research by Mao et al. [49] highlights that this evaporation process is rapid; a droplet with an initial diameter of 10 microns can evaporate to a droplet nucleus of roughly 3 microns in mere milliseconds to seconds, depending on the relative humidity (RH).

This phase change is critical for building operators. A particle that begins its journey as a "heavy droplet" destined for the floor can effectively transform into an "airborne aerosol" destined for the HVAC return grille before it hits the ground [49]. The rate of evaporation is governed by the ambient RH; in dry conditions (<40% RH), evaporation is accelerated, rapidly converting potentially settling droplets into buoyant aerosols that can remain suspended for hours [49]. This underscores the role of humidification not just for comfort, but as a physical intervention to maintain droplet size and encourage gravitational settling, thereby reducing the airborne viral load. Though this must be balanced as it may lead to condensation and become a "magnet" for particles by having droplets on the surface.

1.13 The Ventilation Variable: CO_2 as a Sentinel

1.13.1 The Historical Deficit

The linkage between ventilation rates and human health is well-established in the literature, yet frequently ignored in the design of everyday buildings. A landmark multidisciplinary review by Seppänen et al. [76] analyzed over 20 studies involving 30,000 subjects and found a consistent association: ventilation rates below 10 L/s per person are significantly associated with worsened health outcomes, including respiratory illnesses, sick building syndrome (SBS) symptoms, and perceived air quality dissatisfaction.

Historically, ventilation standards were often driven by the need to dilute body odours rather than (bioeffluent rather than to prevent infection. The "people source and room source" rule used in these standards assumes that pollutant loads are static [42]. However, in the context of an infectious outbreak, the "source" is a biological replicator. The Seppänen review noted that relative risks for respiratory illnesses ranged from 1.1 to 6.0 in low ventilation environments compared to high ventilation environments [76]. This suggests that the energy-saving trend of "tightening" building envelopes since the 1970s has inadvertently created biologically "fragile" environments where infectious agents can accumulate.

1.13.2 Carbon Dioxide (CO_2) as a Proxy for Risk

Because real-time measurement of viral pathogens in the air is technically difficult and expensive, building scientists rely on proxies. Carbon dioxide (CO_2), generated by human respiration, serves as the primary tracer for "rebreathed air." In a fully occupied space, indoor CO_2 levels above outdoor background levels (approx. 400–500 ppm) indicate the fraction of air that has been previously exhaled by someone else.

Recent guidance suggests that maintaining indoor CO_2 levels below 800 ppm (approximately 1% rebreathed air fraction) may be a prudent target proxy for infection control [28]. This value may even be considered as 500 ppm, but the 800 is what multiple experts have proposed. While CO_2 is not a direct measure of viral load—an infected person exhales the same amount of CO_2 as an uninfected one—it is a robust indicator of ventilation sufficiency. If CO_2 levels rise, it indicates that the air exchange rate is insufficient to clear human-generated contaminants, including potential viral aerosols. The "Rebreathed Fraction" (γ) becomes a critical metric; as γ increases, the probability of inhaling a quantum of infection from an index case rises mathematically [42].

1.13.3 The Diminishing Returns of Ventilation

While increasing ventilation is crucial, it may not be considered a panacea. The relationship between ventilation rate and infection risk follows a law of diminishing returns. Li et al. [42] demonstrated that increasing ventilation from 1 to 10 L/s per person results in a massive reduction in infection risk. However, increasing from 10 to 20 L/s may yield a smaller marginal benefit, and beyond a certain point, the energy cost of conditioning vast amounts of outdoor air may eventually outweigh the incremental reduction in risk [42]. This necessitates a "layered" approach to infection control, where ventilation is supplemented by filtration and air disinfection technologies (like UVGI) to achieve high equivalent air change rates (eACH) without the energy penalty of thermal conditioning [83]. Though this is highly contextual and depends upon the setting and the resources.

1.14 Beyond Air: The Water-Aerosol Interface

1.14.1 Wastewater-Based Epidemiology (WBE)

While air is the primary medium of transmission for respiratory pathogens, the building's water and waste systems serve as a critical secondary medium, both as a reservoir and a diagnostic tool. The COVID-19 pandemic accelerated the adoption of wastewater-based epidemiology (WBE) [1]. Infected individuals shed SARS-CoV-2 RNA in their faeces, often days before developing symptoms [38, 64].

For the building manager, the sewage outflow is a continuous stream of biological data. By sampling wastewater at the building level—such as in university dormitories, prisons, or nursing homes—public health officials can detect the presence of an outbreak up to a week before clinical cases appear [24, 41]. This "invisible" surveillance allows for targeted interventions, such as mass testing or isolation of specific floors or wings, effectively turning the building's plumbing infrastructure into a diagnostic device [64].

1.14.2 The Fecal-Aerosol Route

The interaction between plumbing and air quality is not limited to surveillance; it is also a transmission pathway. The "fecal-aerosol" route, famously documented during the 2003 SARS outbreak at Amoy Gardens, remains a potent threat in modern high-rise buildings. When toilet U-traps dry out or seals fail, negative pressure from exhaust fans can draw pathogen-laden sewer gases back into the living space. SARS-CoV-2 has been detected in fecal matter and can remain viable in wastewater environments [4]. This highlights the necessity of a holistic view of "Infection Control in the Built Environment," where plumbing maintenance (keeping water seals filled) is as vital as filter changes in the HVAC system.

1.15 The Hierarchy of Controls in the Built Environment

1.15.1 Adapting Occupational Hygiene to Public Spaces

To organize the myriad interventions available—ventilation, filtration, UVGI, masks, distancing—building professionals must adopt the "Hierarchy of Controls" framework used in occupational hygiene. This hierarchy ranks interventions from most effective (removing the hazard) to least effective (protecting the worker).

1. *Elimination/Substitution:* In a building context, this involves identifying infected individuals (testing, thermal screening) and preventing their entry. While ideal, the prevalence of asymptomatic transmission may render this to be somewhat imperfect [43].
2. *Engineering Controls:* This is the domain of the building professional. It involves physical changes to the environment to isolate people from the hazard. This includes:
   - *Ventilation:* Diluting the contaminant with outdoor air [76].
   - *Filtration:* Removing particulates via HEPA or high-MERV filters. Research shows that HEPA filtration can reduce the concentration of sub-micron particles (which carry viruses) by over 99%, significantly lowering the inhalation dose [62, 66]. Though this only works if it is replaced as per requirements and maintained, else it is reported to become "breeding grounds" for problems.
   - *Disinfection:* Using upper-room ultraviolet germicidal irradiation (UVGI). As reviewed by Thornton et al. [83], UVGI is a highly effective engineering control that inactivates airborne pathogens by damaging their DNA/RNA, offering a high "equivalent" air change rate at a lower energy cost. This claim has been supported by Nyugen et al. [65].
3. *Administrative Controls:* Changing the way people work or occupy the space. This includes de-densification (reducing occupancy), staggering shifts, and directional flow of foot traffic to minimize face-to-face interactions [17]. It also includes source control mechanisms.

4. *Personal Protective Equipment (PPE):* The last line of defense. This includes N95 masks, PPE kits etc. The issue of comfort while wearing this has to looked at and people be conditioned to wear these for their protection.

1.15.2 The Role of Masks as Source Control

While masks are often viewed as a personal choice, in the context of building physics, they function as a *source control device* that fundamentally alters the input parameters of the ventilation equation. By trapping respiratory droplets at the source, masks reduce the *quanta emission rate* (q) of an infector. See Wells-Riley Equation for more elaborate detail.

A systematic review by Chu et al. [13] and subsequent network meta-analyses [35] have quantified the efficacy of various mask types. N95 respirators offer the highest protection, but even surgical and cloth masks significantly reduce the emission of virus-laden aerosols [13, 35]. It is worth noting that N95 is for the wearer, but surgical mask is an administrative control leading to source control. From an engineering perspective, widespread masking reduces the burden on the ventilation system. A building that might be "unsafe" at 2 ACH with unmasked occupants may become "safe" with masked occupants, as the source strength is drastically curtailed [42]. Thus, the definition of an "infection-resilient environment" is not static; it depends on the behavioral protocols (masking) enforced within that environment.

1.16 Vulnerability and Equity in the Built Environment

1.16.1 The Unequal Burden of Indoor Air

The capacity of a building to protect its occupants is not distributed equally across society. "Sick building syndrome" and infection risks are disproportionately concentrated in older, lower-income housing stock and public infrastructure. These buildings often suffer from poor ventilation, overcrowding, and deferred maintenance, creating ideal conditions for bioaerosol accumulation and fungal growth [39, 79]. Spaces that have undergone renovations, or with new carpets and furnitures may also be an issue.

Research indicates that overcrowding is one of the primary drivers of transmission for respiratory diseases like tuberculosis and COVID-19 [39]. In these settings, the "people source" load overwhelms the "room source" ventilation capacity. Furthermore, the lack of some form of mechanical ventilation in many low-income schools and housing units means reliance on natural ventilation (windows), which is often contextual and may work in most situations, but some situations may have issues like outdoor noise, pollution, or security concerns [92]. Addressing infection control in the everyday built environment is therefore a matter of public health equity; it requires prioritizing retrofits and upgrades in the communities that are most structurally vulnerable to airborne disease.

We have established that the "everyday built environment" is a dynamic system where physics, biology, and human behavior intersect. The transmission of infection is governed by the continuum of aerosol dispersion, modulated by ventilation rates, and influenced by the thermodynamic state of the air. We have moved beyond the vague malaise of "sick building syndrome" to a specific understanding of how buildings can act as vectors for specific pathogens through air and water systems. In the final section of this chapter, we will synthesize these concepts into a cohesive framework for "infection resilient design," outlining the future directions for research, policy, and practice that will define the post-pandemic era of building engineering.

1.17 The Economic Calculus: Health vs. Energy

1.17.1 The False Economy of "Tight" Buildings

For the past 50 years, the dominant narrative in facility management and architectural engineering has been cost containment, primarily achieved through energy efficiency. This paradigm, which may have been born from the energy crises of the 1970s, prioritized the sealing of the building envelope to retain conditioned air. As noted by Horvath [27], buildings became "tighter" and ventilation rates were lowered to reduce fuel consumption, inadvertently creating incubators for indoor air pollutants and biological agents. While this strategy successfully lowered utility bills, it may have created a hidden debt paid in human health—a debt foreclosed upon during the COVID-19 pandemic.

The resistance to increasing ventilation rates often stems from the perceived "energy penalty." Conditioning vast amounts of outdoor air—heating it in winter and cooling/dehumidifying it in summer—requires significant power. However, this view ignores the "salary penalty." In a commercial office environment, energy costs typically account for approximately 1% of total operating costs, whereas human salaries and benefits account for approximately 90% [22]. A small improvement in indoor environmental quality (IEQ) that reduces absenteeism or increases cognitive function by even 1% can yield financial returns that dwarf the entire energy budget of the building [74].

1.17.2 The Cost of Sick Leave and Productivity

The economic implications of poor ventilation are empirically robust. In a landmark review, Seppänen et al. [76] analyzed data from over 30,000 subjects and found a consistent association between low ventilation rates (below 10 L/s per person) and increased prevalence of sick building syndrome (SBS) symptoms and respiratory illnesses. These illnesses translate directly into sick leave. Milton et al. [58], in a study of 3720 employees, found, stated in simple generalised terms, that 35% of short-term sick leave was associated with lower ventilation rates.

Furthermore, the cost of "presenteeism"—working while sick or impaired by the building environment—is often higher than absenteeism. Poor air quality, characterized by high CO_2 and bioeffluents, has been linked to "stuffy" air and reduced mental performance [11, 76]. When occupants are suffering from headaches, mucosal irritation, or lethargy caused by the building, their productivity plummets. Therefore, the "infection resilient" building is not an extravagance; it is a fundamental asset management strategy. Investing in ventilation and filtration preserves the most valuable asset inside the building: the human occupants.

1.17.3 Cost-Effectiveness of Interventions: The UVGI Advantage

When evaluating infection control strategies, the metric must shift from "energy per square meter" to "cost per equivalent air change." While mechanical ventilation is effective, it may have certain limitations and tends to follow a law of diminishing returns; one study reported that doubling the air change rate from 10 to 20 ACH requires a massive increase in fan power and thermal conditioning [42]. A more economically viable alternative, where it can be used with high initial capital and regular maintenance for achieving high levels of protection is upper-room ultraviolet germicidal irradiation (UVGI). Research indicates that UVGI in some situations may be somewhat more cost-effective than mechanical ventilation for pathogen removal. A well-designed upper-room UVGI system, when pressed with no other alternative and under favorable controlled conditions, has been reported to provide equivalent air-cleaning effects comparable to approximately 10–20 eACH under favorable design and airflow conditions, for the energy cost of a few light bulbs, bypassing the thermal load of conditioning outdoor air [63]. Though, as mentioned multiple times in the book, the initial capital cost, the maintenance and the health effects of UV (which may still be under research to get a complete picture), may need to be taken into account.

1.18 The Ethical Imperative: Clean Air as a Human Right

1.18.1 The Paradigm Shift

Historically, society has accepted that the water drawn from a tap is free of cholera and the food purchased is free of Salmonella. Yet, there has been a tacit acceptance that the air breathed in a crowded room may be laden with influenza, tuberculosis, or coronaviruses. The scientific consensus is now shifting to view indoor air safety as a fundamental human right, akin to water sanitation [61].

1.18.2 Equity in the Built Environment

Infection control in buildings is also a profound matter of social equity. Low-income populations are disproportionately relegated to "sick buildings"—older structures with poor ventilation, moisture ingress, and overcrowding. These environments act as amplification nodes for infectious diseases. Systematic reviews have consistently linked housing characteristics such as overcrowding and poor ventilation to the incidence of tuberculosis and COVID-19 [39]. In these settings, the lack of mechanical ventilation forces reliance on windows, which may remain closed due to security concerns or outdoor pollution, trapping pathogens indoors [92]. Furthermore, the burden of "energy poverty" means that vulnerable populations cannot afford to run heating or dehumidification systems, leading to dampness and fungal growth (e.g., *Stachybotrys chartarum*), which exacerbates respiratory health issues [79]. Designing infection-resilient environments is not just a luxury for Class-A office towers; it is a public health necessity for public housing, schools, and prisons, where the most vulnerable members of society are confined.

1.18.3 Professional Responsibility

Architects, engineers, and facility managers now bear a heightened professional responsibility. Ignorance of airborne transmission physics is no longer a valid defense. The definition of "standard of care" is evolving. A building designed today that fails to accommodate surge capacity for ventilation or air disinfection may be considered negligent in the face of future pandemics. The built environment professions must move beyond minimum code compliance to a performance-based standard of "health protection."

1.19 Policy and Future Directions: The Sentient Building

1.19.1 From Minimums to Targets

Older, but popular building codes set *minimum* ventilation rates primarily for odour control. The future requires *target* rates based on health outcomes. The Royal Academy of Engineering [72] proposes a shift toward "infection resilience" standards that are dynamic. Buildings should possess a "pandemic mode"—a pre-programmed operational state that maximizes outdoor air, disables demand-controlled ventilation (DCV) reduction, and activates disinfection systems when epidemiological risk is high.

1.19.2 The Role of Sensors and AI

The static building is obsolete. The future is the "sentient" building, equipped with networks of biosensors and environmental monitors. This may be rephrased by stating that the traditional static building paradigm is increasingly challenged by the emergence of responsive buildings.

- *Real-Time Monitoring:* The deployment of low-cost sensors for CO_2, particulate matter (PM2.5), temperature, and humidity allows for the real-time estimation of occupancy and infection risk [56, 91]. These systems can automatically modulate ventilation rates based on the "rebreathed fraction" of air, ensuring that risk thresholds are never breached.
- *Wastewater Surveillance (WBE):* The building's plumbing system serves as a diagnostic tool. As demonstrated during the COVID-19 pandemic, testing building sewage for viral RNA can predict outbreaks days before clinical symptoms appear [38, 50]. Future buildings may integrate automated samplers to serve as an early warning system for a range of pathogens, from SARS-CoV-2 to poliovirus [50].

1.20 Conclusion

The everyday built environment is the primary "battlefield" for respiratory health. We spend 90% of our lives indoors, submerged in an invisible ocean of air that connects the lungs of every occupant. This chapter has dissected the anatomy of this connection, revealing that "infection" is not merely a biological event but an architectural one.

We have established that the distinction between "droplet" and "airborne" is a physical continuum; that for many enveloped viruses, low RH is associated with increased stability; and that our buildings may have largely been designed to trap pollutants rather than purge them. We have moved beyond the vague malaise of "sick building syndrome" to a specific understanding of building-related illness, where the building acts as a vector for pathogens like *Legionella* and SARS-CoV-2.

However, we have also identified the arsenal available to us: the physics of dilution (ventilation), the mechanics of capture (filtration), and the photochemistry of inactivation (UVGI). The challenge moving forward is not technological; the engineering solutions exist. The challenge is cultural and economic. It requires valuing the invisible asset of health over the visible cost of energy. It requires a new pedagogy for designers and a new rigorousness for operators.

By embracing the concept of the *infection-resilient environment*, we can transform our buildings from passive containers of disease into active guardians of public health. The building of the future does not just shelter us from the "storm outside"; it protects us from the "storm within". Non-rhetorically, this means that the building of the future should not only provide shelter and protection against external elements, but actively protect occupants' health by mitigating biological and environmental risks, esp. the ones arising indoors.

Acknowledgments The authors acknowledge the support provided by the institutions including School of Planning and Architecture, New Delhi, All India Institute of Medical Sciences, New Delhi, and Drexel University. Special thanks to Rajshekhar Pullabhatla and Group Captain P Aanand Naidu of ISAC Centre for Built Environment Policy and Tathatara Foundation. Many thanks to Arthur L Frank, MD and Milan Ben for their kind support. Many thanks to all the people who supported this work in many ways.

Declarations The authors Raja Singh, Nirupam Madaan, and Anil Dewan declare no conflict of interests or competing interests in this work. There is no involvement of human participants, animals, human or animal tissue. All authors declare that there was no specific financial support received from any organization for the submitted work. All authors declare that they have no financial relationships at present or within the previous 3 years with any organizations that might have an interest in the submitted work. While all care has been taken in ensuring the accuracy of this work, any inadvertent error may be reported at the earliest. The authors acknowledge the use of supervised language learning models/large language models for enhancement of the work, with responsibility lying with the authors. For more information, the corresponding author may be contacted at email rajaresearch@proton.me.

CRediT Statement The following is the CRediT statement which declares the author credits for this chapter:

Raja Singh: Conceptualization, Methodology, Formal Analysis, Investigation, Data Curation, Writing-Original Draft, Writing-Review & Editing, Visualization, Project Administration.
Nirupam Madaan: Conceptualization, Resources, Validation, Supervision, Project Administration.
Anil Dewan: Resources, Validation Supervision.

References

1. Ahmed W, et al. SARS-CoV-2 surveillance of wastewater: a systematic review. Water Res. 2022;213:118136.
2. Allen JG, Macomber JD. Healthy buildings: how indoor spaces drive performance and productivity. Harvard University Press; 2020.
3. Allen JG, MacNaughton P, Laurent JGC, Flanigan SS, Eitland ES, Spengler JD. Green buildings and health. Curr Environ Health Rep. 2015;2(3):250–8.
4. Anand U, et al. SARS-CoV-2 in municipal wastewater, landfill leachate, and solid waste: a review about virus surveillance, infectivity, and inactivation. Environ Res. 2022;203:111839.
5. Anderson K, Anderson J. Acute toxic effects of fragrance products. Arch Environ Health. 1998;53:138–46.
6. Appleby PH. ABC of work related disorders: building related illnesses. BMJ. 1996;313:674.
7. ASHRAE. Standard 62.1-2019, ventilation for acceptable indoor air quality. American Society of Heating, Refrigerating and Air-Conditioning Engineers; 2019.
8. Bascom R. The upper respiratory tract: mucous membrane irritation. Environ Health Perspect. 1991;95:39–44.
9. Bourouiba L. Turbulent gas clouds and respiratory pathogen emissions. JAMA. 2020;323(18):1837–8.
10. Burge PS. Sick building syndrome. Occup Environ Med. 2004;61(2):185–90.
11. Clements-Croome DJ. Indoor environment and productivity. In: Creating the productive workplace. Taylor & Francis; 2006. p. 35–59.

12. Chen W, Zhang N, Wei J, Yen HL, Li Y. Short-range airborne route dominates exposure of respiratory infection during close contact. Build Environ. 2020;176:106859.
13. Chu DK, et al. Physical distancing, face masks, and eye protection. Lancet. 2020;395(10242):1973–87.
14. Cooley JD, Wong WC, Jumper CA, Straus DC. Fungi and the indoor environment. In: Advances in applied microbiology, vol. 55. Academic; 2004. p. 1–30.
15. Crawford JO, Bolas SM. Sick building syndrome, work factors and occupational stress. Scand J Work Environ Health. 1996;22(4):243–50.
16. Dubey S, Sahoo KC, Dash GC. Housing-related challenges during COVID-19. Front Public Health. 2022;10:1029394.
17. Epton T, et al. Physical distancing interventions. Soc Sci Med. 2022;303:114946.
18. Etzel RA, Montana E, Sorenson WG, Kullman GJ, Allan TM, Dearborn DG. Acute pulmonary haemorrhage in infants. Arch Pediatr Adolesc Med. 1998;152(8):757–62.
19. Evans GW. The built environment and mental health. J Urban Health. 2003;80(4):536–55.
20. Finnegan MJ, Pickering CA, Burge PS. The sick building syndrome. BMJ. 1984;289(6458):1573–5.
21. Fisk WJ, Black DR, Brunner G. Benefits and costs of improved IEQ in US offices. Indoor Air. 2011;21(5):357–67.
22. Fisk WJ, Rosenfeld AH. Estimates of improved productivity and health. Indoor Air. 1997;7(3):158–72.
23. Greenhalgh T, Jimenez JL, Prather KA, Tufekci Z, Fisman D, Schooley R. Ten scientific reasons for airborne transmission. Lancet. 2021;397(10285):1603–5.
24. Harris-Lovett S, et al. Wastewater surveillance on college campuses. IJERPH. 2021;18(9):4455.
25. Hodgson M. Indoor environmental exposures and symptoms. Environ Health Perspect. 2002;110(Suppl 4):663–7.
26. Hoisington AJ, Brenner LA, Kinney KA, Postolache TT, Lowry CA. The microbiome of the built environment and mental health. Microbiome. 2015;3(1):60.
27. Horvath EP. Building-related illness and sick building syndrome. Cleve Clin J Med. 1997;64(6):303–9.
28. Hou D, et al. Bayesian calibration of CO_2 sensors. J Build Eng. 2022;46:103725.
29. Huang J, et al. Airborne transmission of the Delta variant. Build Environ. 2022;219:109212.
30. Husman T. Health effects of indoor-air microorganisms. Scand J Work Environ Health. 1996;22:5–13.
31. Joshi SM. The sick building syndrome. Indian J Occup Environ Med. 2008;12(2):61–4.
32. Kampf G, Todt D, Pfaender S, Steinmann E. Persistence of coronaviruses on surfaces. J Hosp Infect. 2020;104(3):246–51.
33. Kelley ST, Gilbert JA. Studying the microbiology of the indoor environment. Genome Biol. 2013;14(2):202.
34. Kembel SW, et al. Architectural design influences indoor microbiome. ISME J. 2012;6(8):1469–79.
35. Kim MN. What type of face mask is appropriate for everyone-mask-wearing policy amidst COVID-19 pandemic? J Korean Med Sci. 2020;35(20):e186. https://doi.org/10.3346/jkms.2020.35.e186. PMID: 32449327; PMCID: PMC7246185.
36. Kimani TN, et al. Transmission dynamics in the built environment. Public Health Practice. 2021;2:100128.
37. Klepeis NE, et al. The national human activity pattern survey. J Exposure Sci Environ Epidemiol. 2001;11(3):231–52.
38. Larsen DA, Wigginton KR. Tracking COVID-19 with wastewater. Nat Biotechnol. 2020;38(10):1151–3.
39. Lee JY, Kim N, Gwak G. Housing-related risk factors for tuberculosis. BMC Public Health. 2022;22(1):1–13.
40. Letz GA. Sick building syndrome. Allergy Proc. 1990;11(3):109–16.
41. Li X, et al. Modeling SARS-CoV-2 transmission in wastewater. J Hazard Mater. 2022;432:128667.

42. Li Y, Cheng P, Jia W. Poor ventilation worsens short-range airborne transmission. Indoor Air. 2021;32(1):e12946.
43. Li Y, Qian H, Hang J, Chen X, Hong L, Liang P, et al. Probable airborne transmission in a restaurant. Build Environ. 2020;196:107788.
44. Licina D, Nazaroff WW. Clothing as a transport vector. Indoor Air. 2018;28(3):404–14.
45. Lopez RP. The built environment and public health. 1st ed. Jossey-Bass; 2012. ISBN 978-0-470-62003-8
46. Lu J, et al. COVID-19 outbreak associated with air conditioning. Emerg Infect Dis. 2020;26(7):1628.
47. Lyles WB, et al. Sick building syndrome. South Med J. 1991;84(1):65–71.
48. Mahmoudi M, Gershwin ME. Sick building syndrome III. J Asthma. 2000;37(2):191–8.
49. Mao N, et al. Transmission risk of infectious droplets. Build Environ. 2020;185:107307.
50. McCall C, et al. Viral diseases identified via wastewater. Water Res. 2020;184:116160.
51. Meadow JF, et al. Indoor airborne bacterial communities. Indoor Air. 2014;24(1):41–8.
52. Megahed NA, Ghoneim EM. Rethinking building design post-pandemic. Environ Res. 2021;193:110471.
53. Meggs WJ. Neurogenic inflammation. Environ Health Perspect. 1993;101(3):234–8.
54. Meggs WJ. Neurogenic switching. Environ Health Perspect. 1995;103(1):54–6.
55. Meggs WJ. Chemical sensitivity hypothesis. Environ Health Perspect. 1997;105(Suppl 2):473–8.
56. Mena AR, Ceballos HG, Alvarado-Uribe J. Measuring indoor occupancy using sensors. Sensors. 2022;22(10):3770.
57. Mendell MJ. Non-specific symptoms in office workers. Indoor Air. 1993;3(4):227–36.
58. Milton DK, Glencross PM, Walters MD. Risk of sick leave and ventilation. Indoor Air. 2000;10(4):212–21.
59. Miller SL, et al. Negative pressure isolation space. Am J Infect Control. 2020.
60. Morawska L, Milton DK. Addressing airborne transmission. Clin Infect Dis. 2020;71(9):2311–3.
61. Morawska L, et al. Minimising airborne transmission indoors. Environ Int. 2020;142:105832.
62. Nair AN, et al. Strategies to reduce indoor airborne transmission. Environ Res. 2022;213:113579.
63. Nardell EA. Germicidal UV and airborne infection control. Photochem Photobiol. 2021;97(3):493–7.
64. Naughton CC, et al. Global COVID-19 wastewater monitoring. medRxiv. 2021.
65. Nguyen TT, Johnson GR, Bell SC, Knibbs LD. Indoor air disinfection techniques. IJERPH. 2022;19:1197.
66. Oh J, et al. Decontamination of filtering facepiece respirators. Environ Sci Pollut Res. 2022;29:1645–76.
67. Onakpoya IJ, Heneghan CJ, Jefferson T. Viral cultures for fomite transmission. J Hosp Infect. 2022;130:63–94.
68. Patel JA, et al. Poverty, inequality and COVID-19. Public Health. 2020;183:110.
69. Rabenau HF, et al. Efficacy of disinfectants against viruses. J Hosp Infect. 2014;86(3):232–4.
70. Redlich CA, Sparer J, Cullen MR. Sick building syndrome. Lancet. 1997;349(9057):1013–6.
71. Rook GA. Regulation of the immune system by biodiversity. PNAS. 2013;110(46):18360–7.
72. Royal Academy of Engineering. Infection resilient environments: time for a major upgrade. National Engineering Policy Centre; 2022.
73. Runeson R, et al. Psychosocial factors and sick building symptoms. Indoor Air. 2004;16(1):13–21.
74. Sadikin S, Turan I, Chegut A. Financial impact of healthy buildings. MIT Press; 2020.
75. Seppänen OA, Fisk WJ. Ventilation system type and SBS symptoms. Indoor Air. 2002;12(2):98–112.
76. Seppänen OA, Fisk WJ, Mendell MJ. Ventilation rates and health. Indoor Air. 1999;9(4):226–52.
77. Shendell DG, et al. Classroom CO_2 and attendance. Indoor Air. 2004;14(5):333–41.

78. Stanwell-Smith R, Bloomfield SF, Rook GA. Hygiene hypothesis. International Scientific Forum on Home Hygiene; 2006.
79. Straus DC. Fungal contamination in sick building syndrome. Front Biosci. 2011;E3:562–80.
80. Sundell J, et al. Ventilation rates and health. Indoor Air. 2011;21(3):191–204.
81. Svajlenka J, et al. Biomonitoring agricultural indoor environments. Ann Agric Environ Med. 2018;25(2).
82. Tang JW, et al. Dismantling myths on airborne transmission. J Hosp Infect. 2021;110:89–96.
83. Thornton GM, et al. HVAC and ultraviolet radiation. PLoS ONE. 2022;17(4):e0266487.
84. Tran VV, Park D, Lee YC. Indoor air pollution and health. IJERPH. 2020;17(8):2927.
85. Van Doremalen N, et al. Aerosol and surface stability of SARS-CoV-2. NEJM. 2020;382(16):1564–7.
86. Vardoulakis S, Espinoza Oyarce DA, Donner E. Transmission in public washrooms. Sci Total Environ. 2022;803:149932.
87. Viana Martins CP, Xavier CSF, Cobrado L. Disinfection methods against SARS-CoV-2. J Hosp Infect. 2022;119:84–117.
88. Wakayama T, et al. Review of 2-ethyl-1-hexanol as pollutant. J Occup Health. 2019;61(1):19–35.
89. Wargocki P, et al. Outdoor air supply and productivity. Indoor Air. 2000;10(4):222–36.
90. Welch LS. Severity of health effects. Environ Health Perspect. 1991;95:67–9.
91. Wiryasaputra R, et al. IoT-based indoor air quality monitoring. Front Public Health. 2022;10:1022055.
92. Yang L, et al. Urban design and infectious disease transmission. Prog Plan. 2022:100657.

2 Perception of Building Professionals Related to Infection Control: Survey and Pedagogy for Positive Change

Raja Singh, Nirupam Madaan, and Anil Dewan

2.1 A Study on How Architects Perceive Infection Control and the Role They Play

2.1.1 Empirical Evidence from a Perception Survey of Architects in India

To examine how architects themselves perceive their role in infection control, an original perception study was conducted using a structured questionnaire administered through both online and paper-based formats. The respondents included practicing architects, healthcare architects, architecture faculty, research scholars, postgraduate students, and undergraduate students from 5-year degree programs. A total of 246 valid responses were collected, of which 173 respondents were registered architects in India. The overall sample achieved a confidence level of 95% with a margin of error of ±7.45, while the undergraduate subgroup achieved a confidence level of 95% with a margin of error of ±11.51.

The respondents represented a broad cross-section of the architectural ecosystem. Architecture students (undergraduate) constituted 29.3% of respondents, post graduate students 6.9%, architects working in firms 26.1%, architects with independent practice 19.5%, architecture faculty 13.4%, research scholars 3.7%,

R. Singh
Founder/Researcher, The Built, New Delhi, Delhi, India

Former Post Doctoral Fellow, Department of Environmental and Occupational Health, Dornsife School of Public Health, Drexel University, Philadelphia, Pennsylvania, USA

N. Madaan
Department of Hospital Administration, All India Institute of Medical Sciences, New Delhi, Delhi, India

A. Dewan
Department of Architecture, School of Planning and Architecture, New Delhi, Delhi, India

R. Singh et al., *Infection Control in the Everyday Built Environment*,
https://doi.org/10.1007/978-981-95-8624-0_2

and other professional roles 1.1%. This distribution ensured that the findings reflect both emerging professionals and experienced practitioners.

The Invisible Architecture

Imagine standing in the atrium of a modern, glass-encased skyscraper. To the naked eye, it is a marvel of engineering—a testament to human ingenuity, bathed in natural light, climate-controlled to a precise 22 °C, and designed to facilitate the flow of commerce and social interaction. However, to a microbiologist or a building physicist, this same space looks radically different. It is not merely a void filled with air; it is a complex, turbulent fluid dynamic system, a swirling ocean of invisible particulates, respiratory aerosols, and distinct microbial ecosystems. Every cough, every flush of a toilet, and every hum of the HVAC system alters the biological landscape of this environment. For decades, the professionals who design these spaces—architects, engineers, and facility managers—have focused primarily on the visible and the tangible: aesthetics, structural integrity, energy efficiency, and thermal comfort. Yet, the emergence of the SARS-CoV-2 pandemic has violently pulled back the curtain on the invisible architecture of our built environment, forcing a reckoning with a dimension of design that has long been relegated to the background: infection resilience.

The perception of infection control among building professionals may have historically been one of delegation. However, findings from the perception study indicate that this delegation mindset is actively shifting. Among the respondents, 97.6% acknowledged that architects play a direct role in controlling building ventilation, and 95.1% agreed that architects have a role in hospital infection control. Further, 91.5% agreed that ventilation plays a critical role in controlling airborne infections such as tuberculosis.

The architect designs the form; the mechanical engineer handles the air; the facility manager handles the cleaning. However, the scientific literature confirms that the built environment is a primary determinant of health, particularly regarding respiratory infections [4]. We spend approximately 90% of our time indoors, making the indoor environment the principal theatre of exposure to chemical, biological, and physical hazards [4, 44]. Consequently, the building professional is not merely a designer of shelter but a custodian of public health. This chapter explores the evolving perception of this responsibility, dissecting how architects and engineers view their role in mitigating the spread of infectious diseases, and how this perception must shift from reactive intervention to proactive design.

The Historical Disconnect: From Sanitation to Sustainability

To understand the current perception of infection control among architects, we must first look at the historical trajectory of the profession. Urban planning and building design originated in the late nineteenth century largely as a public health intervention. The sanitation movement was a direct response to outbreaks of infectious diseases like cholera and tuberculosis, leading to innovations in sewage systems, lighting, and ventilation to combat overcrowding and 'miasma' [49]. In this era, the architect and the civil engineer may have been the primary lines of defense against epidemics.

However, as the twentieth century progressed, the advent of antibiotics and vaccines allowed the built environment professions to shift their focus. The medical community took over the burden of infection control, allowing architects to prioritize other emerging challenges, specifically the car-dominated urban development and the energy crises of the 1970s [21, 49]. The energy crisis, in particular, was a pivot point. It is believed to have driven a desire to reduce fuel consumption for heating and cooling, leading to the construction of "tighter" building envelopes with lower ventilation rates [21].

This shift created a paradoxical relationship between building performance and human health. While buildings became more energy-efficient, they also became more conducive to the accumulation of indoor pollutants and pathogens. This era birthed the phenomenon known as "sick building syndrome" (SBS). SBS refers to non-specific complaints—headaches, fatigue, mucous membrane irritation—that arc temporally linked to occupancy in a specific building but lack a definitive etiological agent [21, 37]. The architectural perception during this period was often defensive; if a specific toxin couldn't be found, the building was deemed "healthy," even if the occupants were not.

The perception of infection control was further complicated by the distinction between SBS and building-related illness (BRI). BRI describes diagnosable illnesses with identified causative agents, such as Legionnaires' disease or hypersensitivity pneumonitis, which can be directly traced to building systems like cooling towers or humidifiers [21, 37]. For decades, architects perceived BRI as a failure of maintenance or mechanical engineering rather than a failure of architectural form. However, the COVID-19 pandemic has shattered this compartmentalization. The transmission of SARS-CoV-2 is not just a matter of dirty filters; it is a matter of spatial volume, occupant density, airflow patterns, and human behavior—all variables dictated by architectural design [28].

The Modern Perception: Air as a Vector

In the wake of the COVID-19 pandemic, the perception of infection control among building professionals is undergoing a radical transformation. The scientific consensus that SARS-CoV-2 is transmitted via the airborne route—through the inhalation of virus-laden aerosols—has fundamentally redefined the architect's responsibility [31, 42]. Previously, infection control may often be only, in a limited sense, viewed through the lens of surface hygiene (fomites) and large droplets, which required cleaning protocols and physical barriers. However, airborne transmission implies that the air itself is the vector, and the building is the vessel that contains it [3, 30].

Importantly, this awareness does not appear to be limited to COVID-19 alone. In the perception study, 88.6% of respondents correctly identified tuberculosis as an airborne disease. This is particularly significant in the Indian context, where tuberculosis remains a major public health burden and where architectural interventions such as natural ventilation, daylight access, and spatial decongestion have long been recognized as effective preventive measures.

Current studies indicate that building professionals are increasingly recognizing ventilation not just as a tool for odour control or thermal comfort, but as a primary infection control strategy. The Federation of European Heating, Ventilation and Air Conditioning Associations (REHVA) and others have updated guidelines emphasizing that ventilation should be maximized to dilute airborne contaminants [16]. This shift forces architects to perceive "air" as a structural element of the building, as vital as steel or concrete.

However, a critical gap remains in how this is applied. While mechanical engineers primarily focus on air changes per hour (ACH) and filtration efficiency (MERV ratings), architects must also grapple with the spatial implications. For example, the use of displacement ventilation—where fresh air is introduced at floor level and extracted at the ceiling—has been shown to be more effective than mixing ventilation in removing viral plumes from the breathing zone in environments like auditoriums [22]. This has profound implications for the aesthetic and structural design of a room, requiring large plenums and specific floor layouts that architects must integrate early in the design phase.

The Perception of Technology: Silver Bullets vs. Integrated Systems
A major component of how building professionals perceive infection control is their reliance on technology. In the rush to make buildings "safe" during the pandemic, there was a surge in interest regarding add-on technologies such as air cleaners and UV disinfection systems.

Ultraviolet Germicidal Irradiation (UVGI) Architects and engineers may perceive UVGI as a potent tool, particularly in settings where increasing ventilation is difficult or cost-prohibitive. Upper-room UVGI, which creates a zone of UV-C light near the ceiling to inactivate pathogens as air circulates, has been shown by some to be highly effective, providing an equivalent of 10–20 air changes per hour [33]. This technology is not new; it has been used for tuberculosis control for decades [8]. However, its integration requires architectural foresight. The fixtures must be placed correctly to avoid occupant exposure while maximizing the irradiation field [43]. In some developing world contexts, the system may need maintenance and initial capital cost which may be a challenge. Moreover, it may lead to a false sense of relief, of it being installed, but not maintained (tubes not cleaned etc.) and facilities may not use other methods like dilution under influence of an installed but not working system (due to lack of maintenance).

The perception here is shifting from UVGI being a "hospital-only" solution to a potential standard for public spaces like schools and offices. However, professionals must balance efficacy with safety. While Far-UVC (222 nm) shows promise in being safe for human skin and eyes while effectively inactivating airborne coronaviruses [9, 47], the standard germicidal UV (254 nm) poses health risks if not properly shielded [43]. Architects must therefore view these systems not as fixtures to be hung after construction, but as integral components of the lighting and safety design. Plus, the effect of UVGI on fast-moving air needs to be studied as in-duct systems are merely to sanitize the inside surfaces of the systems. Here again, it must be noted that any false sense of relief should not be advertised as the in duct UV may only disinfect the inside of the ducts and not be sanitising the air at high velocities.

Filtration and Air Purifiers The perception of high-efficiency particulate air (HEPA) filters has also evolved. While effective at capturing 99.97% of particles, including virus-laden aerosols, their implementation is often limited by the pressure drop they create in HVAC systems, which can reduce overall airflow if the system is not designed for high-resistance filters [19, 32]. Building professionals are learning that simply upgrading filters in an existing system is not a panacea; it requires a holistic view of the building's mechanical capacity. Plus, filters if not changed regularly and not maintained may do more harm than good. The Indian Public Health Standards of 2012 for district hospitals discourage use of filters for the same purpose (of these becoming breeding grounds on lack of maintenance).

Furthermore, the use of portable air cleaners has become a common visible intervention. While these devices can reduce airborne concentrations of pathogens, their effectiveness depends heavily on their clean air delivery rate (CADR) relative to the room volume [33]. Architects often perceive these as clutter or temporary fixes, yet in the absence of deep retrofits, they are essential tools for resilience. Newer technologies are being made available where these portable systems are being supplied with a small pipe for outdoor filtered air supply. Further, in tuberculosis facilities where fresh air changes are needed, the use of recirculation only based air cleaners may not be an accepted practice and may end up giving false illusion of relief to users of such facilities and they may not use other methods including dilution ventilation.

The Perception of Behavior: Design as a Nudge

Building professionals are increasingly aware that design influences behavior, which in turn influences infection risk. The concept of the "microbiome of the built environment" (MoBE) suggests that occupants are the primary source of indoor bacteria and viruses [20]. Therefore, controlling how people move and interact may be a contributory form of infection control.

Architects perceive the layout of spaces—corridors, waiting rooms, open-plan offices—as mechanisms to enable or inhibit social distancing. For example, the implementation of "anterooms" (vestibules) in hospital wards acts as a buffer zone to maintain pressure differentials and prevent the migration of airborne contaminants [5]. While traditionally limited to isolation wards, the concept of the anteroom is now being considered for broader applications to protect staff and patients.

Furthermore, the design of public washrooms has come under scrutiny. Research indicates that open-lid toilet flushing can generate bioaerosol plumes capable of transmitting pathogens [45]. Architects must now perceive the toilet not just as a sanitary fixture but as a bioaerosol generator, necessitating design changes such as lid requirements, improved exhaust ventilation at the source, and spatial separation from other hygiene activities [45].

The Perception of Equity and Resilience

A profound shift in professional perception concerns the equity of the built environment. The COVID-19 pandemic disproportionately affected those in poor-quality housing with inadequate ventilation and overcrowding [38]. Architects and planners are recognizing that infection resilience may also be a social justice issue. The "compact city" model, often touted for sustainability, raised concerns during the pandemic regarding density and transmission. However, evidence suggests that density itself may not be the main "enemy"; rather, overcrowding and lack of services may be the drivers of risk [49].

Building professionals are now tasked with designing for "resilience"—the ability of a building to function during a crisis. This includes the ability to surge ventilation rates during an outbreak, the flexibility to repurpose spaces (e.g., turning a hotel into a quarantine facility), and the durability of materials to withstand frequent rigorous cleaning [46].

The perception of infection control by building professionals has matured from a reliance on medical intervention to an acknowledgment of architectural agency. Architects and engineers are no longer passive observers of public health; they are active participants. The building is the first line of defense against airborne pathogens. Whether through advanced and basic ventilation strategies like dilution and displacement ventilation [22], the integration of UVGI technologies [33], or the strategic design of spatial layouts to manage human flux, the professional's role is to create an environment that is hostile to pathogens but hospitable to people. This shift requires a new pedagogical approach, ensuring that the next generation of architects is equipped not just with the tools of design, but with the knowledge of microbiology and public health.

Taken together, the findings of the perception study challenge the assumption that architects view infection control as outside their professional remit. On the contrary, there exists a strong baseline awareness and ethical acknowledgment of responsibility. What appears to be missing is not intent, but structured knowledge, institutional reinforcement, and formal integration of public health principles into architectural education and professional practice. This gap between awareness and actionable competence directly informs the pedagogical intervention proposed in the following section.

2.2 Teaching Built Environment and Public Health to Architecture Students Using a Unique Pedagogical Approach Related to Building Laws

2.2.1 Case Study: An Implemented Pedagogy for Teaching Infection Control to Architecture Students

The elective course was offered to undergraduate students in the fourth and fifth years of the 5-year Bachelor of Architecture program at a premier Indian institute. Fourteen students voluntarily enrolled, of whom eleven completed the feedback evaluation at the end of the semester. The course was delivered across a 16-week semester, using weekly sessions supplemented by assignments and applied exercises rather than written examinations. The evaluation was based on continuous coursework, reflecting the intent to prioritize applied understanding over rote theoretical recall.

The Pedagogical Void: From Aesthetics to Aseptics

The transformation of professional perception regarding infection control, as explored in the previous section, necessitates a fundamental shift in how the built environment disciplines are taught. For generations, architectural pedagogy may have primarily prioritized the visual, the structural, and the sustainable, often relegating public health to a niche specialization or a set of minimum compliance standards. However, the COVID-19 pandemic illustrated that the separation of "health" from "architecture" is a dangerous dichotomy. If the built environment is to function as an immune system for society, the education of its creators must evolve from a focus purely on aesthetics and statics to one that encompasses "aseptics"—the capability of a design to interrupt the chain of infection.

This pedagogical shift requires more than simply adding a microbiology lecture to the curriculum; it requires a systemic re-evaluation of how buildings are regulated and how those regulations influence design thinking. The course was developed in direct response to the recognition that architecture students are rarely exposed to infection control as a structured area of knowledge, despite the built environment playing an active role in disease transmission and prevention. The COVID-19 pandemic made this gap visible and urgent. The elective therefore attempted to create both conceptual awareness and practical competence by combining theoretical grounding with design-oriented and investigative exercises, ensuring that infection control principles were internalized rather than memorized [24].

A unique pedagogical approach involves utilizing the framework of *Building Laws and Regulations* not merely as legal hurdles, but as design generators that reveal the invisible interactions between physics, biology, and human behavior. By deconstructing the regulatory landscape, students can understand how historical pandemics shaped current codes (e.g., cholera and the sewage system, tuberculosis and daylighting) and how current codes must evolve to address airborne threats [38].

This pedagogical position is supported by an implemented and evaluated academic intervention. A semester-long elective course titled *Infection Control in the Built Environment* was formally offered to fourth- and fifth-year undergraduate architecture students at the School of Planning and Architecture, New Delhi, between August and December 2020. The course was conceptualized and delivered by the authors as a structured attempt to define an explicit pedagogy for teaching infection control within architectural education. The design, delivery, and evaluation of this elective have been documented here: https://doi.org/10.5281/zenodo.7722712

The feedback data from the elective supports this diagnosis. When students were asked whether there was a general awareness among architects and architecture students regarding infection control in the built environment, a majority of respondents indicated that such awareness was lacking. This directly reinforces the need for formal curricular integration rather than relying on informal or incidental exposure.

The Regulatory Framework as a Didactic Tool

In the United Kingdom and many other jurisdictions, building regulations are complex, distributed across various documents that address specific technical elements (ventilation, sanitation, energy) rather than holistic health outcomes. For architecture students, this fragmentation often obscures the relationship between a building's performance and occupant health. To bridge this gap, a pedagogical exercise involves analyzing the proposal for a new, unified *"Part of the Building Regulations for Health and Wellbeing,"* as suggested by the National Engineering Policy Centre [38].

This proposed regulation creates an explicit functional requirement: the building must provide an adequate indoor environment that protects the health and well-being of users from adverse effects [38]. In a classroom setting, asking students to design against this hypothetical regulation forces them to move beyond minimum compliance (e.g., simply meeting air change rates) to a performance-based understanding of infection resilience.

1. *Ventilation and Air Quality: The "Invisible" Architecture:* Regulations, such as Part F (Ventilation) in the UK or ASHRAE Standard 62.1 (older versions) in the United States, may often be taught as sizing exercises for mechanical engineers. However, the pedagogical challenge is to teach architects that ventilation is a spatial property. Students must understand that while mechanical engineers calculate air changes per hour (ACH), architects define the volume and geometry that determines airflow effectiveness [16].

For example, studies on classrooms have shown that the effectiveness of natural ventilation strategies—a favorite of architectural studios due to their energy efficiency—is highly dependent on window design, room depth, and external climatic conditions [16]. By engaging with literature that analyses the limitations of single-sided versus cross-ventilation in reducing airborne transmission risk, students learn that a window is not just a framing device for a view, but a critical valve for effecting infection control [16]. The "safe" classroom of the future requires integrating CO_2 sensors as proxies for ventilation effectiveness, a concept that merges building physics with active user management [41].

2. *The Sanitary Core: Beyond the "Back of House":* Architectural education often treats washrooms as "back of house" service spaces, usually if not always drawn quickly to meet code requirements. However, the transmission of pathogens in these spaces is complex, involving fecal-oral, surface (fomite), and potential bioaerosol routes [45]. A pedagogical approach focused on infection control brings the washroom to the forefront of design.

Students must examine the microbiology of the "toilet plume"—the aerosolization of pathogens caused by flushing lidless toilets—which can contaminate surfaces and air [45]. This biological reality necessitates architectural responses: the spatial segregation of toilets from sinks, the specification of lid-closure mechanisms, and the design of airflow regimes that extract contaminants at the source rather than mixing them into the breathing zone [17]. Furthermore, the debate between paper towels and jet air dryers serves as a critical case study in evidence-based design. While jet dryers are energy efficient, some studies suggest they disperse viral particulates further than paper towels, highlighting a trade-off between sustainability and hygiene that students must learn to navigate [45].

3. *The Intersection of Energy and Health: Retrofitting for Resilience:* A critical component of modern architectural education is the "Deep Retrofit." With the drive toward Net Zero, students are taught to seal buildings to conserve energy. However, without a concurrent understanding of infection control, this "tightening" of the building envelope can inadvertently create incubators for pathogens by reducing air infiltration [38].

The pedagogical intervention here is to teach the concept of *"Co-benefits."* Students analyze how upgrades to ventilation systems (e.g., Mechanical Ventilation with Heat Recovery—MVHR) can simultaneously improve energy efficiency and reduce viral transmission, provided the filtration is adequate (e.g., HEPA or MERV 13+) [32]. This aligns with the "One Health" approach, viewing the health of the planet and the health of the occupant as interconnected systems rather than competing interests [7].

A defining strength of the elective was the deliberate use of experiential and investigative exercises designed to make the "invisible" dimensions of infection transmission tangible to students. Rather than treating infection control as abstract theory, the pedagogy emphasized measurement, observation, reflection, and application within architectural contexts. Across the semester, students engaged with structured exercises that addressed history of epidemics, modes of transmission, quantification of airborne risk, spatial interventions, and design-based retrofitting strategies.

Simulation and Modeling as Design Drivers

To visualize the "invisible" threat of bioaerosols, architecture students are increasingly introduced to computational fluid dynamics (CFD) and agent-based modeling. These tools allow students to simulate how a cough or sneeze disperses in a space they have designed, transforming abstract viral risks into tangible design parameters.

1. *Agent-Based Modeling for Social Distancing:* Urban design studios now incorporate simulations that predict human movement and interaction. For instance, studies have shown that specific urban configurations and transport node designs can influence the density of crowds and the likelihood of disease transmission [48]. By using agent-based models, students can test how widening a corridor, altering a queueing system, or changing the layout of a lobby impacts the "contact rate" between occupants [48]. This shifts the design intent from purely "flow efficiency" to "hygienic flow."

2. *Visualizing Airflow and Viral Plumes:* Advanced CFD modeling has demonstrated that standard mixing ventilation (where air is mixed to uniform temperature) can inadvertently spread viral aerosols across a room [16]. In contrast, displacement ventilationwhich introduces air at low velocity near the floor and extracts it at the ceiling, can lift contaminants away from occupants [22]. Integrating these simulations into the design studio allows students to see that the placement of a vent is as critical to the architecture as the placement of a door. This is for advanced requirements, and the same is also useful for low resource settings where mixing ventilation may be better than no ventilation.

Integrating Advanced Technologies: UVGI

A significant gap in current architectural pedagogy is the integration of active disinfection technologies, specifically ultraviolet germicidal irradiation (UVGI). Historically viewed as medical equipment, UVGI is moving into the mainstream built environment. Upper-room UVGI, which creates a zone of UV-C light above occupants' heads to kill rising pathogens, is believed by many to be a highly effective engineering control [43]. This is especially useful where ventilation may not be an option (though that is unlikely in most settings), provided that it is integrated safely without harming human health and it is provisioned to be regularly maintained.

Teaching this technology involves understanding complex variables: the susceptibility of different viruses to UV light (which varies by genomic structure), the impact of relative humidity on UV efficacy, and the geometry of the room [43]. For example, students must learn that at higher relative humidity, viruses like influenza may become more resistant to UV inactivation, requiring higher doses or different system configurations [43]. This reinforces the need for architects to design systems that can maintain humidity within optimal ranges (40–60%) not just for comfort, but for infection control—a concept supported by the "40–60% RH" rule for respiratory health [43].

The integration of public health into architectural education requires a paradigm shift. It demands moving beyond the Vitruvian triad of "Commodity, Firmness, and Delight" to include "Health" as a fourth, non-negotiable pillar. By using building regulations as a framework to understand the biological consequences of design decisions, and by employing advanced simulation tools to visualize invisible risks, educators can equip the next generation of architects to build environments that are not only sustainable and beautiful but also resilient against the microbial threats of the future. This prepares the profession for a new role: not just as designers of space, but as custodians of public health.

Within the elective course, students were introduced to the Wells–Riley equation not merely as theory but as a design tool. They applied it to familiar architectural typologies such as auditoriums, cafeterias, libraries, lifts, restaurants, and classrooms. Students conducted iterative calculations by modifying spatial height, volume, occupancy, mask usage, and ventilation rates, and directly observed how architectural decisions altered infection probability. This exercise was repeatedly identified by students as one of the most impactful learning components of the course.

2.3 The Engineering of Immunity: Re-evaluating Ventilation and Air Distribution Strategies

Beyond student satisfaction, the elective highlights an important structural insight: architecture students respond positively when infection control is taught as a design problem rather than as an abstract technical requirement. The study concludes that the subject requires an explicitly interdisciplinary approach and that architectural education represents the most effective stage at which such integration can occur. This supports the argument that infection control should not remain peripheral or elective, but should form part of the foundational knowledge of future building professionals.

The Paradigm Shift: From Comfort to Contagion Control

For the better part of the last century, the professional perception of heating, ventilation, and air conditioning (HVAC) systems is believed to have been dominated by the concept of thermal comfort and odour control. Architects and engineers may have designed systems to maintain temperature set points and keep carbon dioxide (CO_2) levels low enough to prevent drowsiness. However, the emerging understanding of the continuum between short-range and long-range airborne transmission has forced a radical re-evaluation of these design parameters. The building professional must now view the HVAC system not merely as a climate control device, but as an active immune system for the building—a mechanism capable of interrupting the transmission of pathogens through precise fluid dynamics and biological inactivation.

Recent theoretical advancements have challenged the traditional dichotomy between droplet and airborne transmission. The "short-range airborne route," occurring when individuals are in close proximity (less than 2 m), was previously thought to be dominated by large ballistic droplets. However, new macroscopic aerosol balance models suggest that room ventilation rates significantly affect this short-range exposure, a finding that contradicts traditional beliefs held by many building designers [27]. This revelation implies that the architect's responsibility extends beyond general air quality to the specific micro-environments created between interacting occupants.

2.3.1 The Ventilation Rate Debate: The Rule of 10 L/s

A critical point of contention among building professionals is the determination of adequate ventilation rates. Older standards may rely on a "people source and room source" rule, specifying rates based on occupancy and floor area (e.g., 2.5 L/s per person plus 0.3 $L/s{\cdot}m^2$) [27]. While effective for controlling body odors and off-gassing from materials, these standards are increasingly perceived as inadequate for infection control.

Research indicates that a ventilation rate of 10 L/s per person is a critical threshold. Modeling of exhaled gaseous substances demonstrates a "diminishing returns" phenomenon: increasing ventilation from 1 to 10 L/s yields a massive reduction in infection risk, but increasing it further beyond 10 L/s provides relatively little additional benefit in terms of concentration decay profiles [27]. This finding provides a robust scientific justification for the widely adopted, yet often empirically derived, standard of 10 L/s per person [27].

Within the elective course, students were introduced to the Wells–Riley equation not merely as theory but as a design tool. They applied it to familiar architectural typologies such as auditoriums, cafeterias, libraries, lifts, restaurants, and classrooms. Students conducted iterative calculations by modifying spatial height, volume, occupancy, mask usage, and ventilation rates, and directly observed how architectural decisions altered infection probability. This exercise was repeatedly identified by students as one of the most impactful learning components of the course.

However, professionals must now contend with the reality that a constant outdoor air rate is insufficient for respiratory infection control in crowded spaces. The perception that meeting minimum code requirements equals "safety" is dangerous. Evidence suggests that when physical distance between occupants is less than 2 m, the required ventilation rate must increase dynamically to counteract the high concentration of aerosols in the breathing zone [27]. This requires a shift toward "demand-controlled ventilation" (DCV) that is responsive not just to CO_2 levels, but to infection risk probabilities, potentially utilizing sensors to estimate occupant proximity and density [32]. This is not an absolute requirement but a progressive one. For a facility without any measure, the first step may be ventilation, then monitoring of carbon dioxide and then the sensors for proximity as suggested for DCV. The mix in the equation also involves the fact that resources are involved and many parts of the developing world may be under the grip of diseases requiring such mitigation.

2.3.2 The Geometry of Air: Mixing vs. Displacement

Beyond the volume of air supplied, building professionals are increasingly focused on the *geometry* of airflow. The conventional approach in most commercial and educational buildings is mixing ventilation (MV), where fresh air is introduced at high velocity to dilute contaminants uniformly throughout the space [16]. While efficient for thermal uniformity, MV has a fatal flaw in the context of infection control: it keeps viral particles suspended and disperses them throughout the room, potentially exposing occupants far from the source [16].

Displacement Ventilation (DV) Architects and engineers are now re-examining displacement ventilation (DV) as a potential strategy for pathogen removal. In DV systems, cool fresh air is introduced at low velocity near the floor. As the air warms upon contact with occupants, it rises due to thermal buoyancy, carrying bio-effluents and aerosols upward to extraction points at the ceiling [16, 22]. This creates a "thermal stratification" that effectively locks contaminants in the upper zone of the room, away from the breathing zone of other occupants [16]. It must be noted that displacement ventilation has shown in some configurations to reduce cross-infection compared to mixing ventilation.

Studies utilizing computational fluid dynamics (CFD) in auditoriums have shown that DV can significantly reduce the horizontal spread of viral plumes compared to mixing ventilation [22]. However, the implementation of DV requires early architectural integration. It necessitates higher floor-to-ceiling heights to allow for stratification and specific plenum designs that cannot be easily retrofitted [16]. This reinforces the concept that infection control is a fundamental architectural constraint, not a mechanical add-on.

Under-Floor Air Distribution (UFAD) A variation of DV, the under-floor air distribution (UFAD) system, creates a similar vertical flow pattern. Research indicates that UFAD systems may be more effective at diluting virus concentrations in rows where no infected person is present compared to mixing systems [16]. However, the perception of UFAD is nuanced; if air outlets are positioned directly beneath a seated occupant, the high-velocity jet can disrupt the thermal plume and mix exhaled droplets into the breathing zone of neighbors [16]. Thus, the precise placement of diffusers—a detail that may often be left to contractors—is now a critical design decision for the architect and engineer.

2.3.3 The Renaissance of Ultraviolet Germicidal Irradiation (UVGI)

As building professionals grapple with the energy penalties of increasing outdoor air intake (conditioning cold or hot air requires significant energy), ultraviolet germicidal irradiation (UVGI) is experiencing a renaissance. Historically used for tuberculosis control, UVGI uses UV-C light (typically 254 nm) to damage the DNA or RNA of microorganisms, preventing replication [8, 43].

Upper-Room UVGI Upper-room UVGI systems generate a controlled zone of UV-C radiation near the ceiling. Natural or mechanical air currents lift airborne pathogens into this "kill zone," where they are inactivated before circulating back down to occupants [8]. Studies have shown that a properly designed upper-room UVGI system can provide the equivalent safety like that of multiple air changes per hour (ACH) in terms of disinfection, far exceeding what is typically possible with mechanical ventilation alone [8].

The professional perception of UVGI is shifting from a specialized hospital technology to a general public health utility. However, efficacy is highly dependent on environmental variables. Systematic reviews indicate that the susceptibility of viruses to UV radiation (the Z-value) is significantly influenced by relative humidity (RH) [43]. For enveloped viruses like coronaviruses and influenza, increasing RH is generally associated with decreased susceptibility to UV inactivation [43]. This implies that architects must design HVAC systems capable of maintaining RH within specific ranges (e.g., 40–60%) not just for comfort, but to maximize the efficiency of UVGI systems [43].

In-Duct UVGI For buildings where upper-room fixtures are aesthetically or spatially unfeasible, in-duct UVGI offers an invisible solution. By placing UV lamps within the air handling unit or ducts, recirculated air is disinfected before re-entry. However, the perception of "kill rates" in these systems must be grounded in physics. The air in a duct moves at high velocities (thousands of feet per minute), meaning the pathogen residence time in the irradiation zone is fractions of a second [8]. This means it may actually just be disinfecting the inside surfaces of the HVAC systems. Therefore, in-duct systems require high-intensity lamps and reflective duct materials (like aluminum) to ensure a lethal dose is delivered [8]. Recent modeling confirms that increasing the airflow rate (ACH) decreases the survival fraction of pathogens, provided the UV dose is sufficient [43]. But this is to be studied further before prescription.

2.3.4 Filtration: The First Line of Defense

While UVGI inactivates pathogens, filtration removes them physically. The perception of high-efficiency particulate air (HEPA) filters has transitioned from "clean room only" to a gold standard for infection resilience. HEPA filters capture at least 99.97% of particles 0.3 microns in diameter, which includes the droplet nuclei that carry viruses [32].

However, the integration of HEPA filters into existing building systems presents a significant engineering challenge: pressure drop. High-efficiency filters create resistance to airflow, which can strain fans and reduce overall ventilation rates if the system is not designed for the load [32]. This trade-off forces building professionals to consider alternative filtration strategies, such as minimum efficiency reporting value (MERV) 13 filters, which capture a significant percentage of viral aerosols (70–85%) with a lower pressure penalty [16, 32].

The use of portable air cleaners with HEPA filters has also gained traction as a supplementary measure. These devices are particularly effective in "dead zones" of a room where air stagnation occurs [32]. However, their effectiveness is limited by their clean air delivery rate (CADR) relative to the room volume. A critical review of portable air filters indicates that while they reduce particle counts, their ability to significantly reduce clinical infection rates in real-world settings (outside of controlled chambers) requires rigorous placement strategies to ensure they do not create cross-drafts that pull infectious aerosols past susceptible occupants [19]. Further, it must be noted that these portable devices may end up recirculating the same indoor air and may be unfit for tuberculosis related situations. The solution is to have new portable filters with outdoor fresh air supply.

2.3.5 The Role of Surface and Materiality in Infection Control

While airborne transmission is the primary focus of this chapter, the perception of surface hygiene (fomites) remains a component of the holistic infection control strategy. The persistence of SARS-CoV-2 on inanimate surfaces varies significantly by material type, with viability lasting longer on smooth surfaces like steel and plastic compared to porous surfaces [46].

This has led to renewed interest in antimicrobial surfaces. Materials containing copper or silver ions have shown efficacy in reducing bacterial and viral loads [45]. However, the "deep cleaning" paradigm that emerged early in the COVID-19 pandemic is being scrutinized. Frequent application of potent chemical disinfectants (e.g., quaternary ammonium compounds, chlorine) can lead to the formation of secondary indoor pollutants and respiratory irritants, potentially exacerbating the very health issues they aim to prevent [46].

Consequently, the professional perception is shifting toward "no-touch" disinfection technologies. Automated systems using hydrogen peroxide vapor or pulsed xenon UV light can decontaminate surfaces without leaving toxic residues, provided the space is unoccupied [35]. These technologies require architects to design spaces that can be sealed off for disinfection cycles, further integrating operational protocols into the physical design of the building.

The integration of advanced ventilation, air distribution, and disinfection strategies represents a fundamental maturation of the building professions. No longer passive containers for human activity, buildings are being reimagined as active participants in public health. UVGI is a potent, underutilized tool that depends heavily on humidity control [43]; and ventilation rates must be dynamic, responding to occupancy density to be effective against short-range transmission [27].

As we move to the next section, we will explore how these engineering principles are applied in specific high-risk environments, examining case studies that highlight the successes and failures of design in the face of biological threats.

2.4 The Clinical Fortress: Isolation, Pressurization, and the Laminar Flow Paradox

Defining the Line of Defense

In the hierarchy of the built environment, the hospital represents the fortress—a structure designed not merely for shelter, but for active defense against biological aggression. For the architect and the building services engineer, the perception of the clinical environment is fundamentally different from that of a commercial office. Here, the invisible architecture of airflow patterns, pressure differentials, and filtration efficiencies dictates the boundary between safety and contamination. The COVID-19 pandemic, alongside the persistent threat of multidrug-resistant organisms (MDROs), has forced a rigorous re-evaluation of these defenses, particularly concerning the design of isolation rooms and the efficacy of specialized ventilation systems like laminar air flow (LAF).

2.4.1 The Anteroom: The Airlock of Infection Control

The structural perception of an isolation ward relies heavily on the concept of the "anteroom" (or vestibule). Architecturally, this is often viewed as a buffer zone—a transitional space between the corridor and the patient room. However, from an infection control perspective, the anteroom is a dynamic airlock essential for maintaining pressure gradients and preventing the migration of airborne pathogens [5].

Recent systematic reviews have highlighted that the mere presence of an anteroom significantly enhances the efficiency of isolation systems by preventing pressure loss during door usage [5]. The engineering challenge lies in maintaining precise pressure differentials. Studies suggest that a pressure difference of −8 to −15 Pa may be optimal for preventing the escape of infectious aerosols from a patient room to the corridor [5]. However, building professionals must navigate the complex physics of "door pumping"—the phenomenon where the opening of a hinged door can drag contaminated air out of a negative pressure room, effectively reversing the protective airflow momentarily.

Research indicates that sliding doors may be superior to hinged doors in minimizing this leakage and maintaining the integrity of the pressure gradient [5]. Furthermore, the thermal environment plays a surprising role; a temperature difference of more than 2 °C between the anteroom and the isolation room may generate convective currents strong enough to transport contaminants against the designed airflow direction [5]. Thus, the architect's perception of the anteroom must evolve from a simple spatial buffer to a tightly controlled thermodynamic zone equipped with hands-free sinks, mirrors for personal protective equipment (PPE) checks, and distinct zoning for clean and dirty workflows [5].

2.4.2 The Operating Theatre: The Laminar Flow Paradox

Perhaps the most contentious debate in hospital design concerns the ventilation of operating theatres. For decades, the professional consensus was that laminar air flow (LAF)—a unidirectional stream of ultra-clean air—was the gold standard for preventing surgical site infections (SSIs). The visual intuition is compelling: a curtain of clean air descending over the surgical wound should theoretically sweep away all contaminants.

However, recent meta-analyses have challenged this perception, revealing a counterintuitive reality. While high-efficiency particulate air (HEPA) filters undeniably reduce bioaerosol concentrations, the LAF system itself may not be as effective as previously believed when compared to conventional turbulent ventilation equipped with HEPA filters [12]. A systematic review found that while HEPA filters reduced bacterial counts by an average of 113.14 CFU/m^3, the specific use of LAF systems was associated with only a moderate reduction in bacterial counts compared to turbulent systems, and in some fungal assessments, LAF rooms actually showed higher counts [12].

This "Laminar Flow Paradox" arises from the behavior of fluids and heat. The thermal plumes generated by the surgical team and the patient can disrupt the unidirectional flow of the LAF, creating turbulence that entrains contaminants from the floor or periphery back into the surgical site [12]. Furthermore, the physical presence of surgical lamps and heads of personnel can block the "clean" air stream. Consequently, building professionals are urged to reconsider the heavy capital investment in LAF systems, as HEPA-filtered turbulent airflow may offer a more cost-effective and equally reliable solution for general bioaerosol removal [12]. But this may require further study and observations.

2.5 The Sanitary Nexus: Washrooms, Plumes, and Wastewater

The Bathroom as a Bioaerosol Generator

If the hospital room is the fortress, the public washroom is the breach. For architects and facility managers, washrooms have historically been designed for privacy, ease of cleaning, and odour control. However, the transmission dynamics of SARS-CoV-2 and other enteric pathogens have shifted the focus toward the washroom as a generator of bioaerosols. The "toilet plume"—the aerosolization of fecal matter and water droplets during flushing—has moved from a theoretical concern to a documented environmental hazard [45].

2.5.1 The Flush and the Fomite

Evidence confirms that toilet flushing, particularly with the lid open, generates a plume of bioaerosols that can remain suspended in the air and contaminate surrounding surfaces [45]. While viral RNA, including SARS-CoV-2, has been detected in hospital toilet areas, a systematic review of public washrooms found no direct evidence of airborne transmission of COVID-19 to users in these settings; however, the risk of surface (fomite) contamination remains significant [45]. Yet, at other places like in Hong Kong there was further evidence (see Sect. 2.5.3 below).

This distinction is crucial for building professionals. The primary risk in washrooms appears to be the deposition of pathogens on high-touch surfaces—flush handles, door latches, and taps—rather than inhalation of the plume itself, provided ventilation is adequate [45]. Consequently, design interventions are shifting toward "touchless" technologies. Yet, even this solution has nuances: early designs of non-touch taps with low water pressure and standing columns of warm water were found to promote the growth of *Pseudomonas aeruginosa* and *Legionella*, necessitating a return to conventional fittings in some hospitals [45]. This highlights the complexity of engineering out infection; solving one problem (touch) can inadvertently create another (bacterial growth). Copper based surfaces may be the step ahead.

2.5.2 The Hand Drying Debate

The method of hand drying in public washrooms represents a collision between sustainability goals and infection control. Electric hand dryers, particularly high-speed jet air dryers (JAD), are favored for reducing paper waste. However, from a microbiological perspective, they are viewed with skepticism. JADs have been shown to disperse droplets and microbial markers up to 3 m from the unit, significantly further than paper towels [45].

While no outbreaks have been definitively traced to hand dryers, the mechanism of dispersal creates a potential route for cross-contamination. Building professionals are therefore advised to consider the placement of these units carefully, avoiding locations near open food (in cafeterias) or sensitive patient areas, and considering retrofitting units with HEPA filters to scrub the air used for drying [45].

2.5.3 The Vertical Threat: Plumbing and Wastewater

The built environment extends beyond the visible room to the infrastructure hidden behind the walls. The transmission of SARS-CoV-2 via drainage pipes in high-rise buildings—reminiscent of the Amoy Gardens SARS outbreak in 2003—remains a critical concern. Dry U-traps in floor drains can allow sewer gases containing viral aerosols to enter living spaces [45]. This “vertical” transmission route emphasizes the need for hydraulic sanitary design that ensures water seals are maintained, a responsibility that falls squarely on the plumbing engineer and the facility manager.

Furthermore, wastewater surveillance has emerged as a powerful tool for monitoring community infection levels. The detection of SARS-CoV-2 RNA in sewage serves as an early warning system for outbreaks, often preceding clinical case data [40]. This integrates the building’s waste output into the broader public health surveillance infrastructure, transforming the sewer from a disposal system into a diagnostic tool.

2.6 Congregate Settings: Schools and Transport

The High-Density Challenge

Moving beyond the controlled environments of hospitals, building professionals face the chaotic reality of schools and public transport. These settings are characterized by high occupant density, variable ventilation capacities, and the presence of susceptible populations.

2.6.1 Classrooms: Natural vs. Mechanical Ventilation

In educational settings, the debate often centres on natural versus mechanical ventilation. A systematic review of ventilation strategies in classrooms confirms that while mechanical systems provide consistency, natural ventilation (opening windows) remains a critical, albeit variable, intervention [16]. The efficacy of natural ventilation is highly dependent on architectural features such as window size, cross-ventilation capabilities, and external weather conditions.

The use of CO_2 sensors as proxies for ventilation effectiveness has gained traction. While CO_2 levels do not directly measure viral load, they serve as a reliable indicator of "rebreathed air." However, relying solely on CO_2 setpoints (e.g., 1000 ppm) may be insufficient. Recent evidence suggests that in high-risk scenarios, even meeting standard ventilation rates may not prevent short-range transmission if occupants are in close proximity [27]. This suggests that architects must design classrooms not just for air change rates, but for spatial volume and layout that allow for physical distancing and the rapid dilution of exhaled plumes.

2.6.2 Public Transport: The Mobile Vector

Public transport vehicles—buses, trains, and subways—present a unique challenge: they are mobile, enclosed volumes with high transient occupancy. Systematic reviews of transmission in these settings have identified risks associated with proximity and duration of travel [23]. Engineering controls such as high-efficiency filtration in re-circulated air systems (e.g., in aircraft and modern trains) are effective, but ground transport often lacks such sophistication.

The perception of risk in these settings is often higher than the documented evidence of transmission, partly due to the difficulty of contact tracing in transient populations [23]. However, the "close contact" nature of transit necessitates a multi-layered approach: improved ventilation rates where possible, but heavily reliant on source control (masking) to mitigate the limitations of the engineering systems [23].

The perception of infection control among building professionals is shifting from a passive reliance on code compliance to an active engagement with fluid dynamics and microbiology. Whether designing the pressure gradients of a hospital anteroom [5], selecting the hand-drying method for a public toilet [45], or configuring the ventilation of a classroom [16], the professional is now an active participant in the chain of infection prevention. The building is no longer just a container for people; it is a technological immune system.

2.7 The Domestic Sphere: Housing, Density, and the "Stay at Home" Paradox

Redefining Safe Harbor

For most of the twentieth century, the home was viewed by architects and urban planners as a sanctuary—a private retreat from the noise, pollution, and frenetic energy of the public realm. However, the implementation of non-pharmaceutical interventions (NPIs) such as "lockdowns" and "stay-at-home" orders during the COVID-19 pandemic inverted this paradigm. The home suddenly became the primary site of transmission, particularly in multigenerational households and high-density living arrangements. This phenomenon challenged the building professional's perception of residential design, shifting the focus from aesthetic comfort to biological isolation capacity.

The professional community has had to grapple with the distinction between *population density* (a measure of urban planning) and *household overcrowding* (a measure of architectural interior volume). Systematic reviews indicate that while compact cities with high population density do not inherently facilitate viral spread if public health measures are robust, household overcrowding—defined by the number of occupants per room—is a consistent and potent driver of infection [2, 49].

2.7.1 The Overcrowding Factor and TB Parallels

The link between inadequate housing and respiratory infection is not unique to SARS-CoV-2; it mirrors the historical and ongoing battle against *Mycobacterium tuberculosis* (TB). A systematic review of housing conditions revealed that inadequate housing, characterized by overcrowding, poor ventilation, and lack of sunlight, significantly increases the risk of TB exposure, transmission, and recurrence [26].

For architects, this highlights a critical failure in low-cost housing design: the prioritization of shelter quantity over environmental quality. The data suggests that housing affordability is inextricably linked to infection resilience; when housing is unaffordable, density increases as families double up, directly compromising the "air volume per person" required to dilute infectious aerosols [26]. Consequently, building professionals must perceive housing policy not merely as an economic issue but as a fundamental component of the engineered immune system of a city.

2.7.2 Household Transmission Dynamics

In the context of SARS-CoV-2, household transmission rates have been closely studied, revealing that the architecture of the home dictates the attack rate. Studies indicate that secondary attack rates (SAR) within households are significantly higher than in other community settings due to the duration and intensity of contact [11]. Interestingly, research has shown that while children are often index cases, the transmissibility within a household varies by age and the specific viral variant, with Omicron showing higher household transmissibility than Delta [11].

This biological reality necessitates an architectural response: the concept of "isolation within the home." Traditional open-plan residential designs fail to provide the compartmentalization necessary to isolate an infected family member. Future residential design criteria must evaluate the inclusion of "sick rooms" or flexible partitioning systems that allow for temporary bio-exclusion zones within a dwelling unit [11]. This implies a need for separate ventilation zones within apartments, similar to the compartmentalization used in hospital wards, to prevent the migration of viral aerosols from a sick bedroom to common living areas.

2.8 Inequalities in the Built Environment: Informal Settlements and WASH

The Architecture of Neglect

The disparity in infection control capacity is most visible in the urban slums and informal settlements of low- and middle-income countries (LMICs). Here, the professional perception of "building standards" collides with the reality of survival. In these settings, the built environment often actively facilitates transmission through the lack of water, sanitation, and hygiene (WASH) infrastructure [36].

2.8.1 The WASH Crisis and Gendered Space

A systematic review of WASH in schools across LMICs revealed a catastrophic lack of infrastructure to support basic hand hygiene, a primary defense against fomite transmission [36]. In many urban poor settlements, water is accessed through communal standpipes, and sanitation is provided by shared community latrines. During a pandemic, these shared facilities become high-risk vector points. The architecture of these spaces often ignores gendered needs; women and girls bear a disproportionate burden of water collection and household hygiene, increasing their exposure time in these high-risk communal zones [14].

Building professionals working in development contexts must recognize that installing a tap is insufficient if the spatial design does not allow for physical distancing or if the supply chain does not guarantee water continuity. The "urban advantage"—the idea that city dwellers have better health outcomes than rural populations—disappears in slum environments where overcrowding makes "stay at home" orders practically impossible and potentially dangerous [14]. The solution requires a radical rethinking of urban infrastructure to decentralize WASH facilities, reducing the user-to-latrine ratio and integrating touchless technologies that are robust enough for high-intensity public use [14].

2.9 Institutional Vulnerability: Schools, Prisons, and Shelters

Designing for the Vulnerable

Beyond the home, specific institutional settings present unique engineering challenges due to the density of occupants and the inability of those occupants to control their own environment.

2.9.1 Schools: The Ventilation Deficit

Schools represent a high-density environment where prolonged exposure is mandatory. Systematic reviews of school reopenings during the pandemic highlighted that while children may have lower susceptibility to severe disease, schools can act as transmission hubs if mitigation strategies are lax [13, 39]. Engineering controls in schools have historically been neglected, with many classrooms relying only on window opening, which is a great start, but needs optimisation of window size, direction and may also be subject to weather constraints.

Effective strategies identified include the reorganization of spatial layouts to ensure the option for unidirectional seating, the installation of CO_2 monitors as proxies for ventilation efficacy, and the use of hybrid learning models to de-densify classrooms [13, 39]. However, the literature also points to a significant gap in WASH infrastructure in schools, with many lacking basic soap and water, rendering hygiene education theoretical rather than practical [36]. The architect's role in school design must evolve to prioritize "breathing buildings"—structures that passively maximize air exchange rates without compromising thermal comfort or acoustic performance required for learning.

2.9.2 Prisons and Shelters: Carceral and Congregate Risks

Prisons and homeless shelters are perhaps the most challenging built environments for infection control. Inmates and shelter clients share air and sanitation facilities with no option for self-isolation. A systematic review of COVID-19 in prisons identified overcrowding and poor ventilation as primary drivers of massive outbreaks [25]. The architectural rigidity of prisons—designed for containment rather than health—creates so to say "incubation chambers."

Similarly, homeless shelters have required rapid restructuring. Interventions identified as effective include the physical spacing of beds (head-to-toe configuration), the installation of physical barriers (partitions), and the use of "satellite" isolation sites such as hotels [50]. However, a critical engineering intervention in these spaces is the *anteroom*. Research indicates that the inclusion of anterooms (vestibules) at the entrance of isolation areas in congregate settings significantly maintains pressure differentials and reduces the migration of airborne particles into corridors [5]. While standard in hospitals, the retrofitting of anterooms into shelters and prisons represents a necessary evolution of these building typologies to handle respiratory pathogens.

2.10 The Underground Sentinel: Wastewater-Based Epidemiology (WBE)

The Sewer as a Diagnostic Tool

While architects focus on the visible structure, a critical component of building performance lies underground. Wastewater-based epidemiology (WBE) has emerged as a powerful tool for monitoring community infection levels. The detection of SARS-CoV-2 RNA in sewage provides an early warning system, often preceding clinical case data by several days [40].

2.10.1 The Plumbing System as a Transmission Route

Building professionals must also perceive the plumbing system not just as a waste removal mechanism, but as a potential transmission route. The "fecal-oral-aerosol" pathway, famously documented in the Amoy Gardens SARS outbreak, remains a threat. Defective sanitary plumbing—specifically dried-out U-traps—can allow sewer gases containing aerosolized pathogens to enter living spaces [18, 45]. This vertical transmission route links the health of one apartment unit to the biological waste of another.

The presence of viral RNA in wastewater confirms that buildings are constantly shedding biological data [6]. For the building engineer, this implies a responsibility to design hydraulic systems that maintain trap seals under pressure fluctuations and to view the building's waste output as a valuable stream of public health information. The integration of sampling ports for WBE into building design could become a standard feature of future "pandemic-resilient" infrastructure [10].

The perception of infection control by building professionals has shifted from a passive reliance on medical solutions to an active engagement with the physical determinants of transmission. From the high-tech filtration systems of hospitals to the humble U-trap in a residential high-rise, every component of the built environment plays a role in either propagating or interrupting the chain of infection. The integration of microbiology, fluid dynamics, and social science into the architectural curriculum and professional practice is no longer optional; it is a prerequisite for designing a resilient future.

2.11 The Convergence of Sustainability and Health: Beyond Net Zero

The False Dichotomy

For decades, the dominant narrative in the building industry may have been pegged to energy efficiency. The drive toward "Net Zero" carbon emissions has dictated architectural form, leading to the construction of tightly sealed building envelopes designed to minimize thermal loss. However, the professional perception of sustainability is undergoing a critical expansion. The COVID 19 pandemic has laid bare a tension that has long existed but was frequently ignored: the trade-off between energy efficiency and infection control. Historically, reducing ventilation rates may have been a primary method for saving energy; today, it is recognized as one of the leading risk factor for airborne transmission [38].

Building professionals are now tasked with reconciling these competing demands. The new paradigm posits that a building cannot be truly "sustainable" if it is not "healthy." This realization necessitates a systems approach where infection resilience is not an optional add-on but a fundamental functional requirement, akin to structural stability or fire safety [38].

2.11.1 The Energy Penalty and Heat Recovery

Increasing outdoor air supply to dilute airborne pathogens inevitably increases the energy load required to condition that air. This "energy penalty" is a significant concern for engineers and facility managers. However, recent reviews suggest that energy efficiency and indoor air quality (IAQ) need not be mutually exclusive. The integration of heat recovery systems—which capture thermal energy from exhaust air to condition incoming fresh air—can reduce the heat lost by approximately 80%, enabling high ventilation rates without the prohibitive energy costs associated with unconstrained winter heat losses [38].

Furthermore, professionals are increasingly viewing air cleaning technologies as energy-saving devices. By using high-efficiency particulate air (HEPA) filters or ultraviolet germicidal irradiation (UVGI) to recirculate cleaned air, buildings can achieve high "equivalent air changes per hour" (eACH) without the thermal load of conditioning 100% outside air [32, 33]. This shift in perception transforms the HVAC system from a simple air mover into a complex "pathogen processing plant".

2.11.2 Retrofitting for Resilience

A major challenge facing the built environment is the existing building stock. While new hospitals can be designed with state-of-the-art isolation rooms, the vast majority of transmission may actually occur in existing schools, offices, and homes. The concept of "retrofitting for resilience" has emerged as a priority. This involves aligning infection control upgrades with national decarbonization programs [38].

For example, when retrofitting a building for energy efficiency (e.g., adding insulation and double glazing), there is a risk of reducing air permeability to the point where pollutants and pathogens accumulate—a phenomenon that contributed to the "sick building syndrome" of the late twentieth century [37, 38]. Professionals must now ensure that any energy retrofit includes a concurrent ventilation strategy. This might involve installing mechanical ventilation with heat recovery (MVHR) in homes that were previously naturally ventilated, or deploying upper-room UVGI systems in older public buildings where increasing mechanical ventilation is structurally unfeasible [33, 38].

2.12 The Digital Turn: Smart Buildings and Sentinel Systems

Making the Invisible Visible

One of the greatest hurdles in infection control is the invisibility of the threat. Unlike a structural crack or a water leak, a high viral load in the air is imperceptible to the human senses. Consequently, building professionals are turning to digital technology to render the invisible visible. The integration of the Internet of Things (IoT) and smart sensors into the built environment represents a profound shift in how we manage biological risk.

2.12.1 Carbon Dioxide (CO_2) as a Proxy

While real-time detection of viral RNA in the air remains technologically complex and expensive for general application, carbon dioxide (CO_2) monitoring has emerged as a robust, low-cost proxy for ventilation effectiveness and infection risk [32, 34]. Since humans exhale both CO_2 and potentially virus-laden aerosols, high indoor CO_2 levels indicate a high fraction of "rebreathed air."

Recent studies have derived CO_2-based risk proxies, suggesting that maintaining lower CO_2 levels (e.g., below 700–800 ppm) significantly increases the efficiency of ventilation measures in reducing relative infection risk [16, 32]. Building professionals are increasingly specifying CO_2 sensors not just for demand-controlled ventilation (DCV) to save energy, but as "traffic light" systems to warn occupants when ventilation is insufficient. In the event of a pandemic, the logic of DCV systems must be inverted: rather than reducing ventilation when occupancy is low to save energy, systems should be programmed to maximize fresh air intake regardless of CO_2 levels, or the setpoints must be drastically lowered [32].

2.12.2 Occupancy Sensing and Crowd Management

The risk of airborne transmission is inextricably linked to occupant density. To manage this, building automation systems are utilizing advanced occupancy sensors. These include passive infrared (PIR) sensors, ultrasonic sensors, and camera-based systems that can estimate the number of people in a room [29].

Data from these sensors can drive "Smart Ventilation" strategies. For instance, if a meeting room exceeds a certain occupancy threshold, the building management system (BMS) can automatically surge the ventilation rate or activate supplementary air purification units [29]. Furthermore, these data streams allow facility managers to identify "hot spots" of congestion in real-time, enabling administrative controls such as redirecting foot traffic or closing specific areas for cleaning [1]. This represents a move toward "precision building management," where resources are dynamically allocated based on real-time biological risk rather than static schedules [29].

2.12.3 Computational Modeling and Digital Twins

At the urban and building design stage, computational fluid dynamics (CFD) and agent-based modeling are becoming standard tools for "pandemic-resilient" design [48]. These models allow designers to simulate the release of pathogen-laden droplets in a virtual environment (a "Digital Twin") and observe their dispersion under different ventilation scenarios [22].

For example, simulations in auditoriums have demonstrated that thermal plumes from the audience can drive aerosols upward, and that displacement ventilation is believed to be superior to mixing ventilation in removing these contaminants

[22]. Similarly, agent-based models can predict how urban design features—such as street width or the location of transport hubs—influence social contact rates and disease propagation [48]. These tools empower architects to test the "immune system" of a building before a single brick is laid.

2.13 Policy and Regulation: From Voluntary Standards to Functional Requirements

The Regulatory Gap

Currently, building regulations in many jurisdictions prioritize safety (structural integrity, fire resistance) and sustainability (energy conservation). Health, particularly regarding infection control, may have historically been a secondary consideration, often addressed through vague requirements for "adequate" ventilation without defining what is adequate for pathogen control [38].

The COVID-19 pandemic has highlighted the need for a regulatory paradigm shift. Voluntary standards like LEED or WELL have paved the way by incentivizing healthy building features, but they cover only a fraction of the building stock. There is a growing consensus among engineering bodies that infection resilience must be codified into mandatory building regulations [38].

2.13.1 A New "Part" for Health

The UK National Engineering Policy Centre has proposed the establishment of a new "Part" of the Building Regulations dedicated explicitly to health and wellbeing [38]. This regulation would set a functional requirement that a building must provide an indoor environment that protects the health of its users from adverse effects, including airborne infection.

This would involve:

1. *Defining Best Practice:* Moving beyond minimum ventilation rates for odour control to rates defined by infection risk models (e.g., 10 L/s/person or higher) [27, 38].
2. *Commissioning and Testing:* Ensuring that ventilation systems perform as designed at handover. Currently, performance gaps between design intent and operational reality are common; rigorous commissioning is essential to ensure infection resilience [38].
3. *In-Use Regulation:* Unlike fire safety, which is monitored throughout a building's life, ventilation performance is rarely checked after construction. New regulations would require periodic assessments of IAQ and ventilation performance in existing buildings, similar to elevator safety inspections [38].

2.13.2 Standardization of Air Cleaning Technologies

The market for air cleaning technologies (portable HEPA filters, ionizers, ozone generators) exploded during the pandemic. However, the lack of standardized testing protocols may have led to confusion and the marketing of ineffective or potentially harmful devices (e.g., those emitting ozone and may not be tested) [19]. There is an urgent need for independent certification standards that verify the efficacy of these technologies in real-world settings, not just in small test chambers [19, 38]. This would provide building managers with the confidence to invest in technologies that genuinely enhance infection resilience.

2.14 The Human Factor: Behavior, Psychology, and Perception

The Building User as an Active Participant
Even the most perfectly engineered building can fail if the human element is ignored. Infection control is a sociotechnical challenge. The perception of safety by building occupants is crucial for the economic and social recovery of cities [38]. If people do not feel safe entering an office or a theatre, the building becomes obsolete.

2.14.1 Nudging Behavior Through Design

Architectural design can subtly influence behavior to reduce transmission risk—a concept known as "nudging." For example, the placement of hand hygiene dispensers in direct sight lines and along natural paths of movement significantly increases usage rates [35]. Widening corridors and stairwells reduces the density of momentary contacts. In open-plan offices, visual cues and furniture arrangements can define personal space boundaries, encouraging physical distancing without the need for draconian enforcement [15, 48].

2.14.2 The Psychology of Visible Hygiene

There is a distinction between hygiene theatre (measures that look good but do little, like deep cleaning surfaces for an airborne virus) and visible indicators of effective control. However, visibility is important for psychological reassurance. While ventilation is invisible, CO_2 monitors with visual displays make air quality tangible to occupants, empowering them to open windows or reduce occupancy when levels rise [32]. This transparency builds trust between the facility manager and the occupant, transforming the user from a passive recipient of air to an active participant in their own health protection.

2.15 Conclusion

The professional perception of infection control in the built environment has traversed a significant arc. It began with the sanitary movement of the nineteenth century, which used engineering to conquer waterborne diseases like cholera. It then receded during the antibiotic era, where health was viewed as the exclusive domain of medicine, and buildings focused on energy efficiency, often to the detriment of air quality. The COVID-19 pandemic has violently swung the pendulum back, re-establishing the architect, the engineer, and the facility manager as frontline public health workers.

The perception study presented in this chapter further demonstrates that this shift is already occurring within the profession itself, with overwhelming agreement among architects regarding their responsibility toward ventilation design and infection prevention.

We have learned that the building is not merely a container for human activity; it is a dynamic biological system. The air we share indoors is a vector for transmission, governed by the laws of fluid dynamics and thermodynamics. Through the sections of this chapter, we have explored the invisible architecture of aerosols (Sect. 2.1), the necessity of integrating microbiology into architectural pedagogy (Sect. 2.2), and the technical evolution of ventilation from simple mixing to sophisticated displacement and disinfection strategies (Sect. 2.3). We have examined the specific vulnerabilities of clinical fortresses (Sect. 2.4), the bioaerosol risks of the sanitary core (Sect. 2.5), and the challenges of congregate settings like schools and transport (Sect. 2.6).

The synthesis of this knowledge points to a future where buildings are "infection resilient." This resilience is built on four pillars:

1. *Enhanced Ventilation:* Prioritizing displacement ventilation and dynamic airflow rates that respond to infection risk, not just odor control [22, 27]. If displacement not feasible, start with any form of increased air changes.
2. *Integrated Technology:* Utilizing UVGI and advanced filtration as standard components of HVAC systems, where such a system does not harm health and will be maintained, supported by smart sensors that make air quality visible and manageable [29, 33].
3. *Regulatory Robustness:* Moving from voluntary wellness standards to mandatory building codes that treat air quality with the same gravity as fire safety [38].
4. *Human-Centric Design:* Creating spaces that intuitively encourage hygienic behavior and provide psychological reassurance to occupants [35].

The empirical evidence presented through the implemented elective course further demonstrates that when infection control is introduced through applied, design-integrated pedagogy, students not only grasp the concepts effectively but actively express intent to carry these principles into professional practice.

As we move forward, the siloed approach to building design—where energy, aesthetics, and health are treated separately—must be abandoned. The building of the future is a unified system designed to protect its occupants from the microbial threats of a hyper-connected world, ensuring that our indoor environments remain sanctuaries for life, work, and recovery.

Acknowledgements Many thanks to Dr Gurkirpal Singh, HoD, IKG PTU Mohali Campus 2 for support. The authors acknowledge the support provided by the institutions including School of Planning and Architecture, New Delhi, All India Institute of Medical Sciences, New Delhi, and Drexel University. Special thanks to Rajshekhar Pullabhatla and Group Captain P Aanand Naidu of ISAC Centre for Built Environment Policy and Tathatara Foundation. Many thanks to Dr Arthur L Frank, MD. Many thanks to all the people who supported this work in many ways.

Declarations The authors Raja Singh, Nirupam Madaan, and Anil Dewan declare no conflict of interests or competing interests in this work. There is no involvement of human participants, animals, human or animal tissue. All authors declare that there was no specific financial support received from any organization for the submitted work. All authors declare that they have no financial relationships at present or within the previous 3 years with any organizations that might have an interest in the submitted work. While all care has been taken in ensuring the accuracy of this work, any inadvertent error may be reported at the earliest. The authors acknowledge the use of supervised language learning models/large language models for enhancement of the work, with responsibility lying with the authors. For more information, the corresponding author may be contacted at email rajaresearch@proton.me.

CRediT Statement The following is the CRediT statement which declares the author credits for this chapter:

Raja Singh: Conceptualization, Methodology, Formal Analysis, Investigation, Data Curation, Writing-Original Draft, Writing-Review & Editing, Visualization, Project Administration.
Nirupam Madaan: Conceptualization, Resources, Validation, Supervision, Project Administration.
Anil Dewan: Resources, Validation Supervision.

References

1. Abusaada H, Elshater A. COVID-19 challenge, information technologies, and smart cities: considerations for well-being. Int J Community Well-Being. 2020;3:417–24.
2. Alidadi M, Sharifi A. Effects of the built environment and human factors on the spread of COVID-19: a systematic literature review. Sci Total Environ. 2022;850:158056.
3. Allen JG, Marr LC. Recognizing and controlling airborne transmission of SARS-CoV-2 in indoor environments. Indoor Air. 2020;30(4):557–8.
4. Allen JG, MacNaughton P, Cedeno Laurent JG, Flanigan SS, Eitland ES, Spengler JD. Green buildings and health. Curr Environ Health Rep. 2015;2(3):250–8.
5. Andalib S, Faghani M, Zia Ziabari SM, Shenagari M, Salehiniya H, Keivanlou MH, Rafat Z. The effectiveness of the anteroom on hospital infection control: a systematic review. Front Public Health. 2022;10:828845.
6. Anand U, Nandy S, Mundhra S, Das N, Tripathi V, Bontempi E. A review of molecular mechanisms and transmission dynamics of SARS-CoV-2: the role of the environment. Environ Res. 2022;203:111839.
7. Asif Z, Chen Z, Coghlan A, Sadiq R. Dynamics of SARS-CoV-2 spreading under the influence of environmental factors and strategies to tackle the pandemic. Sustain Cities Soc. 2022;81:103840.

8. Brickner PW, Vincent RL, First M, Nardell E, Murray M, Kaufman W. The application of ultraviolet germicidal irradiation to control transmission of airborne disease: bioterrorism countermeasure. Public Health Rep. 2003;118(2):99–114.
9. Buonanno M, Welch D, Shuryak I, Brenner DJ. Far-UVC light (222 nm) efficiently and safely inactivates airborne human coronaviruses. Sci Rep. 2020;10:10285.
10. Chau KK, Barker L, Budgell E, Vihta KD, Sims N, Kasprzyk-Hordern B, et al. Systematic review of wastewater surveillance of antimicrobial resistance in human populations. Environ Int. 2022;162:107171.
11. Chen F, Tian Y, Zhang L, Shi Y. The role of children in household transmission of COVID-19: a systematic review and meta-analysis. Int J Infect Dis. 2022;122:266–75.
12. Dai R, Liu S, Li Q, Wu H, Wu L, Ji C. Indoor bioaerosols in hospitals and the influence of HVAC: a systematic review and meta-analysis. PLoS ONE. 2021;16(12):e0259996.
13. Dewan M, Sharma N, Panda PS, Banerjee P. School reopening strategies during COVID-19. J Family Med Prim Care. 2022;11(5):1618–25.
14. Dubey S, Sahoo KC, Dash GC, Sahay MR, Mahapatra P, Bhattacharya D, et al. Housing-related challenges during COVID-19. Front Public Health. 2022;10:1029394.
15. Epton T, Ghio D, Ballard LM, Allen SF, Kassianos AP, Hewitt R, et al. Impact of COVID-19 isolation on nursing care. J Adv Nurs. 2022;78(5):1229–49.
16. Ferrari S, Blázquez T, Cardelli R, Puglisi G, Suárez R, Mazzarella L. Ventilation strategies to reduce airborne transmission in classrooms. Build Environ. 2022;222:109366.
17. Gormley M, Aspray TJ, Kelly DA, Rodriguez-Gil C. Pathogen cross-transmission via sanitary plumbing systems. PLoS ONE. 2017;12(2):e0171556.
18. Gormley M, Aspray TJ, Kelly DA. Aerosol and bioaerosol dynamics from defective plumbing systems. Indoor Air. 2021;31(2):332–45.
19. Hammond A, Khalid T, Thornton HV, Woodall CA, Hay AD. Portable air filters for SARS-CoV-2. PLoS ONE. 2021;16(4):e0251049.
20. Hoisington AJ, Brenner LA, Kinney KA, Postolache TT, Lowry CA. The microbiome of the built environment and mental health. Microbiome. 2015;3:60.
21. Horvath EP. Building-related illness and sick building syndrome. Cleve Clin J Med. 1997;64(6):303–9.
22. Huang J, Hao T, Liu X, Jones P, Ou C, Liang W, Liu F. Airborne transmission of Delta variant in an auditorium. Build Environ. 2022;219:109212.
23. Jefferson T, Spencer EA, Onakpoya IJ, Plüddemann A, Conly JM, Heneghan CJ. Transmission of SARS-CoV-2 in non-healthcare settings. J Infect. 2022;84:361–82.
24. Khorram-Manesh A, Dulebenets M, Goniewicz K. Public health strategies and educational initiatives. IJERPH. 2021;18(11):5888.
25. Kim H, Hughes E, Cavanagh A, Norris E, Gao A, Bondy SJ, McLeod KE, Kanagalingam T, Kouyoumdjian FG. The health impacts of the COVID-19 pandemic on adults who experience imprisonment globally: a mixed methods systematic review. PLoS One. 2022;17(5):e0268866. https://doi.org/10.1371/journal.pone.0268866. PMID: 35594288; PMCID: PMC9122186.
26. Lee JY, Kwon N, Goo G, Cho SI. Inadequate housing and pulmonary tuberculosis. BMC Public Health. 2022;22:622.
27. Li Y, Cheng P, Jia W. Poor ventilation worsens short-range airborne transmission. Indoor Air. 2022;32(1):e12946.
28. Megahed NA, Ghoneim EM. Rethinking building design strategies post-pandemic. Environ Res. 2021;193:110471.
29. Mena AR, Ceballos HG, Alvarado-Uribe J. Measuring indoor occupancy using sensors. Sensors. 2022;22:3770.
30. Morawska L, Milton DK. Airborne transmission of COVID-19. Clin Infect Dis. 2020;71(9):2311–3.
31. Morawska L, Tang JW, Bahnfleth W, Bluyssen PM, Boerstra A, Buonanno G, et al. Minimising airborne transmission indoors. Environ Int. 2020;142:105832.
32. Nair AN, Anand P, George A, Mondal N. Strategies to reduce airborne transmission. Environ Res. 2022;213:113579.

33. Nardell EA. Germicidal UV and airborne infection control. Photochem Photobiol. 2021;97:493–7.
34. Peng Z, Jimenez JL. Exhaled CO_2 as COVID-19 risk proxy. Environ Sci Technol Lett. 2021;8(5):392–7.
35. Peters A, Schmid MN, Parneix P, Lebowitz D, de Kraker M, Sauser J, Zingg W, Pittet D. Environmental hygiene interventions. Antimicrob Resist Infect Control. 2022;11:38.
36. Poague KIHM, Blanford JI, Anthonj C. WASH in schools during COVID-19. IJERPH. 2022;19:3124.
37. Redlich CA, Sparer J, Cullen MR. Sick-building syndrome. Lancet. 1997;349:1013–6.
38. Royal Academy of Engineering. Infection resilient environments: time for a major upgrade. National Engineering Policy Centre; 2022.
39. Sakti AMT, Ajis SZM, Azlan AA, Kim HJ, Wong E, Mohamad E. Impact of COVID-19 on school populations. IJERPH. 2022;19:4024.
40. Shah S, Gwee SXW, Ng JQX, Lau N, Koh J, Pang J. Wastewater surveillance of SARS-CoV-2 variants. Sci Total Environ. 2022;804:150060.
41. Stabile L, Pacitto A, Mikszewski A, Morawska L, Buonanno G. Ventilation procedures in classrooms. Build Environ. 2021;202:108042.
42. Tang JW, Bahnfleth WP, Bluyssen PM, Buonanno G, Jimenez JL, Kurnitski J, Li Y, Miller S, Sekhar C, Morawska L, Marr LC, Melikov AK, Nazaroff WW, Nielsen PV, Tellier R, Wargocki P, Dancer SJ. Dismantling myths on the airborne transmission of severe acute respiratory syndrome coronavirus-2 (SARS-CoV-2). J Hosp Infect. 2021;110:89–96.
43. Thornton GM, Fleck BA, Fleck N, Kroeker E, Dandnayak D, Zhong L, Hartling L. HVAC and ultraviolet radiation. PLoS ONE. 2022;17(4):e0266487.
44. Tran VV, Park D, Lee YC. Indoor air pollution and health. IJERPH. 2020;17:2927.
45. Vardoulakis S, Espinoza Oyarce DA, Donner E. Transmission risks in public washrooms. Sci Total Environ. 2022;803:149932.
46. Viana Martins CP, Xavier CSF, Cobrado L. Disinfection methods against SARS-CoV-2. J Hosp Infect. 2022;119:84–117.
47. Welch D, Buonanno M, Grilj V, Shuryak I, Crickmore C, Bigelow AW, et al. Far-UVC light. Sci Rep. 2018;8:2752.
48. Yang L, Iwami M, Chen Y, Wu M, van Dam KH. Urban design and modelling post-COVID. Prog Plan. 2022:100657.
49. Zhang X, Sun Z, Ashcroft T, Dozier M, Ostrishko K, Krishan P, et al. Compact cities and COVID-19 transmission. Health Place. 2022;76:102827.
50. Zhu A, Bruketa E, Svoboda T, Orkin AM. Mitigation measures in homeless shelters. Ann Epidemiol. 2023;77:127–35.

Introduction to Infection in Buildings

3

Raja Singh, Nirupam Madaan, and Anil Dewan

3.1 The Biological Soup: Defining the Indoor Pathosphere

The Invisible Occupants When we walk into a room—be it a high-rise office in Shanghai, a classroom in London, or a residential apartment in New York—we are never truly alone. We share our built environments with a vast, invisible, and dynamic ecosystem of biological agents [4]. For the better part of the twentieth century, building physics focused principally on thermal comfort, lighting, and acoustic privacy, treating the air simply as a fluid medium for heat transfer. However, the paradigm has shifted violently. We must now recognize that the indoor environment is a "pathosphere"—a complex biological suspension where viruses, bacteria, and fungi drift, settle, resuspend, and infect [32, 46]. The concept of a pathosphere is a heuristic framework.

The classification of infections within the built environment has historically been divided into rigid categories based on the size of the carrier particle and the distance it travels. These categories—contact (fomite), droplet, and airborne—were treated as distinct silos in medical textbooks for decades. However, recent scrutiny of fluid dynamics and microbiology, accelerated by the SARS-CoV-2 pandemic, has revealed that these boundaries are artificial and scientifically porous [22, 26]. To control infection in the everyday built environment, we must first dissect these

R. Singh
Founder/Researcher, The Built, New Delhi, Delhi, India

Former Post Doctoral Fellow, Department of Environmental and Occupational Health, Dornsife School of Public Health, Drexel University, Philadelphia, Pennsylvania, USA

N. Madaan
Department of Hospital Administration, All India Institute of Medical Sciences, New Delhi, Delhi, India

A. Dewan
Department of Architecture, School of Planning and Architecture, New Delhi, Delhi, India

R. Singh et al., *Infection Control in the Everyday Built Environment*,
https://doi.org/10.1007/978-981-95-8624-0_3

transmission modes not as abstract medical concepts, but as physical phenomena governed by the laws of gravity, evaporation, and airflow.

The Three Pillars of Transmission: A Re-evaluation Classically, the transmission of respiratory pathogens in buildings is understood through three primary routes:

1. *Contact/Fomite Transmission:* The pathogen survives on inanimate surfaces (fomites). A susceptible host touches the surface and then touches their mucous membranes (eyes, nose, mouth).
2. *Droplet Transmission:* The pathogen is expelled in large, heavy fluid particles (>5–10 microns) that follow a ballistic trajectory, succumbing to gravity within 1–2 m of the source.
3. *Airborne (Aerosol) Transmission:* The pathogen is carried in small droplet nuclei (<5 microns) that remain suspended in the air for extended periods, traveling distances greater than 2 m on air currents [32, 34].

While this classification remains the bedrock of infection control guidelines, the reality within a building is far more fluid. A "droplet" can become an "aerosol" through evaporation before it hits the ground; an "aerosol" can deposit on a surface to become a "fomite"; and a "fomite" can release secondary aerosols when disturbed [14, 26].

3.1.1 The Fomite Fallacy: Surface vs. Air

For years, surface hygiene was the primary focus of building cleaning protocols. The logic was visually intuitive: we see dirt on surfaces, therefore surfaces must be the vector. Research confirms that pathogens like methicillin-resistant *Staphylococcus aureus* (MRSA), *Clostridium difficile*, and various coronaviruses can persist on dry surfaces for days or even months [36, 37]. For instance, SARS-CoV-2 RNA has been extensively detected on high-touch surfaces in hospitals, such as bed rails, door handles, and computer keyboards [36, 42].

However, the detection of viral RNA may not directly equate to the presence of a viable, infectious virus. A systematic review and meta-analysis of viral cultures found that while SARS-CoV-2 RNA is frequently found on surfaces, the rate of successful live viral culture from these fomites is low, often below 10% [36]. This suggests that while surfaces play a role, particularly in healthcare settings where viral loads are extreme, in the *everyday* built environment (offices, schools, homes), the risk of fomite transmission likely plays a secondary role compared to airborne transmission in most everyday settings [36, 50].

The built environment professional must understand that while cleaning surfaces is necessary for hygiene, it may be insufficient for infection control on its own [16]. A building with sparkling floors but stagnant air is a biological trap. The primary vector for respiratory pandemics is not the door handle; it is the air we share.

3.2 Focus on Airborne Infection: The Physics of the Plume

The "5-Micron" Dogma The most contentious and critical debate in modern building science centres on the definition of "airborne." For decades, the medical community adhered to a dichotomy: particles larger than 5 microns were "droplets" (safe beyond 2 m), and those smaller were "aerosols" (requiring isolation) [22, 26]. This threshold was not based on empirical physics but may have been an arbitrary historical carryover.

In reality, humans exhale a continuum of particle sizes during breathing, speaking, singing, and coughing. Physics dictates that a particle of 5 microns, or even 20 microns, does not immediately drop to the floor. It is subject to drag forces and air currents. As noted in recent reviews of transmission risk, particles up to 100 microns can remain suspended for extended periods under realistic indoor airflow conditions, depending on the ambient air velocity and humidity [26, 32]. The "5-micron" cutoff is physically flawed; aerosols should be viewed as any respirable particle capable of remaining suspended in the air long enough to be inhaled by another person, regardless of an arbitrary size limit [34].

The Short-Range Airborne Route One of the most profound realizations to emerge from recent aerodynamic studies is the concept of "short-range airborne transmission." Historically, if transmission occurred between two people standing 1 m apart, it was attributed to "droplets" spraying onto the recipient's face. However, detailed modeling and tracer gas experiments have proven this to be an oversimplification.

When two people converse, they are enveloped in each other's thermal and respiratory plumes. Within this "conversation distance" (<1.5 m), the concentration of aerosols is orders of magnitude higher than in the general room air [22]. This is not just because of large droplets; it is because the exhaled jet of air contains a high density of fine aerosols that have not yet diluted into the room volume.

A pivotal study by Li et al. [22] demonstrated that poor ventilation exacerbates this short-range transmission. Counter-intuitively, one might assume ventilation only affects long-range (room-scale) buildup. However, the study showed that when the background room air is not cleared, the "cone" of concentrated aerosols between two people dissipates much more slowly. In poorly ventilated spaces (<10 L/s/person), the exhaled jet penetrates further and lingers longer, effectively bridging the physical distance between occupants [22, 32]. This reveals that social distancing is not a substitute for ventilation; rather, ventilation is a prerequisite for social distancing to work effectively.

Evaporation and the "Droplet Nuclei" The behavior of an infectious particle is dictated by the psychrometric chart. When a droplet leaves the warm, saturated environment of the human respiratory tract (~30 ° C, 100 % *RH*) and enters the drier, cooler air of a building (~22 ° C, 50 % *RH*), it immediately begins to evaporate.

Physics dictates that a 10-micron droplet will evaporate to roughly half its diameter (and one-eighth its volume) on the order of fractions of a second to a few seconds depending on conditions, becoming a "droplet nucleus" [26]. This evaporation process transforms what might have started as a ballistic "droplet" into a buoyant "aerosol" before it travels even a few centimeters.

- *High Humidity:* In very humid environments, evaporation is slowed, and droplets stay larger and settle faster.
- *Low Humidity:* In dry environments (common in heated buildings in winter), droplets evaporate rapidly into small nuclei that remain airborne for hours [26, 45].

This physical reality means that the "dry air" often found in energy-efficient, tight buildings during winter acts as a catalyst for airborne transmission. It converts heavy, short-range projectiles into light, long-range explorers. Consequently, humidity control is not merely a comfort parameter; it is an infection control parameter. The "Goldilocks zone" of 40–60% relative humidity is critical not just for human mucosal health but for destabilizing the physics of aerosol travel ([45]; Ahlawat et al. 2020 cited in [32]).

3.3 The Policy View on Airborne Infection: A Slow Awakening

The Resistance to "Airborne" Classification The recognition of airborne transmission in building policy has been characterized by significant inertia. During the early stages of the COVID-19 pandemic, major health organizations, including the WHO, maintained that SARS-CoV-2 was primarily a contact and droplet pathogen [32]. This policy stance had massive implications for the built environment: it prioritized deep cleaning (fomite control) and glass/acrylic barriers (droplet control) over ventilation upgrades (airborne control).

It was not until overwhelming evidence from "superspreading events"—such as the Skagit Valley Chorale rehearsal and the Guangzhou restaurant outbreak—that the scientific consensus forced a policy shift. In the Guangzhou restaurant case, viral transmission occurred between tables that were physically distant but connected by the airflow stream of an air conditioning unit [22]. There was no direct contact, and large droplets could not have bridged the gap. The vector was the air itself, propelled by a recirculating HVAC system with inadequate fresh air supply ([22]; Lu et al. 2020 cited in [32]).

Current Policy Landscape Today, the policy view is shifting toward "infection-resilient environments" [39]. This acknowledges that buildings must be designed to mitigate airborne risk. Key policy shifts include:

1. *Ventilation Rates:* Moving beyond older versions of older codes, minimums equivalent to roughly 7–10 L/s/person in many occupancies when area and people components are combined to be designed for body odour control, toward higher rates (>10–14 L/s/person) explicitly for infection control [22, 32].

2. *CO_2 Monitoring:* The acceptance of carbon dioxide (CO_2) as a proxy for "rebreathed air" and infection risk. Policies are increasingly recommending CO_2 monitors in classrooms and offices, with thresholds of 800–1000 ppm indicating a need for intervention [32].
3. *Filtration:* A move from protecting equipment (MERV 8) to protecting people (MERV 13/F7 or higher). Policies now emphasize that recirculated air must be filtered to a high efficiency to prevent the distribution of pathogens from one zone to another [17, 32].

3.4 Other Infections and Interventions

While viral respiratory pathogens (SARS-CoV-2, Influenza, MERS) dominate the current discourse, the built environment is also a reservoir for bacterial and fungal infections.

Bacterial Bioaerosols Bacterial infections such as tuberculosis (TB) and Legionnaires' disease are classic building-related illnesses. TB is the archetype of obligate airborne transmission; it relies entirely on functionally obligate airborne transmission in real-world epidemiology as the air currents to move from host to host [33]. Unlike viruses, which often require a living host to multiply, some bacteria (like *Legionella*) can amplify within the building's own infrastructure—specifically within cooling towers and stagnant water pipes—before becoming aerosolized and inhaled [32].

Furthermore, a systematic review of indoor air disinfection for bacterial pathogens identified that technologies such as ultraviolet germicidal irradiation (UVGI) (Subject to safety, cost and maintenance) may be highly effective against airborne bacteria like *Pseudomonas aeruginosa* and *Staphylococcus aureus* [34]. This highlights that interventions designed for viruses often have co-benefits for bacterial control.

Fungal Bioaerosols Fungal contamination is primarily associated with moisture damage. Fungi like *Aspergillus* and *Stachybotrys* release spores that are easily airborne. While often discussed in the context of allergies or sick building syndrome (SBS), fungal spores can cause severe infections (aspergillosis) in immunocompromised individuals. The interventions here differ slightly: while ventilation helps, the root cause—moisture control—is the primary engineering intervention [46].

Intervention Hierarchy The management of these diverse infections requires a hierarchy of engineering controls:

1. *Source Control:* preventing the release (masks, plumbing maintenance, moisture control).
2. *Ventilation:* Diluting the contaminant with fresh air [22, 32].

3. *Filtration/Purification:* Removing the contaminant from the air [17, 34]. Subject to conditions.
4. *Inactivation:* Killing the pathogen in the air using UV-C or Far-UVC light [33, 45]. Subject to conditions.

3.5 Quantifying the Invisible: The Concept of "Quanta"

Defining the Infectious Dose To engineer a building against infection, we must first measure the threat. However, unlike a chemical pollutant where we can measure concentration in parts per million (ppm), biological pathogens are discrete, replicating entities. Their infectivity varies wildly depending on the strain, the host's immune system, and environmental conditions. To bridge the gap between biology and building physics, researchers utilize a theoretical unit known as the *"quanta."*

A "quanta" is not a single virus particle. It is defined as the infectious dose required to induce infection in 63% of susceptible persons in an enclosed space [19, 22]. This definition is derived from the Poisson probability distribution, acknowledging the randomness of inhaling infectious particles. One quantum might contain hundreds of viral copies for a highly infectious variant like SARS-CoV-2 Delta or Omicron, or thousands for a less efficient pathogen [50].

For the building professional, the quanta emission rate (q) is the critical design parameter. It represents the "source strength" of an infected occupant.

- *Speaking vs. Breathing:* Research indicates that the rate of quanta emission is not static. Loud speaking or singing can increase aerosol emission by orders of magnitude compared to quiet breathing [6].
- *The Variant Variable:* The evolution of the virus fundamentally alters this metric. For instance, in a detailed forensic analysis of an outbreak in an auditorium involving the Delta variant, the back-calculated quanta emission rate was estimated at roughly 31 quanta/hour for masked individuals, a figure significantly higher than estimates for the original Wuhan strain [19].

The Wells-Riley Equation: The Architect's Formula The relationship between the building and the infection is mathematically codified in the *Wells-Riley equation*. This formula calculates the probability of infection (P) based on the number of infectors (I), the quanta production rate (q), the pulmonary ventilation rate of the occupants (p), the duration of exposure (t), and—crucially for architects—the volume of clean air supplied to the room (Q) [22].

$$P = 1 - e^{-\frac{Iqpt}{Q}}$$

where:

- P is the probability of infection.
- Q is the room ventilation rate (dilution).

This equation reveals a stark truth: *dilution is the only variable in the denominator that building operators can fully control.* To halve the risk of infection, one must essentially double the clean air supply, assuming other factors remain constant. However, recent modifications to this classic model suggest it may underestimate risk in "short-range" scenarios. Li et al. [22] proposed a "continuum model" which accounts for the high concentration of quanta in the jet plume of exhaled breath before it is fully mixed into the room air. Their findings suggest that when people are in close proximity (<1.5 m), the ventilation rate required to protect them skyrockets, challenging standard displacement ventilation designs [22].

3.6 The Silent Threat: Asymptomatic and Presymptomatic Transmission

The Non-success of Symptomatic Screening Historically, infection control in buildings relied on a "reactive" model: identify the sick person (coughing, fever) and remove them from the environment. The SARS-CoV-2 pandemic dismantled this strategy by revealing the dominance of *asymptomatic and presymptomatic transmission*.

- *Asymptomatic cases* never develop symptoms but shed virus.
- *Presymptomatic cases* shed virus at high levels days before symptoms appear.

A systematic review of transmission clusters found that children, in particular, act as silent reservoirs. While secondary attack rates from children in school settings were initially thought to be lower than adults (0.7% vs 7.6% in households), children often manifest milder or no symptoms, making them undetected vectors in poorly ventilated classrooms [48]. In household settings, where contact is prolonged and ventilation is typically poor, asymptomatic individuals have been documented to trigger significant outbreaks [38].

Implications for Building Design The prevalence of silent transmission means buildings must move from "symptom-based defenses" (like thermal scanners at lobbies) to *"universal precautions."*

1. *The Building as a Mask:* Since we cannot reliably identify who is infected, the building must assume *everyone* is a potential source. This necessitates continuous high-efficiency filtration (MERV-13+) and increased air change rates (ACH) regardless of whether occupants "look" sick [39].
2. *The Bathroom Hazard:* Asymptomatic shedding is not limited to the respiratory tract. Viral RNA has been frequently detected in fecal matter and subsequently in wastewater systems [5, 38]. High titers of virus in septic tanks and sewage implicate the plumbing system as a potential vector for fecal-aerosol transmission, particularly in high-rise buildings with defective U-traps, reminiscent of the Amoy Gardens SARS outbreak [5].

3.7 The Reinfection Reality: Permanence of the Threat

The End of "One and Done" Early in the pandemic, there was hope that infection would confer lasting immunity, allowing buildings to return to pre-pandemic operational modes once "herd immunity" was reached. However, the emergence of variants (Alpha, Delta, Omicron) and the documentation of reinfections have shattered this notion.

A systematic review of reinfection cases identified that immunity wanes and that new variants can escape neutralization [38]. For example, the Omicron variant showed a marked ability to reinfect individuals who had recovered from previous strains or were vaccinated [50].

- *Genetic Drift:* The mutations in the Spike protein (e.g., D614G, N501Y) not only increase transmissibility but also alter the viral load [50].
- *Operational Consequence:* This biological reality dictates that "Infection Control Mode" in building management systems (BMS) cannot be a temporary setting. The capacity to surge ventilation and disinfection must be a permanent, resilient feature of the built environment infrastructure, ready to be deployed against seasonal waves of reinfection or novel pathogens.

3.8 Moving Ahead

We have established that the indoor environment is a dynamic pathosphere where invisible "quanta" of infection are generated by often-asymptomatic occupants. These infectious particles defy the simple gravity-based models of the past, lingering in the air and exploiting low ventilation rates to find new hosts. As we move into the next sections, we will examine the specific engineering controls—ventilation strategies, filtration technologies, and air disinfection—that can intercept these quanta and break the chain of transmission.

3.9 The Thermodynamic Envelope: Temperature, Humidity, and Viral Fate

The Building as a Biological Incubator If ventilation provides the "transport mechanism" for airborne pathogens, the thermodynamic condition of the indoor air constitutes the "life support system" for the virus. For decades, building managers have manipulated temperature and humidity primarily for human thermal comfort and energy efficiency, adhering to popular global standards. However, microbiology does not always align with human comfort. The indoor climate creates a specific thermodynamic envelope that dictates the stability of the viral lipid membrane, the rate of droplet evaporation, and ultimately, the viability of the pathogen.

To understand infection control, we must view the air not merely as a void to be filled with heat or cold, but as a chemically active medium. The survival of enveloped viruses like SARS-CoV-2, influenza, and RSV is heavily dependent on the hygrothermal properties of the air they inhabit [45].

The "Goldilocks Zone" of Relative Humidity One of the most scientifically robust yet operationally neglected interventions in building health is the management of relative humidity (RH). Research has consistently identified a "Goldilocks zone" of approximately 40–60% RH where the infectivity of many respiratory viruses is minimized [45].

1. *Low Humidity (<40%): The Preservation Effect.* In dry air, typical of heated buildings in winter, respiratory droplets expelled by an infector undergo rapid evaporation. According to physical modeling reviewed by Mao et al. [26], a 10-micron droplet can evaporate to a fraction of its size in milliseconds. This rapid desiccation transforms a heavy, settling droplet into a buoyant "droplet nucleus" or aerosol, which remains suspended in the air for hours, traveling on thermal plumes far beyond the 2-m social distancing perimeter [26]. Biologically, low humidity promotes viral survival. When the water content of a droplet evaporates quickly, the solute concentration (salts and proteins) within the droplet rises. For some viruses, this crystallization creates a protective shield around the virion, preserving its integrity. Furthermore, dry air may impair the human immune defense; it is believed to desiccate the mucous membranes of the nose and throat, reducing mucociliary clearance and making the host more susceptible to infection [45].
2. *High Humidity (>60%): The Settling Effect.* In very humid environments, droplets evaporate slowly. They remain large and heavy, succumbing to gravity more quickly. While this reduces the range of airborne transmission, extremely high humidity can support the survival of bacteria and fungi (molds), creating a different set of indoor air quality (IAQ) problems, such as sick building syndrome (SBS) or mold-induced hypersensitivity [43].
3. *Intermediate Humidity (40–60%): The Kill Zone.* In this mid-range, the physics and chemistry of the droplet work against the virus. The evaporation rate is such that the salt and solute concentrations within the droplet reach levels that can be toxic to the virus or disrupt its lipid envelope before it fully dries out. A systematic review by Thornton et al. [45] analyzing the impact of HVAC design features on virus transmission concluded that maintaining RH between 40% and 60% is associated with decreased viral viability and transmission rates. For example, studies on Influenza A have shown that increasing RH from low levels (20%) to mid-levels (50%) may significantly reduce viral transmission and infectivity [45].

The Energy-Health Trade-Off in Humidification Implementing this "Goldilocks zone" in the everyday built environment presents a significant engineering challenge. In cold climates, heating outdoor air (which has low absolute humidity) causes the indoor RH to plummet, often below 20%. To maintain 40% RH requires active humidification, which is energy-intensive and water-consuming. Furthermore, poorly maintained humidifiers can become breeding grounds for bacteria (e.g., *Legionella*) and fungi, potentially trading a viral risk for a bacterial one [18, 43]. Therefore, infection control in buildings requires a nuanced approach where humidification is viewed as a medical intervention, requiring the same rigor in maintenance and hygiene as ventilation systems.

Temperature: The Cold Storage Effect Temperature also plays a critical, albeit secondary, role. Generally, enveloped viruses survive longer at lower temperatures. This is the principle of "cold storage." In the built environment, air-conditioned spaces that are kept very cold may inadvertently extend the half-life of viral aerosols [45]. However, the use of heat as a disinfection strategy—known as *thermal inactivation*—has been explored for personal protective equipment (PPE) and surfaces. Research indicates that SARS-CoV-2 infectivity decreases significantly as temperatures rise. For example, exposure to 70 °C can effectively inactivate the virus on surfaces within minutes [47]. While we cannot heat occupied rooms to these temperatures, this principle underlies the efficacy of steam cleaning and high-temperature laundering for infection control in linen and soft furnishings.

3.10 Materiality and Persistence: The Surface Paradox

From Fomites to Reservoirs While the airborne route has gained prominence, the role of surfaces (fomites) in the everyday built environment cannot be ignored. The "high-touch surface" (door handles, elevator buttons, handrails) has long been the target of cleaning protocols. However, recent evidence requires us to distinguish between the *presence* of the virus and the *risk* of infection.

RNA vs. Viable Virus: The Detective's Dilemma During the COVID-19 pandemic, researchers swabbed thousands of surfaces in hospitals, cruise ships, and public transport. They frequently found SARS-CoV-2 RNA. On the *Diamond Princess* cruise ship, for instance, viral RNA was identified on surfaces in cabins of infected passengers up to 17 days after the cabins were vacated [31, 36]. Similarly, studies in hospitals have detected viral RNA on bed rails, floors, and computer mice [42].

However, a critical distinction must be made between detecting viral genetic material (RNA) and detecting a viable, infectious virus. A systematic review and meta-analysis by Onakpoya et al. [36] found that while RNA contamination is common, the successful culture of live virus from these surfaces is rare. In their review of 29 studies attempting to culture SARS-CoV-2 from fomites, only a small fraction successfully grew the virus. This suggests that while the "fingerprint" of the virus lingers, the "threat" degrades relatively quickly.

The Persistence Hierarchy of Materials Not all building materials are equal in their capacity to harbour pathogens. The persistence of a virus on a surface depends on the material's porosity, surface energy, and chemical composition.

- *Non-porous surfaces* (stainless steel, plastic, glass) tend to allow viruses to persist longer than porous surfaces (fabric, paper). Viana Martins et al. [47] reviewed data showing that SARS-CoV-2 can remain infectious on plastic and stainless steel for up to 72 h, whereas on cardboard or copper, viability drops significantly within 4–24 h.
- *Copper and Its Alloys:* Copper possesses intrinsic antimicrobial properties (the oligodynamic effect). Copper ions released from the surface can disrupt the viral envelope and degrade genomic DNA/RNA. Studies reviewed by Viana Martins et al. [47] indicate that copper surfaces can inactivate SARS-CoV-2 in as little as 4 h. This has profound implications for architectural hardware specifications; replacing stainless steel door furniture with copper alloys could serve as a passive, permanent infection control measure.

The Re-aerosolisation Phenomenon The danger of surface contamination is not limited to touch. A less discussed but physically significant mechanism is *re-aerosolisation*. Viruses that have settled on floors or horizontal surfaces can be lofted back into the air by human activity (walking, sweeping) or air currents. Research in hospital wards has detected SARS-CoV-2 RNA in air samples collected in hallways and rooms where no aerosol-generating procedures were taking place, suggesting that the movement of staff and the resuspension of floor dust contributed to the airborne viral load ([11]; Santarpia et al. 2020 cited in [36]). In a study of the *Diamond Princess*, traces of the virus were found in air handling units, suggesting that aerosolised and potentially re-aerosolised particles could be transported through ventilation systems [31].

This re-aerosolization risk challenges the standard "spray and wipe" cleaning protocols. If cleaning staff use high-pressure sprays or vigorous dry sweeping, they may inadvertently aerosolize settled pathogens, increasing the inhalation risk for themselves and others. This advocates for the use of damp dusting, wet mopping, vacuum cleaners with HEPA filtration, and floor cleaning machines that capture liquid immediately. Re-aerosolization is a plausible secondary mechanism supported by environmental sampling studies.

3.11 Disinfection Technologies in the Built Environment

Given the persistence of pathogens in the air and on surfaces, the built environment must employ active disinfection technologies. These interventions move beyond passive ventilation to active neutralization.

1. *Ultraviolet Germicidal Irradiation (UVGI)*, particularly UV-C light (200–280 nm), is a potent tool for inactivating microorganisms by damaging their nucleic acids (DNA/RNA), preventing replication.
   - *Upper-Room UVGI:* This involves installing shielded UV-C fixtures that irradiate the air in the upper zone of a room. Natural convection and mechanical fans circulate air from the lower occupied zone to the upper irradiated zone. As reviewed by Thornton et al. [45], upper-room UVGI can provide an "equivalent air change rate" (eACH) of 10–20 ACH, far exceeding what is typically achievable with mechanical ventilation alone. It is particularly cost-effective; Nardell [33] estimated that UVGI is approximately 9 times more cost-effective than mechanical ventilation for equivalent pathogen removal. Care must be taken that in low resource settings capital cost, maintenance and safety risks due to lack of training may be concerns.
   - *Far-UVC (222 nm):* A promising advancement is the use of Far-UVC light (222 nm). Unlike conventional 254 nm UV-C, which is harmful to human skin and eyes, 222 nm light has a shorter range of penetration in biological tissue and appears promising under controlled exposure limits, though long-term safety and regulatory standards are still under evaluation, while remaining lethal to viruses. Studies reviewed by Welch et al. [49] and Thornton et al. [45] demonstrate that 222 nm light effectively inactivates airborne influenza and coronaviruses without inducing the DNA damage associated with skin cancer in mammalian models. This technology could theoretically allow for "continuous disinfection" of occupied spaces, a holy grail for infection control in high-density areas like buses or lobbies.
2. *Chemical Disinfection: Ozone and Hydrogen Peroxide:* Chemical disinfection methods such as vaporized hydrogen peroxide (VHP) and ozone have been widely used for decontamination, particularly of N95 respirators and hospital rooms during the pandemic.
   - *Hydrogen Peroxide Vapor (HPV/VHP):* This method is highly effective, achieving greater than 6-log reduction of spores and viruses [35]. It breaks down into water and oxygen, leaving no toxic residue. However, it requires the space to be unoccupied and sealed, making it a "terminal cleaning" solution rather than a continuous one.
   - *Ozone:* Ozone is a powerful oxidant that destroys viral capsids. While effective against SARS-CoV-2 on surfaces [47], it is toxic to humans and causes degradation of building materials like rubber and certain plastics. Its use is therefore limited to unoccupied spaces with rigorous safety controls.
3. *Filtration Technologies:* Filtration remains the workhorse of indoor air cleaning. The efficacy of a filter is defined by its minimum efficiency reporting value (MERV).
   - *MERV 13 and HEPA:* For effective capture of the droplet nuclei (<5 microns) that carry viruses, filters rated MERV 13 or higher are generally recommended [32]. High efficiency particulate air (HEPA) filters capture at least 99.97% of particles at 0.3 microns.

- *Portable Air Cleaners (PACs):* In older buildings where the HVAC system cannot handle high-resistance filters, portable HEPA units offer a flexible solution. A systematic review by Nair et al. [32] confirms that PACs can significantly reduce aerosol concentrations in classrooms and offices, provided they are sized correctly for the room volume (clean air delivery rate, CADR). However, their placement is critical; poorly placed units can alter airflow patterns to draw infectious breath plumes *across* occupants rather than away from them [22].

3.12 Moving Ahead

The dynamics of transmission are further complicated by the biology of the virus itself—specifically, the emergence of variants like Delta and Omicron, which have demonstrated increased transmissibility and the ability to cause reinfections [19, 38]. This biological evolution means that building defenses must be robust and adaptable.

3.13 The Bacterial Persistence: Tuberculosis and the Built Environment

The Archetype of Airborne Disease While the COVID-19 pandemic forced a re-evaluation of airborne transmission for respiratory viruses, *Mycobacterium tuberculosis* (TB) has long stood as the irrefutable evidence of building-mediated infection. Unlike SARS-CoV-2, which utilizes an "opportunistic" airborne route (capable of droplet and contact transmission), TB is an obligate airborne pathogen. It relies entirely on the built environment's air currents to transport droplet nuclei (<5 microns) from the deep lungs of an infectious host to the alveoli of a susceptible occupant [33].

For the building professional, TB represents the "stress test" for ventilation design. Historical data illustrates that standard ventilation rates, often deemed sufficient for comfort (odour removal), are frequently inadequate to prevent TB transmission. Analyses of actual TB exposures in office buildings and intensive care units (ICUs) demonstrate that the probability of infection follows the Wells-Riley prediction curves; however, these curves also reveal a disturbing reality: to achieve high levels of protection against a potent emitter of TB quanta, ventilation rates may often exceed practical engineering limits (e.g., requiring >20 air changes per hour) [33].

Multidrug-Resistant TB (MDR-TB): The High-Stakes Variant The challenge of TB control in the built environment is compounded by the prevalence of multidrug-resistant TB (MDR-TB). A systematic review of MDR-TB prevalence in East Africa highlighted that pooled prevalence rates can be as high as 21% among previously treated cases [28]. In dense urban environments or healthcare facilities where undiagnosed MDR-TB patients congregate, the building itself becomes the primary line of defense. If the HVAC system recirculates air without adequate filtration (HEPA) or disinfection (UVGI), it essentially creates a loop of antibiotic-resistant biological hazards. The persistence of MDR-TB underscores the necessity for engineering controls that are agnostic to the drug resistance profile of the pathogen; a UV photon inactivates a drug-resistant bacterium just as effectively as a drug-susceptible one [33].

The Particle Physics of Bacterial Deposition Understanding the fate of bacterial aerosols requires an appreciation of particle physics within the respiratory tract and the room volume. Models such as the multiple path particle dosimetry (MPPD) allow researchers to predict where particles of different sizes—ranging from 0.01 to 10 microns—deposit within the human lung [23].

- *Tracheobronchial Deposition:* Larger bacterial aggregates often deposit in the upper airways, where mucociliary clearance can remove them.
- *Alveolar Deposition:* The critical danger zone for TB is the alveolar region. Droplet nuclei in the 1–3 micron range are small enough to navigate the bronchial tree but large enough to settle in the alveoli by sedimentation [23].

Building ventilation strategies must therefore be tuned to remove these specific particle sizes. While Brownian motion dominates the removal of ultrafine particles (<0.1 micron) and gravitational settling removes large droplets (>10 microns), the "accumulation mode" particles (0.1–1.0 micron)—which include many bacterial bioaerosols—are the most persistent in indoor air and the most difficult to capture with low-efficiency filters [23].

3.14 The Fungal Frontier: Mold, Moisture, and Mycotoxins

The "Damp Building" Ecosystem Beyond bacteria and viruses, the built environment hosts a complex kingdom of fungi. Unlike obligate pathogens that require a human host, fungi require only moisture and a carbon source—often provided by building materials like drywall, ceiling tiles, and insulation. The presence of excess moisture turns a building into a cultivator of fungal biomass, leading to what is clinically and structurally defined as a "Damp Building" [20, 25].

Specific Agents of Concern Research into the microbiome of HVAC systems and water-damaged interiors has identified specific fungal genera that pose significant health risks:

1. *Stachybotrys chartarum* (Black Mold): Perhaps the most notorious building-associated fungus, *S. chartarum* requires high water activity ($a_w > 0.9$) and cellulose-rich substrates. It produces potent trichothecene mycotoxins (satratoxins)

which inhibit protein synthesis [25]. Studies have isolated these mycotoxins from building materials in homes where infants suffered from acute pulmonary hemorrhage, suggesting a potential link between airborne toxin exposure and severe respiratory pathology [25].

2. *Cladosporium* and *Penicillium*: These are the most common genera recovered from HVAC insulation and cooling coils. In a study of fungal contamination in "sick buildings," *Cladosporium cladosporioides* and *Cladosporium sphaerospermum* were frequently recovered from blower wheels and duct liners [43]. These fungi are prolific spore producers; when the HVAC system starts up, mechanical vibration can release bursts of spores into the occupied zone, triggering allergic rhinitis, asthma, and hypersensitivity pneumonitis (HP) in sensitized occupants [20].
3. *Aspergillus* species: *Aspergillus fumigatus* and *Aspergillus versicolor* are significant sources of indoor allergens and mycotoxins (sterigmatocystin). *Aspergillus* spores are small (2–3 microns) and easily respirable, allowing them to penetrate deep into the lungs [1].

Mechanisms of Illness: Infection vs. Intoxication vs. Inflammation Fungal exposure in buildings triggers health effects through three distinct mechanisms, often confusing the diagnosis of "mold illness":

- *IgE-Mediated Allergy:* Immediate hypersensitivity reactions (asthma, rhinitis) to fungal proteins (e.g., Alt a 1 from *Alternaria*) [1].
- *Infection (Mycosis):* Direct colonization of tissue, such as Aspergillosis. This is rare in healthy individuals but a critical concern in hospital environments with immunocompromised patients [20].
- *Toxicosis and Inflammation:* Inhalation of mycotoxins and glucans (cell wall components). Research suggests that even non-viable fungal fragments can trigger powerful innate immune responses via Toll-like receptors, leading to chronic inflammation. A theoretical model proposes that this "chemical irritant" pathway may induce neurogenic inflammation, where environmental chemicals trigger sensory nerves to release inflammatory neuropeptides (Substance P), resulting in the multi-system symptoms characteristic of sick building syndrome (SBS) and multiple chemical sensitivity (MCS) [7, 27].

The HVAC System as a Fungal Amplifier A critical failure point in modern buildings is the internal lining of HVAC ducts. Porous insulation used for acoustic damping can trap organic dust and moisture, creating an ideal niche for fungal growth. Once established, these colonies are protected from cleaning and can continuously seed the building with spores and microbial volatile organic compounds (MVOCs), which manifest as the characteristic "musty" odour associated with SBS [43].

3.15 The Water-Air Interface: Aerosolization from Plumbing

The Toilet Plume Phenomenon While respiratory aerosols are generated by humans, another class of infectious aerosols is generated by the building's plumbing system. The "toilet plume"—the aerosolisation of toilet bowl water during flushing—is a recognized vector for enteric and potentially respiratory pathogens [15].

Recent reviews of transmission risks in washrooms have quantified the bioaerosol load generated by flushing. Studies indicate that a single flush can generate thousands of droplets, many of which are small enough to remain airborne and be inhaled or settle on surfaces (fomites) like door handles and toilet seats [15]. In one study, bacterial counts exceeding 100 $\frac{CFU}{m^3}$ were detected in the air after flushing, and enteric viruses such as adenovirus and norovirus have been recovered from washroom air and surfaces [15].

Wastewater Surveillance: The Building as a Diagnostic Tool The pathogen load in a building's wastewater is not just a hazard; it is data. The COVID-19 pandemic accelerated the adoption of wastewater-based epidemiology (WBE). Because infected individuals (including asymptomatic ones) shed SARS-CoV-2 RNA in their faeces, sampling sewage at the building level (e.g., university dormitories, nursing homes, cruise ships) can provide an early warning of an outbreak days before clinical symptoms appear ([2]; Sherchan et al. 2020 cited in [2]).

Systematic reviews of WBE have shown a strong correlation between viral RNA concentrations in wastewater and the number of clinical cases in the catchment area [2]. For building managers, this offers a proactive tool: detecting a spike in viral load in a building's sewage outflow can trigger targeted clinical testing and isolation protocols, potentially arresting an outbreak in its infancy (high certainty of evidence) [2].

The indoor pathosphere is not limited to the viruses we exhale. It is a polymicrobial environment where bacteria like TB exploit ventilation failures, fungi like *Stachybotrys* exploit moisture failures, and enteric pathogens exploit plumbing mechanics. The "infection-resilient" building must therefore be defended on multiple fronts: air distribution systems that dilute droplet nuclei, envelope designs that prevent moisture ingress, and plumbing systems that contain bioaerosols. In the next section, we will turn our attention to the specific engineering interventions—such as advanced filtration and air cleaning technologies—that serve as the active immune system of the built environment.

3.16 The Mechanical Immune System: Filtration and Purification

The Building's Kidneys If ventilation represents the respiratory system of a building—inhaling fresh air and exhaling contaminants—then filtration represents its renal system. It is the mechanism by which the built environment actively cleanses its own circulatory fluid of particulate impurities. In the context of the "pathosphere," where viral aerosols and bacterial spores drift on thermal plumes, the air filter (if maintained and regularly replaced) is often the single most critical line of defense against the recirculation of disease.

Historically, filtration standards in commercial and residential buildings were driven by the need to protect HVAC equipment from dust accumulation, rather than protecting occupants from biological agents. The standard MERV-8 (minimum efficiency reporting value) filter, ubiquitous in many pre-pandemic offices and schools, captures pollen and carpet lint but is largely "transparent" to the droplet nuclei (<5 microns) that carry SARS-CoV-2, influenza, and tuberculosis. The shift toward *infection-resilient environments* demands a recalibration of our filtration philosophy, prioritising the interception of the sub-micron viral fraction.

The Physics of Capture: Beyond the Sieve A common misconception among building professionals is that air filters work solely like sieves, trapping only particles larger than the gaps between fibers. In reality, high-efficiency filtration relies on four distinct physical mechanisms that allow them to capture particles far smaller than the pore size of the filter media:

1. *Inertial Impaction:* Larger particles (>1 micron) cannot follow the airstream as it bends around a fiber; they crash into the fiber due to inertia.
2. *Interception:* Mid-sized particles follow the streamline but come within one particle radius of a fiber, adhering to it.
3. *Diffusion (Brownian Motion):* The smallest particles (<0.1 micron) behave like gas molecules, zig-zagging randomly due to collisions with air molecules. This erratic motion increases the probability that they will bump into a filter fiber.
4. *Electrostatic Attraction:* Synthetic media often carry a charge that pulls particles from the airstream like a magnet [45].

This physics explains the "most penetrating particle size" (MPPS), typically around 0.3 micron, where neither diffusion nor impaction is maximally effective. This is precisely why HEPA (high-efficiency particulate air) filters are rated on their ability to capture 99.97% of particles at this specific 0.3 micron size—the hardest size to catch.

HEPA vs. MERV: The Evidence Base The efficacy of upgrading filtration has been empirically validated. A systematic review of ventilation strategies in schools found that upgrading to MERV 13 filters resulted in a significant reduction in infection risk, estimated at roughly 30% relative to baseline scenarios with lower efficiency filters [13]. However, the review also noted a plateau effect; utilizing filters more efficient than MERV 13 (such as HEPA) in a standard central HVAC system often incurred a massive pressure drop penalty—requiring stronger fans and more energy—without yielding a proportional reduction in risk, unless the system was specifically designed for high-resistance filtration [13].

In healthcare settings, the stakes are higher. A meta-analysis comparing operating theatres with laminar air flow (LAF) versus conventional ventilation found that HEPA filters were instrumental in reducing bacterial colony-forming units (CFU) in the air. Specifically, HEPA-filtered environments reduced bacterial counts by approximately 113 $\frac{CFU}{m^3}$ compared to environments without such stringent filtration [10]. This finding underscores that for high-risk zones, HEPA is non-negotiable.

Portable Air Cleaners (PACs): The Retrofit Solution For the vast majority of existing buildings where HVAC systems cannot handle the pressure drop of HEPA filters, *portable air cleaners (PACs)* have emerged as a vital stopgap. These standalone units, equipped with HEPA filters and fans, essentially scrub the air within a room. Evidence suggests that PACs can significantly reduce aerosol concentrations, but their placement is critical. Improperly placed PACs can create cross-drafts that pull infectious aerosols *across* the breathing zone of other occupants before filtering them [13]. Therefore, the "mechanical immune system" must be spatially aware; simply adding a machine is insufficient without considering the airflow topology it creates. Further, there are now available PACs which have a small inlet pipe for outdoor air which also enables dilution of the indoor air.

3.17 Light as a Weapon: Ultraviolet Germicidal Irradiation (UVGI)

Inactivation vs. Capture While filtration captures pathogens, *ultraviolet germicidal irradiation (UVGI)* kills them. Specifically, UV-C light (wavelength 200–280 nm) penetrates the pathogen and is absorbed by its DNA or RNA, causing the formation of pyrimidine dimers. This damage prevents the microorganism from replicating, rendering it non-infectious. In the fight against airborne transmission, UVGI offers a unique advantage: it does not impede airflow.

Susceptibility and the "Z" Value Not all pathogens are equally vulnerable to UV light. The sensitivity of a microorganism is defined by its *Z-value* (susceptibility constant, $\frac{m^2}{J}$). A systematic review by Thornton et al. [45] aggregated susceptibility data for coronaviruses, finding that SARS-CoV-2 and its surrogates are highly susceptible to UV-C. For example, studies indicated that a UV dose as low as 12 $\frac{m^2}{J}$ could achieve significant inactivation of viral surrogates like Phi6 [45].

Crucially, environmental conditions modulate this susceptibility. The review highlighted that increasing relative humidity (RH) is generally associated with *decreasing* susceptibility (lower Z-values). For the bacteriophage MS2, the Z-value dropped from 0.81 $\frac{m^2}{J}$ at 55% RH to 0.64 $\frac{m^2}{J}$ at 85% RH [45]. This implies that in humid environments (e.g., tropical climates or swimming pools), UVGI systems must be sized to deliver higher doses to achieve the same kill rate.

Upper-Room UVGI: The Air Disinfection Workhorse The most effective application for occupied spaces is *Upper-Room UVGI*. Fixtures shield the occupants below while irradiating the air in the upper 30–50 cm of the room. Natural convection and mechanical fans lift warm, exhaled aerosols into this "kill zone," where they are neutralized before cooling and settling back down. Research indicates that a well-designed upper-room system can provide an "equivalent air change rate" (eACH) of 10–20 changes per hour, far exceeding what mechanical ventilation can typically provide (often 2–6 ACH) and at a fraction of the energy cost [45]. It acts as a silent, invisible sanitizing ceiling.

The Frontier: Far-UVC (222 nm) A major limitation of traditional UV-C (254 nm) is its potential to damage human eyes (photokeratitis) and skin (erythema). This necessitates strict shielding and limits its use to the upper room. However, emerging research into *Far-UVC (222 nm)* suggests a game-changing possibility. Light at 222 nm cannot penetrate the dead outer layer of human skin (stratum corneum) or the tear layer of the eye, but it can still easily penetrate bacteria and viruses [12]. Studies show that 222 nm irradiation effectively inactivates airborne pathogens without inducing the DNA damage associated with skin cancer in mammalian models [12]. This technology could theoretically allow for "whole-room" irradiation, where lights continuously disinfect the air *and* surfaces around occupants, providing a persistent level of sterility previously impossible in occupied spaces. For many settings in India, exposure to natural sunlight may also serve the same function. This is esp. mentioned as some settings may have issues with respect to the initial capital cost, safety issues and the need for maintenance in UVGI.

3.18 The Chemical Additives: Ozone and Ionization

The Risks of "Additive" Cleaning In the desperation of the pandemic, many building managers turned to "additive" air cleaning technologies—devices that release substances like ozone, hydrogen peroxide, or ions into the air to attack pathogens. While these methods can be effective surface disinfectants, their safety in occupied air is highly contentious.

Ozone (O_3) Ozone is a potent oxidant known to destroy viral capsids. A scoping review of ozone disinfection confirmed its efficacy against SARS-CoV-2 on surfaces, noting that it can degrade viral proteins and lipids [9]. However, ozone is also a respiratory irritant regulated by agencies like the EPA. The concentrations required to rapidly kill viruses in the air may often exceed safe exposure limits for humans. Furthermore, ozone reacts with indoor VOCs (from carpets, cleaners, or furniture) to create harmful secondary byproducts, including formaldehyde and ultrafine particles [9]. Therefore, ozone is largely restricted to "terminal cleaning" of unoccupied rooms (e.g., between patients in a hospital) rather than continuous air cleaning.

Hydrogen Peroxide Vapor (HPV) Similarly, systems using vaporized hydrogen peroxide are highly effective for decontamination. Studies involving N95 respirator decontamination demonstrated that HPV could achieve a 6-log reduction in bioburden without compromising the filter's integrity [35]. Like ozone, however, this is an unoccupied-state intervention.

The consensus among building scientists leans heavily toward *subtractive* technologies (filtration) and *contained inactivation* (UVGI) rather than additive chemistries, due to the principle of "first, do no harm" regarding indoor air chemistry.

3.19 Source Control: The Building Policy Interface

Masks as Engineering Controls While masks are personal protective equipment (PPE), from a building physics perspective, they function as *source control*. They reduce the "source term" (q, quanta generation rate) in the Wells-Riley equation.

A comprehensive network meta-analysis by Kim et al. [21] compared the effectiveness of N95, surgical, and non-medical masks. The study found that N95 respirators reduced the risk of SARS-CoV-2 infection by approximately 70% compared to no mask, while surgical masks provided statistically significant but slightly lower protection [21]. Crucially, the study highlighted that in community settings, even non-medical masks provided a protective benefit, although the certainty of evidence was lower [21].

For the building designer, this implies that the required ventilation rate is dependent on mask policy. A building designed for a "masked" population can achieve safety targets with lower air change rates than one designed for an unmasked population. For example, modelling of an auditorium outbreak showed that if the index cases had worn effective masks (outward protection efficiency of 75%), the estimated quanta emission rate would have dropped from ~31 q/h to ~8 q/h, drastically reducing the ventilation required to prevent secondary infections [19].

Behavioral Adherence However, engineering cannot assume 100% compliance. A review of physical distancing interventions found that while instructions (like floor decals) can influence behavior, they are not foolproof [12]. Similarly, mask adherence varies by demographic and setting. A systematic review on mask use in children found that while feasible, adherence is influenced by age and comfort [8]. Consequently, "infection-resilient" buildings must be designed with a safety factor that accounts for imperfect human behavior—essentially, the building must compensate for the unmasked occupant.

3.20 The Intelligent Building: Sensors and Demand Control

Visualizing the Invisible The final frontier in infection control is the integration of sensor networks to make invisible risks visible. Traditional demand control ventilation (DCV) uses CO_2 sensors to *reduce* ventilation when occupancy is low to save energy. The new paradigm requires inverting this logic: using sensors to *increase* ventilation when risk is high.

Sensor Deployment A systematic review by Mena et al. [29] analyzed the deployment of environmental sensors for occupancy estimation. The study found that CO_2 sensors, combined with temperature and humidity data, can accurately predict the number of occupants in a room [29].

The CO_2 Proxy Strategy Since we cannot measure real-time viral load, CO_2 remains the best proxy for "rebreathed air." [44]. As established in previous sections, a specific CO_2 threshold (e.g., 800 ppm) can serve as a trigger point. An intelligent building management system (BMS) would continuously monitor these levels. Upon approaching the threshold, the system would automatically open outdoor air dampers, increase fan speeds, or activate upper-room UVGI systems. This creates a dynamic immune response: the building "senses" the congestion (pathogen potential) and "fevers" (activates defenses) to clear the threat [29, 40].

3.21 Moving Forward

We have moved from understanding the "biological enemy" to deploying the "mechanical arsenal". The engineering interventions available—high-efficiency filtration, specific ventilation strategies, and UVGI—are robust and scientifically proven. They transform the building from a passive container into an active defense system. However, these technologies are not silver bullets; they are part of a complex ecosystem that includes human behavior (masks) and operational policies.

In the final section of this chapter, we will synthesize these biological, physical, and engineering insights into a cohesive framework for the future, discussing the economic and ethical implications of "infection-resilient design" and finalising the policy recommendations for the everyday built environment.

3.22 The Economic Calculus: Health vs. Energy

The False Economy of "Tight" Buildings For decades, the dominant narrative in facility management has been cost containment, primarily achieved through energy efficiency. This often meant reducing air exchange rates to the minimums allowed by code, effectively sealing the "thermodynamic envelope" to retain heat or cooling. While this strategy successfully lowered utility bills, it created a hidden debt paid in human health. The COVID-19 pandemic acted as a foreclosure on this debt, revealing that buildings optimized solely for energy are biologically fragile [39].

The resistance to increasing ventilation often stems from the perceived "energy penalty." Conditioning vast amounts of outdoor air requires significant power. However, this view ignores the "salary penalty." In a commercial office, energy costs typically account for approximately 1% of total operating costs, while human salaries and benefits account for 90% [3]. A small improvement in indoor environmental quality (IEQ) that reduces absenteeism or increases cognitive function by even 1% may yield financial returns that dwarf the entire energy budget of the building [40].

Cost-Effectiveness of Interventions When evaluating infection control strategies, the metric must shift from "energy per square meter" to "cost per equivalent air change."

3.23 The Ethical Imperative: Clean Air as a Human Right

The Paradigm Shift Historically, we have accepted that the water we drink from a tap is free of cholera and the food we buy is free of salmonella. Yet, we have accepted that the air we breathe in a crowded room may be laden with influenza or coronaviruses. The scientific consensus is shifting to view indoor air safety as a fundamental human right, akin to water sanitation [30].

Equity in the Built Environment Infection control in buildings is also a matter of social equity. Low-income populations often inhabit "sick buildings"—older structures with poor ventilation, moisture problems, and overcrowding. These environments act as amplification nodes for diseases like tuberculosis and COVID-19. Studies have shown that during the pandemic, secondary attack rates were significantly higher in households with higher density and poorer infrastructure [24, 38]. Designing infection-resilient environments is not just a luxury for Class-A office towers; it is a public health necessity for schools, public housing, and public transport systems where the most vulnerable congregate.

Professional Responsibility Architects, engineers, and facility managers now bear a heightened professional responsibility. Ignorance of airborne transmission physics is no longer a valid defense. The definition of "standard of care" is evolving. A building designed today that fails to accommodate surge capacity for ventilation or air disinfection may increasingly be viewed as falling below emerging expectations of professional duty of care in the face of future pandemics. The "infection control plan" (ICCP) discussed in previous chapters must become a standard deliverable, ensuring that the building's "immune system" is as robust as its "structural skeleton."

3.24 Policy and Future Directions

From Minimums to Targets Popular Building codes set *minimum* ventilation rates. The future requires *target* rates based on health outcomes. The Royal Academy of Engineering [39] proposes a shift toward "infection resilience" standards that are dynamic. Buildings should have a "pandemic mode"—a pre-programmed operational state that maximizes outdoor air, disables demand-controlled ventilation (DCV) reduction, and activates disinfection systems when epidemiological risk is high [39].

The Role of Sensors and AI The static building is obsolete. The future is the "sentient" building, equipped with networks of biosensors and CO_2 monitors. These systems will not just react to temperature but to biological risk.

- *Wastewater Surveillance:* As demonstrated during the pandemic, testing building sewage for viral RNA can predict outbreaks days before symptoms appear [41]. Future buildings may have automated samplers in the plumbing infrastructure to serve as an early warning system.
- *Real-time Risk Displays:* Just as we see a "speedometer" in a car, occupants may soon expect to see an "Air Safety Index" displayed in lobbies, derived from real-time CO_2, particulate matter, and humidity data [29]. The easiest being the CO_2 measure which is a proxy for ventilation.

3.25 Conclusion

The everyday built environment is the primary battlefield for respiratory health. We spend upto 90% of our lives indoors, submerged in an invisible ocean of air that connects us to the lungs of everyone around us. This chapter has dissected the anatomy of this connection, revealing that "infection" is not merely a biological event but an architectural one.

We have learned that the distinction between "droplet" and "airborne" is physically flawed; that dry air preserves viruses while humid air inactivates them; and that our buildings have largely been designed to trap pollutants rather than purge them. However, we have also identified the arsenal available to us: the physics of dilution (ventilation), the mechanics of capture (filtration), and the photochemistry of inactivation (UVGI).

The challenge moving forward is not technological; it is cultural and economic. It requires valuing the invisible asset of health over the visible cost of energy. It requires a new pedagogy for designers and a new rigorousness for operators. By embracing the concept of the *infection-resilient environment*, we can transform our buildings from passive containers of disease into active guardians of public health. The building of the future does not just shelter us from the storm outside; it protects us from the "storm" within.

Acknowledgments The authors acknowledge the support provided by the institutions including School of Planning and Architecture, New Delhi, All India Institute of Medical Sciences, New Delhi, and Drexel University. Special thanks to Rajshekhar Pullabhatla and Group Captain P Aanand Naidu of ISAC Centre for Built Environment Policy and Tathatara Foundation. Many thanks to Dr Arthur L Frank, MD. Many thanks to all the people who supported this work in many ways.

Declarations The authors Raja Singh, Nirupam Madaan, and Anil Dewan declare no conflict of interests or competing interests in this work. There is no involvement of human participants, animals, human or animal tissue. All authors declare that there was no specific financial support received from any organization for the submitted work. All authors declare that they have no financial relationships at present or within the previous 3 years with any organizations that might have an interest in the submitted work. While all care has been taken in ensuring the accuracy of this work, any inadvertent error may be reported at the earliest. The authors acknowledge the use of supervised language learning models/large language models for enhancement of the work, with responsibility lying with the authors. For more information, the corresponding author may be contacted at email rajaresearch@proton.me.

CRediT Statement The following is the CRediT statement which declares the author credits for this chapter:

Raja Singh: Conceptualization, Methodology, Formal Analysis, Investigation, Data Curation, Writing-Original Draft, Writing-Review & Editing, Visualization, Project Administration.
Nirupam Madaan: Conceptualization, Resources, Validation, Supervision, Project Administration.
Anil Dewan: Resources, Validation Supervision.

References

1. Abel-Fernández E, Martínez MJ, Galán T, Pineda F. Going over fungal allergy: *Alternaria alternata* and its allergens. J Fungi. 2022;8:542.
2. Ahmed W, et al. SARS-CoV-2 surveillance of wastewater: a systematic review. Water Res. 2022;213:118136.
3. Allen JG, MacNaughton P, Laurent JGC, Flanigan SS, Eitland ES, Spengler JD. Green buildings and health. Curr Environ Health Rep. 2015;2(3):250–8.
4. Amoatey P, Omidvarborna H, Baawain MS, Al-Mamun A. Indoor air pollution and exposure assessment of the gulf cooperation council countries: a critical review. Environ Int. 2018;121:491–506.
5. Anand U, et al. SARS-CoV-2 in municipal wastewater, landfill leachate, and solid waste. Environ Res. 2022;203:111839.
6. Asadi S, et al. Efficacy of masks and face coverings in controlling outward aerosol emission. Sci Rep. 2020;10:15665.
7. Bascom R, et al. Neurogenic inflammation. Environ Health Perspect. 1997;105(Suppl 2):531–7.
8. Braga PP, et al. Use of masks by children. Revista da Escola de Enfermagem da USP. 2022;56.
9. Câmara AB, et al. Ozone disinfection for viruses. J Hosp Infect. 2022;130:63–94.
10. Dai Z, et al. Systematic review of HVAC in hospitals. PLoS ONE. 2021;16(11):e0259996.
11. Dinoi A, Feltracco M, Chirizzi D, et al. Airborne microorganism inactivation using UV-C systems. Int J Environ Res Public Health. 2022;19:1559.
12. Epton T, et al. Physical distancing interventions. Soc Sci Med. 2022;303:114946.

13. Ferrari S, Blázquez T, Cardellino P, Borgstein EH. Ventilation strategies to reduce airborne transmission in classrooms. Build Environ. 2022;222:109366.
14. Gholipour S, et al. Occurrence of viruses in sewage sludge. Sci Total Environ. 2022;824:153886.
15. Gormley M, Aspray TJ, Kelly DA. Bioaerosols in the built environment. Infect Prevent Pract. 2021;3(4):100186.
16. Gozdzielewska L, et al. Hand hygiene interventions. BMC Public Health. 2022;22:1283.
17. Hammond A, et al. Portable air filters for SARS-CoV-2. PLoS ONE. 2021;16(4):e0251049.
18. Horvath EP. Building-related illness and sick building syndrome. Cleve Clin J Med. 1997;64(6):303–9.
19. Huang J, Hao T, Liu X, Jones P, Ou C, Liang W, Liu F. Airborne transmission of Delta variant in an auditorium. Build Environ. 2022;219:109212.
20. Husman T. Health effects of indoor-air microorganisms. Scand J Work Environ Health. 1996;22(1):5–13.
21. Kim MS, et al. Comparative effectiveness of masks. Rev Med Virol. 2022;32(5):e2336.
22. Li Y, Cheng P, Jia W. Poor ventilation worsens short-range airborne transmission. Indoor Air. 2022;32(1):e12946.
23. Luo K, et al. Distribution of inhaled aerosol particles. J Aerosol Sci. 2022;164:105995.
24. Madewell ZJ, Yang Y, Longini IM, Halloran ME, Dean NE. Household transmission of SARS-CoV-2. JAMA Netw Open. 2020;3(12):e2031756.
25. Mahmoudi M, Gershwin ME. Sick building syndrome III. J Asthma. 2000;37(2):191–8.
26. Mao N, An CK, Guo LY, Wang M, Guo L, Guo SR, Long ES. Transmission risk of infectious droplets. Build Environ. 2020;185:107307.
27. Meggs WJ. Neurogenic inflammation and chemical sensitivity. Environ Health Perspect. 1993;101(3):234–8.
28. Mekonnen F, et al. Multidrug-resistant tuberculosis in East Africa. PLoS ONE. 2022;17(6):e0270272.
29. Mena AR, Ceballos HG, Alvarado-Uribe J. Measuring indoor occupancy using sensors. Sensors. 2022;22(10):3770.
30. Morawska L, et al. Minimising airborne transmission indoors. Environ Int. 2020;142:105832.
31. Moriarty LF, et al. COVID-19 outbreaks on cruise ships. MMWR. 2020;69:347–52.
32. Nair AN, Anand P, George A, Mondal N. Strategies to reduce airborne transmission. Environ Res. 2022;213:113579.
33. Nardell EA. Air disinfection and germicidal UV. Photochem Photobiol. 2021;97(3):493–7.
34. Nguyen TT, Johnson GR, Bell SC, Knibbs LD. Review of indoor air disinfection techniques. Int J Environ Res Public Health. 2022;19:1197.
35. Oh J, Thaper R, Fagen B. Decontamination of respirators. Environ Sci Pollut Res. 2022;29:1645–76.
36. Onakpoya IJ, Heneghan CJ, Jefferson T. Viral cultures and fomite transmission. J Hosp Infect. 2022;130:63–94.
37. Peters A, et al. Environmental hygiene interventions. Antimicrob Resist Infect Control. 2022;11:38.
38. Ren X, et al. Reinfection and recurrence of COVID-19. J Med Virol. 2022;94:44–53.
39. Royal Academy of Engineering. Infection resilient environments: time for a major upgrade. National Engineering Policy Centre; 2022.
40. Seppänen O, Fisk WJ. Ventilation rates and CO_2. Indoor Air. 1999;9(4):226–52.
41. Shah S, et al. Wastewater surveillance for SARS-CoV-2 variants. Sci Total Environ. 2022;804:150060.
42. Silverberg SL, Zhang BY, Li SNJ, et al. SARS-CoV-2 on environmental surfaces. BMC Infect Dis. 2022;22:172.
43. Straus DC. Fungal contamination and sick building syndrome. Front Biosci. 2011;E3:562–80.
44. Sundell J, et al. Ventilation rates and health. Indoor Air. 2011;21(3):191–204.
45. Thornton GM, Fleck BA, Fleck N, Kroeker E, Dandnayak D, Zhong L, Hartling L. HVAC design and ultraviolet radiation. PLoS ONE. 2022;17(4):e0266487.

46. Tran VV, Park D, Lee YC. Indoor air pollution and human disease. Int J Environ Res Public Health. 2020;17:2927.
47. Viana Martins CP, et al. Stability of SARS-CoV-2 on surfaces. J Hosp Infect. 2022;119:84–117.
48. Viner R, et al. Transmission by children and young people. J Infect. 2022;84:361–82.
49. Welch D, et al. Far-UVC light. Sci Rep. 2022;8:2752.
50. Zhang Y, et al. Bibliometric analysis of SARS-CoV-2 variant research. Front Public Health. 2022;10:966847.

Dilution Ventilation as the Means for Airborne Infection Control

4

Raja Singh, Nirupam Madaan, and Anil Dewan

4.1 The Physics of the Invisible: Introduction to Airborne Contaminant Removal

To understand the imperative of dilution ventilation, we must first visualize the invisible. Imagine a quiet room, perhaps a library or a shared office space. To the naked eye, the air is empty, a transparent void through which we move and breathe. However, to the physicist and the microbiologist, this air is a chaotic, gelatinous soup of fluid dynamics (air is a complex turbulent fluid containing suspended particulate matter, among other things), thermal plumes, and suspended particulate matter. Every occupant within this space is a biological engine, continuously emitting thermal energy and, crucially, bioaerosols. When a human breathes, speaks, coughs, or sings, they are not merely expelling gas; they are atomizing respiratory fluids into a mist of droplets ranging from the macroscopic to the microscopic.

For decades, infection control was dominated by a binary dogma: the distinction between "droplets" (large, ballistic projectiles that fall within 1–2 m) and "airborne" (small particles that remain suspended). This dichotomy, largely based on antiquated work from the 1930s and 1940s, suggested that unless a pathogen was classified as "airborne" (like measles or tuberculosis), spatial

R. Singh
Founder/Researcher, The Built, New Delhi, Delhi, India

Former Post Doctoral Fellow, Department of Environmental and Occupational Health, Dornsife School of Public Health, Drexel University, Philadelphia, Pennsylvania, USA

N. Madaan
Department of Hospital Administration, All India Institute of Medical Sciences, New Delhi, Delhi, India

A. Dewan
Department of Architecture, School of Planning and Architecture, New Delhi, Delhi, India

R. Singh et al., *Infection Control in the Everyday Built Environment*, https://doi.org/10.1007/978-981-95-8624-0_4

separation was sufficient protection [52, 85]. However, the SARS-CoV-2 pandemic dismantled this simplistic view, revealing that respiratory exhalations form a turbulent gas cloud containing clusters of droplets of a continuum of sizes [13, 48].

The fundamental challenge in indoor environments is the persistence of the "droplet nucleus." Upon exhalation, a respiratory droplet immediately encounters the ambient environment, which typically has a lower relative humidity than the respiratory tract. Driven by the laws of thermodynamics, rapid heat and mass transfer occur. The water content of the droplet evaporates, shrinking the particle to a fraction of its original size—often down to 20–40% of the initial diameter—leaving behind a residue of salts, proteins, and potential pathogens [48, 59]. These resulting droplet nuclei are light enough that gravitational settling becomes negligible compared to the forces of air currents and thermal buoyancy. A particle smaller than 5 micrometers can remain suspended in stagnant air for hours, traveling on convection currents generated by computers, heating systems, and even the body heat of the occupants themselves [36, 58].

Therefore, the enclosed space becomes a trap. Without intervention, the concentration of these infectious quanta—defined as the dose required to infect 63% of susceptible persons—accumulates over time, much like smoke filling a sealed room [16, 51]. The primary, and often most accessible, mechanism to counteract this accumulation is dilution ventilation.

Dilution ventilation is the engineering process of introducing "clean" air (usually outdoor air) into a space and removing stale, contaminated air, thereby lowering the concentration of internally generated pollutants. Ideally, this process reduces the probability that an occupant will inhale a critical infectious dose. The efficacy of this mechanism is governed by the principles of mass balance, often modeled using the Wells-Riley equation, which posits that the probability of infection is a function of the number of infectors, the quanta generation rate, the pulmonary ventilation rate of susceptibles, the duration of exposure, and, critically, the volume of fresh air supply [14, 75].

However, ventilation is not merely about opening a window or turning on a fan. It is a complex interplay of air change rates (ACH), ventilation effectiveness (how well the fresh air mixes with the room air), and airflow patterns (directional flow). If ventilation is poorly designed, it can inadvertently transport pathogens from an infector to a susceptible host before dilution occurs—a phenomenon observed in restaurant outbreaks where air conditioning units created a focused stream of viral aerosols [42, 44, 45].

In this chapter, we will dissect the mechanics of dilution ventilation, placing it in rigorous comparison with other airborne infection control methodologies. We will explore why, despite the advent of advanced air cleaning technologies, the simple act of replacing stale air with fresh air remains the cornerstone of healthy building design, yet why it simultaneously faces critical limitations in the era of energy efficiency and high-occupancy urban living.

4.2 Comparing Dilution Ventilation to Other Methods of Airborne Infection Control

To appreciate the role of dilution ventilation, we must situate it within the broader hierarchy of controls for airborne pathogens. The objective of any engineering control in this context is to interrupt the chain of transmission at the level of the environment, specifically after the pathogen has left the reservoir (the infected host) and before it enters the portal of entry (the respiratory tract) of the susceptible host. The primary methods available to building engineers and industrial hygienists include:

1. *Dilution Ventilation:* Replacing contaminated indoor air with fresh outdoor air.
2. *Filtration (In-duct and Portable):* Removing particulate matter, including bioaerosols, via mechanical or electrostatic interception.
3. *Ultraviolet Germicidal Irradiation (UVGI):* Inactivating the pathogen's DNA or RNA, rendering it unable to replicate.
4. *Chemical Disinfection:* Using agents like ozone, hydrogen peroxide vapor, or bipolar ionization to chemically neutralize pathogens.

4.2.1 The Thermodynamic and Economic Battle: Ventilation vs. Filtration

Ventilation and filtration are often discussed in the same breath, frequently conflated under the umbrella of "HVAC" (heating, ventilation, and air conditioning). However, their mechanisms of action and economic implications differ fundamentally.

Dilution ventilation operates on the principle of *removal* via exchange. When outdoor air is introduced, it displaces an equal volume of indoor air (assuming balanced pressure). This removes not only biological particulates but also gaseous contaminants like carbon dioxide (CO_2), volatile organic compounds (VOCs), and body odours [80, 84]. This broad-spectrum efficacy is the primary advantage of ventilation. A building ventilated to popular older standards for acceptable indoor air quality relies on this mechanism to manage the "bioeffluents" of occupants [9, 67].

However, dilution ventilation carries a significant thermodynamic penalty. The outdoor air introduced must be conditioned to thermal comfort levels. In the sweltering heat of a Mumbai summer or the freezing cold of a Canadian winter, the energy required to cool or heat this massive volume of air constitutes a significant portion of the building's energy load [43, 59]. Furthermore, in highly polluted urban environments, "fresh" outdoor air may introduce particulate matter ($PM_{2.5}$, PM_{10}), nitrogen oxides (NO_x), and ozone (O_3), necessitating rigorous intake filtration to prevent trading a biological hazard for a chemical one [4, 7]. Yet, for the sake of infection control, these have to be disregarded.

In contrast, filtration—specifically recirculation through high-efficiency particulate air (HEPA) filters or high-MERV (minimum efficiency reporting value) filters—focuses on *capture* rather than exchange. A HEPA filter is defined by its ability to capture at least 99.97% of particles at the most penetrating particle size (MPPS), typically around 0.3 micrometers [31, 55]. Since viruses like SARS-CoV-2 (approx. 0.1 micron) and *Mycobacterium tuberculosis* (approx. 1–5 micron droplet nuclei) travel on larger respiratory particles or cluster together, they are efficiently intercepted by mechanisms of diffusion, interception, and impaction within the filter media [37, 62].

The advantage of filtration over dilution ventilation lies in energy conservation. By recirculating and cleaning indoor air, the system retains the thermal energy already invested in the air mass. Azimi and Stephens [10] and Stephens et al. [83] demonstrated that high-efficiency filtration could reduce the risk of infectious disease transmission at a lower operational cost than equivalent levels of outdoor air ventilation, specifically because of the energy savings associated with not conditioning outdoor air [10, 42, 44]. Yet, in the developing world context, it must be noted that simply opening the window may be more viable as there may not be HEPA filtration, or the filters once used may not be maintained or not regularly replaced. This creates more harm than benefit.

Further, filtration has more limitations. It does not remove gaseous pollutants like CO_2. Consequently, a room relying solely on recirculating filtration might achieve low particle counts but accumulate metabolic CO_2 to levels that impair cognitive function [6, 78]. Furthermore, the efficacy of in-duct filtration depends on the air actually reaching the filter. In a room with poor mixing, a pathogen emitted by a source might circulate in the breathing zone of other occupants for extended periods before being drawn into the return duct and filtered. This "short-circuiting" or local stagnation limits the effectiveness of central filtration compared to distributed ventilation or in-room air cleaning [39, 59].

4.2.2 The Speed of Inactivation: Ventilation vs. UVGI

While ventilation and filtration are mechanical removal methods, ultraviolet germicidal irradiation (UVGI) is a biological inactivation method. Specifically, UV-C light (wavelength 200–280 nm, peak germicidal efficiency near 265 nm) penetrates the pathogen and is absorbed by the nucleic acids (DNA or RNA). This absorption causes the formation of pyrimidine dimers (in DNA) or uracil dimers (in RNA), distorting the genetic helix and preventing replication [14, 37].

When comparing dilution ventilation to upper-room UVGI, the metric of comparison is often "equivalent air changes per hour" (eACH). Mechanical ventilation in a typical office or school might provide 2–6 ACH (air changes per hour). To control highly infectious airborne pathogens like measles or tuberculosis, guidelines often recommend 6–12 ACH [17, 80]. Achieving 12 ACH via mechanical ventilation in an existing building may sometimes if not often be structurally and economically less feasible due to duct size limitations and fan capacities [23, 59].

Upper-room UVGI, however, creates a "kill zone" in the upper portion of the room. As natural convection currents (from body heat) and mechanical air currents lift contaminated air into the upper room, the pathogens are rapidly inactivated. Nardell and colleagues have demonstrated that a well-designed upper-room UVGI system can provide an eACH of 10–20 or more, vastly exceeding what is may be typically achievable by mechanical ventilation alone, and at a fraction of the energy cost [56, 60].

The limitation of UVGI is that it does not remove the particle itself, nor does it remove gases. It kills the biological activity but leaves the biomass. Furthermore, it requires careful commissioning to ensure safety from ocular or cutaneous exposure [26]. Thus, UVGI is rarely a standalone solution but a powerful adjunct to ventilation, particularly in high-risk settings like tuberculosis wards or during pandemics [11, 59]. There has been some further research on this [91]. Dilution ventilation remains necessary to remove the non-biological components of the air and to provide the air movement required to bring pathogens into the UVGI field [38, 63]. UVGI in many developing world settings was seen as not maintained and creating a false safety syndrome, as the systems were switched on but were never maintained (lamps not cleaned and therefore not effective). In such situations, simply opening windows may be better advice. And in the developing world, not all cities may have outdoor pollution (and the fear of outdoor pollution entering indoors due to open windows).

4.2.3 The Risk of Chemistry: Ventilation vs. Chemical Cleaning

Recent years have seen a proliferation of electronic air cleaners utilizing ionization, hydroxyl radicals, or hydrogen peroxide vapor. These technologies aim to clean the air in the occupied space, theoretically offering the benefits of dilution without the energy cost. However, the scientific consensus on these technologies remains cautious. Unlike dilution which simply removes contaminants, chemical cleaning methods rely on chemical reactions that can generate unintended byproducts.

For example, ozone generators and some ionizers can react with terpenes (chemicals found in cleaning products and air fresheners) to produce formaldehyde and ultrafine particles, which are respiratory irritants [15, 93]. A study by Zeng et al. [97] and earlier work by Waring and Siegel [89] highlight that the "net health effect" of such additive technologies must be carefully evaluated against the proven safety profile of dilution ventilation [89, 97]. Dilution ventilation, assuming clean outdoor air, introduces no new chemistry into the indoor environment; it resets the chemical baseline, making it the gold standard for safety, even if it is not always the most energy-efficient.

4.3 Central Idea of Dilution Ventilation

The central idea of dilution ventilation is predicated on the concept of the *concentration decay*. In a perfectly mixed room (an idealization where contaminant concentration is uniform throughout), the relationship between the concentration of a contaminant and the ventilation rate is governed by a first-order differential equation. If a source emits contaminants at a rate G (generation), and fresh air is supplied at a rate Q, the steady-state concentration C_{ss} (above outdoor levels) is given by:

$$C_{ss} = \frac{G}{Q}$$

This simple equation reveals the fundamental power and the fundamental limitation of dilution ventilation. The concentration is inversely proportional to the flow rate. To halve the risk (assuming risk is linear with concentration), one must double the ventilation rate [43, 71].

4.3.1 The Concept of "Quanta" and Infection Probability

In microbiology and epidemiology, we cannot always count the exact number of virions required to cause infection, as this varies by host immunity and pathogen virulence. Instead, we utilize the concept of "quanta," developed by Wells and Riley. A quantum is a hypothetical infectious dose—not a single virus, but the amount of infectious material required to infect $1 - e^{-1}$ of susceptible persons in an enclosed space [73, 92].

The central idea of dilution ventilation in infection control is to increase the volume of virus-free air (Q) to such a degree that the concentration of quanta (quanta/m^3) drops below the threshold required to trigger a transmission event within the exposure time (t). This relationship is non-linear regarding infection probability (P), as described by the Wells-Riley equation:

$$P = 1 - e^{-\frac{Iqpt}{Q}}$$

where:

- I is the number of infectors.
- q is the quanta generation rate (quanta/h).
- p is the pulmonary ventilation rate of susceptibles (m^3/h).
- t is the exposure time (h).
- Q is the absolute ventilation rate (m^3/h).

This mathematical framework illustrates why dilution ventilation is the "means" of control. By manipulating Q, we directly manipulate the exponent. If Q is very low (poor ventilation), the exponent approaches zero, and P approaches $1 - 1 = 0$? No, if Q is low, the fraction $\frac{Iqpt}{Q}$ becomes large. As the exponent becomes a large negative number, $e^{-\text{large}}$ approaches zero, so P approaches $1 - 0 = 1$ (100% infection probability). Conversely, as Q approaches infinity (like being outdoors), the fraction approaches zero, $e^0 = 1$, and P approaches $1 - 1 = 0$ (0% infection).

4.3.2 The "Rebreathed Air" Fraction

A more tangible way to conceptualize the central idea of dilution ventilation for the layperson is through the "rebreathed air" fraction. Every time humans breathe in an indoor space, they are inhaling a certain percentage of air that has recently exited the lungs of others. This fraction is a direct proxy for infection risk for airborne pathogens [66, 75].

Carbon dioxide (CO_2) serves as the natural tracer for this rebreathed fraction. Since outdoor air contains approximately 400–420 ppm of CO_2, and human exhalation contains approximately 38,000 ppm, the elevation of indoor CO_2 levels above outdoor background levels indicates the balance between occupancy and ventilation [68].

If the CO_2 level in a room is 800 ppm, the excess is 400 ppm. Since exhaled breath is ~38,000 ppm above ambient, the fraction of rebreathed air is roughly $\frac{400}{38,000} \approx 1\%$. If the CO_2 is 2400 ppm (excess 2000), the rebreathed fraction is $\frac{2000}{38,000} \approx 5.2\%$. While these percentages seem small, they represent a massive difference in exposure to airborne pathogens. A change from 1% to 5% rebreathed air quintuples the intake of potential viral aerosols [22, 75].

Thus, the central operational goal of dilution ventilation is to minimize this rebreathed fraction. It is a race against time and biology: the ventilation system must extract the droplet nuclei containing the pathogen faster than the occupants can inhale them or the pathogen can settle on surfaces (though settling is slow for fine aerosols).

4.3.3 Limitations of the "Perfect Mixing" Assumption

A critical nuance in the central idea of dilution ventilation is the assumption of perfect mixing. The Wells-Riley equation assumes that once a pathogen is released, it is instantly and uniformly distributed throughout the room volume. In reality, ventilation creates airflow patterns—plumes, jets, and stagnant zones. If an infected person is located in an air stream upwind of a susceptible person, the local concentration of quanta in the susceptible person's breathing zone may be significantly higher than the room average [43, 65].

This leads to the concept of *Ventilation Effectiveness*. Displacement ventilation, for instance, supplies cool clean air at the floor level which rises as it warms up from body heat, carrying contaminants upward to ceiling extracts. This can theoretically achieve better removal of bioaerosols than mixing ventilation, which deliberately churns the air to homogenize temperature and contaminants [12, 70]. Therefore, dilution is not just about the *amount* (Q) of air, but the *path* of the air.

In the following sections, we will delve deeper into the mechanics of achieving these dilution rates, the specific standards required for different risk settings, and the integration of dilution with energy recovery systems to make high ventilation rates sustainable.

4.4 Mechanical Ventilation: The Engine of Dilution

In the modern built environment, where sealed windows and deep floor plans often render natural ventilation insufficient or impossible, mechanical ventilation systems become the lungs of the building. These systems are not merely air movers; they are complex thermodynamic engines designed to condition, transport, and distribute air to maintain thermal comfort and indoor air quality (IAQ). However, in the context of airborne infection control, the design intent of these systems—often prioritized for energy efficiency and thermal homogeneity—frequently clashes with the biological imperative of pathogen removal. To understand how dilution ventilation functions as a primary defense against airborne disease, we must dissect the physics of airflow patterns and the engineering strategies that govern them.

4.4.1 The Dichotomy of Airflow: Mixing vs. Displacement

The effectiveness of dilution ventilation is not determined solely by the volume of air supplied but fundamentally by how that air moves through the occupied space. This concept, known as *Ventilation Effectiveness*, dictates how efficiently a system removes bioaerosols generated by an infector before they can be inhaled by a susceptible occupant. Two dominant paradigms govern mechanical airflow strategies: mixing ventilation (MV) and displacement ventilation (DV).

Mixing Ventilation (MV): The Dilution Engine Mixing ventilation is the ubiquitous standard in most commercial and educational buildings. The operational principle of MV is straightforward: supply air is introduced at a high velocity (typically from ceiling diffusers) to induce turbulence. This turbulence promotes the rapid entrainment of room air, creating a homogeneous mixture of temperature and contaminants [24, 79]. Ideally, in a perfectly mixed room, the concentration of a contaminant (such as viral quanta) is uniform throughout the space.

From a thermal comfort perspective, MV is advantageous because it prevents stratification and cold drafts. However, from an infection control perspective, MV has a critical flaw: it actively disperses contaminants. If an infectious individual coughs or breathes in one corner of a room, a mixing system will diligently spread those viral aerosols to every other corner, exposing all occupants to a diluted, yet non-zero, concentration of the pathogen [33, 57].

Recent computational fluid dynamics (CFD) studies and outbreak investigations have highlighted the limitations of MV during the COVID-19 pandemic. For instance, in an investigation of a Delta variant outbreak in an auditorium in China,

Huang et al. [33] found that increased air mixing offered limited protection. While increasing the mixing rate reduced the peak viral concentration near the index case, it simultaneously spread the viral plume further into the occupied zone, potentially increasing the number of medium-risk seats. This phenomenon contradicts the intuitive assumption that "more air movement is better." In reality, strong air currents generated by MV can transport pathogen-laden droplets over distances far exceeding the traditional 1–2 m social distancing guidelines [43, 53]. But what happens in an auditorium may not be the same as a single-room TB clinic in a remote part of India, where mixed ventilation by using ceiling fans/exhaust fans and an open window may be pertinent.

Displacement Ventilation (DV): The Buoyancy-Driven Purge Displacement ventilation operates on a fundamentally different principle. Instead of mixing, DV relies on thermal stratification and buoyancy. Cool, clean air is supplied at low velocity near the floor. As this air encounters heat sources—such as human bodies or computers—it warms up and rises, creating thermal plumes. These plumes carry heat and bioeffluents (including respiratory aerosols) upward toward the ceiling, where they are extracted [24, 57].

In theory, DV provides superior infection control because it creates a single-pass flow regime in the breathing zone. The fresh air displaces the contaminated air rather than mixing with it. Studies comparing DV and MV have consistently shown that DV removes exhaled droplets more effectively, maintaining a lower concentration of contaminants in the breathing zone [24]. In the auditorium study mentioned previously, simulation results indicated that switching from MV to DV could significantly reduce the horizontal spread of the viral plume, thereby lowering the infection risk for the audience [33].

However, DV is not a panacea. Its effectiveness is highly sensitive to the vertical temperature gradient. If the supply air is too cold or the velocity too high, it can cause drafts or revert to a mixing regime. Furthermore, a phenomenon known as "lock-up" or "stratification lock" can occur if the thermal plume is not strong enough to reach the ceiling extraction points, causing contaminants to accumulate in a stratified layer that may coincide with the breathing zone of standing occupants [57, 69].

4.4.2 The Physics of the "Perfect Mix": A Flawed Assumption?

The mathematical models used to predict infection risk, such as the Wells-Riley equation, rely heavily on the assumption of "perfect mixing." This assumption simplifies the complex fluid dynamics of a room into a single tank reactor where the concentration of infectious quanta is uniform. While mathematically convenient, this assumption is physically flawed in most real-world scenarios.

In reality, indoor air is rarely perfectly mixed. Stagnant zones, thermal plumes, and directional airflows created by HVAC systems or moving bodies create heterogeneous distributions of pathogens. A study on the transmission of SARS-CoV-2 in a hospital administration building found that DNA-barcoded aerosol particles released in specific locations (like a cubicle or bathroom) did not disperse uniformly; instead, they were detected in specific sampling sites, often those in proximity or along specific airflow paths, while other areas remained relatively clear [34].

This heterogeneity implies that the calculated "average" risk often underestimates the danger for individuals located in high-concentration zones (e.g., downwind of an infector) while overestimating it for others. Consequently, dilution ventilation strategies must move beyond simple air change rates (ACH) and consider *air change efficiency* (ACE) and *contaminant removal effectiveness* (CRE). A system with high ACH but poor CRE (e.g., short-circuiting where supply air flows directly to the exhaust without mixing) will fail to protect occupants [81].

4.4.3 Advanced Distribution: Downward, Piston, and Personalized Ventilation

Beyond the standard MV and DV, specialized ventilation strategies offer enhanced protection, particularly in high-risk environments.

Downward and Piston Ventilation Often used in cleanrooms and operating theatres, piston ventilation (or unidirectional airflow) supplies air across the entire ceiling (or a large section of it) acting as a piston to push air downward to floor-level extracts. This creates a "clean zone" with minimal turbulence and cross-contamination. While highly effective at removing particles, the energy cost and structural requirements make it impractical for general building applications [57]. However, variations such as "downward ventilation," where air is supplied from ceiling diffusers and extracted near the floor, have been explored for general wards and have shown potential in reducing cross-infection compared to traditional mixing systems [24].

Personalized Ventilation (PV) Personalized ventilation represents a paradigm shift from conditioning the entire room to conditioning the micro-environment of the occupant. PV systems deliver clean air directly to the breathing zone of the individual, often through desk-mounted nozzles or integrated headset devices. By supplying fresh air where it is inhaled, PV minimizes the mixing of inhaled air with the contaminated room air [57, 80].

Research indicates that PV can reduce the intake fraction of infectious aerosols significantly. In simulated office environments, PV has been shown to reduce the risk of infection by preventing the inhalation of "rebreathed" air from neighbors. When combined with localized exhaust systems (personalized exhaust), the efficacy is further enhanced by capturing exhaled contaminants at the source before they disperse into the room [24, 57]. While promising, the implementation of PV requires significant infrastructure changes and may face acceptance challenges regarding acoustic comfort (noise) and draft sensation [80].

4.5 The Critical Role of Air Change Rates (ACH)

The metric most commonly used to quantify dilution ventilation is the air change per hour (ACH). Mathematically, one ACH occurs when a volume of air equal to the room's volume is supplied and removed.

4.5.1 Defining "Clean" Air and the Clearance Curve

In the context of infection control, "clean" air refers to virus-free air. This can be outdoor air, recirculated air that has been passed through high-efficiency (HEPA) filters, or air that has been disinfected (e.g., by UVGI) [98]. The total clean air delivery rate (CADR) determines the effective ACH of a space.

The relationship between ACH and pathogen removal is exponential. In a well-mixed room, the concentration of a contaminant $C(t)$ decaying from an initial concentration C_0 follows the equation:

$$C(t) = C_0 e^{-Nt}$$

where N is the air change rate (time^{-1}) and t is time.

- 1 ACH removes ~63% of airborne contaminants in 1 h ($1 - e^{-1} \approx 0.63$).
- 3 ACH removes ~95% in 1 h.
- 5 ACH removes ~99.3% in 1 h.

This logarithmic decay illustrates why increasing ventilation is so critical during events where aerosols are continuously generated. However, it also reveals a thermodynamic reality: achieving 99% removal via ventilation alone requires significant airflow, which carries substantial energy penalties for heating, cooling, and dehumidification [81].

4.5.2 The Law of Diminishing Returns in Ventilation

While increasing ventilation reduces infection risk, the benefit is not linear. Seppänen et al. [81] and subsequent reviews have identified a "diminishing returns" phenomenon.

- *0–10 L/s/person:* In this range, increases in ventilation yield dramatic improvements in health outcomes, including reductions in sick building syndrome (SBS) symptoms and respiratory infections. This range corresponds to moving from a "suffocating" room to a "decent" room.
- *10–20 L/s/person:* Further improvements are observed, but the slope of the benefit curve begins to flatten.

- *Above 25 L/s/person:* The incremental health benefit of adding more ventilation becomes difficult to detect epidemiologically (or rather marginal gains become progressively harder to detect above ~20–25 L/s/person), while the energy cost continues to rise linearly.

For airborne infection control, however, the target may need to be higher than for general IAQ. The World Health Organization (WHO) and CDC recommend 6–12 ACH for healthcare settings to control pathogens like measles and tuberculosis [59, 61]. Achieving 12 ACH in a standard office or school (which typically operates at 2–3 ACH) is may often be structurally less feasible with existing HVAC infrastructure, necessitating supplementary strategies like in-room air cleaners or upper-room UVGI [59]. This is subject to budgetary, safety and long term maintenance concerns.

4.6 Ventilation and the Short-Range Transmission Paradox

A pervasive misconception in infection control is that dilution ventilation only mitigates "long-range" airborne transmission (infection across a room) and has no effect on "short-range" transmission (close contact, <1–2 m). This dichotomy has been challenged by recent mechanistic modeling.

4.6.1 The Continuum of Transmission

Transmission is a continuum. When two people converse, the "infector" exhales a turbulent jet of air containing droplets of various sizes.

1. *Large droplets:* Ballistic trajectories, fall quickly.
2. *Short-range aerosols:* High-concentration plume that has not yet dispersed into the room volume.
3. *Long-range aerosols:* Dispersed, diluted background concentration.

Li et al. [42, 44] developed a macroscopic model linking these modes. They demonstrated that the distinction between short- and long-range is fluid. As droplets evaporate, they shrink into droplet nuclei (aerosols). The "jet" of exhaled air entrains the surrounding room air as it travels. This entrainment is the key mechanism linking general ventilation to short-range risk.

4.6.2 How Background Ventilation Affects Close Contact

If the surrounding room air is stagnant and contaminated (low ventilation), the exhaled jet entrains this dirty air, maintaining a high concentration of pathogens. Conversely, if the room air is clean (high ventilation), the jet entrains clean air, rapidly diluting the concentration of pathogens within the jet itself before it reaches the face of the susceptible person [42, 44].

Using a mass balance model, Li et al. [42, 44] showed that at a distance of 0.5 m, the exposure risk is significantly higher in a poorly ventilated room (1 L/s/person) compared to a well-ventilated one (10 L/s/person). Specifically, the study found that insufficient ventilation increases the risk of *both* short- and long-range airborne transmission. A ventilation rate of 10 L/s per person was found to provide a concentration decay profile similar to outdoor settings, effectively substantially reducing the "indoor penalty" and meaningfully lowers short-range risk compared with poorly ventilated spaces [42, 44]. This finding is profound: it implies that general dilution ventilation is a protective measure even for close-contact interactions, reinforcing the need for higher ventilation standards not just for "airborne" diseases but for all respiratory infections.

4.7 Natural Ventilation: The Unpredictable Ally

While mechanical ventilation represents the triumph of engineering control over the environment, natural ventilation represents a negotiation with it. Before the advent of cheap electricity and air conditioning, hospital wards and schoolrooms were designed with high ceilings and large operable windows to harness the forces of nature for infection control. In the era of energy efficiency, these passive strategies were largely abandoned in favor of sealed envelopes. However, the resurgence of airborne pathogens like *Mycobacterium tuberculosis* and SARS-CoV-2 has forced a re-evaluation of these ancient techniques.

4.7.1 The Physics of Wind and Buoyancy

Natural ventilation is driven by two fundamental physical forces: wind pressure and thermal buoyancy (the stack effect). Wind-driven ventilation relies on pressure differences across the building envelope created by external wind velocity. When wind strikes a building, it creates positive pressure on the windward side and negative pressure (suction) on the leeward side. If windows are open on both sides, this pressure differential drives cross-ventilation, which can generate massive airflow rates [18].

The second force, the stack effect, is driven by temperature differences and the resulting density gradients between indoor and outdoor air. Warm air is less dense than cold air. In a heated building during winter, warm indoor air rises and escapes through high openings (like clerestory windows or chimneys), creating a vacuum that draws cool outdoor air in through lower openings. This mechanism is particularly valuable when wind speeds are low, yet it is highly dependent on the temperature gradient (ΔT) and the vertical distance between inlets and outlets [40, 71].

4.7.2 The Escombe Study: Rediscovering High-Volume Dilution

The potential of natural ventilation to far exceed the capabilities of standard mechanical systems was dramatically illustrated in a landmark study by Escombe et al. [23] in Lima, Peru. The researchers compared the risk of airborne tuberculosis transmission in old-fashioned, naturally ventilated hospital wards (with high ceilings and large windows) against modern, mechanically ventilated respiratory isolation rooms.

The results were counterintuitive to the modern engineering mindset. The naturally ventilated rooms, when windows and doors were open, achieved air change rates (ACH) ranging from 28 to 40 ACH, with peaks exceeding 70 ACH. In stark contrast, the mechanically ventilated rooms, designed specifically for infection control, struggled to maintain the recommended 12 ACH [23, 59]. The study calculated that the naturally ventilated spaces reduced the probability of infection by approximately 70% compared to the mechanical rooms. This finding underscores a critical reality: achieving the massive dilution rates necessary to render highly infectious aerosols harmless is often economically and structurally feasible only through natural means [59].

4.7.3 The Reliability Paradox

Despite its immense potential capacity, natural ventilation suffers from a fatal flaw in the context of safety-critical environments: unreliability. Its effectiveness is entirely at the mercy of meteorological conditions. On a still, hot day where the indoor and outdoor temperatures are equal

$$\Delta T \approx 0$$

and wind speed is negligible, the air exchange rate in a naturally ventilated room can drop to near zero. In such a "stagnant" event, infectious aerosols accumulate rapidly, creating a high-risk environment [28, 59]. In such situations reliance is made to diffusion of air.

Furthermore, natural ventilation introduces uncontrolled externalities. Opening windows in urban environments may invite noise, outdoor air pollution ($PM_{2.5}$, NO_2), and allergens into the indoor space, potentially trading an infection risk for a chronic respiratory or cardiovascular risk [24, 76]. In healthcare settings, it also disrupts pressure differentials required to maintain isolation zones (e.g., keeping a TB ward at negative pressure relative to the corridor) [2, 69].

Therefore, while natural ventilation is a powerful tool—particularly in resource-limited settings or temperate climates—it cannot be the sole strategy for high-risk environments. It requires "hybrid" or "mixed-mode" systems where mechanical fans assist natural forces when meteorological drivers are insufficient [18, 40].

4.8 The Metric of Safety: Standards and Guidelines

If dilution ventilation is the "medicine" for sick buildings, then the ventilation rate is the dosage. Determining the correct dosage has been a subject of evolving scientific debate for over a century. The history of ventilation standards reveals a tension between two competing goals: energy conservation and occupant health.

4.8.1 The Evolution of Popular Global Standard

In 1981, it is believed that, following the energy crisis, the minimum outdoor air rate ware set at a 2.5 L/s/person (5 cfm/person) probably to conserve fuel. This reduction is widely and generally correlated with accelerating the rise of "sick building syndrome" (SBS) in the 1980s [81, 84]. Recognizing the scope of improvement, raise was made to the standard in 1989 to 7.5 L/s/person (15 cfm/person), later refining this to a formula based on both occupancy and floor area [9, 67].

However, it is crucial to understand that these standards were designed primarily for *comfort* (odour control) and the dilution of generic bioeffluents, not for the control of airborne infectious diseases during a pandemic. The "acceptable" air quality defined by such type of standards is air that satisfies 80% of occupants in terms of perceived freshness—a metric that has little correlation with the absence of viral pathogens [84, 90].

4.8.2 The 10 L/s Threshold and the "Indoor Penalty"

In the wake of the COVID-19 pandemic, researchers have sought to define a ventilation rate that specifically mitigates infection risk. A converging body of evidence suggests that 10 L/s/person is a critical threshold. Seppänen et al. [81] and Sundell et al. [84], in extensive multidisciplinary reviews, found that ventilation rates below 10 L/s/person are consistently associated with significantly higher rates of respiratory infections, sick leave, and SBS symptoms. Increasing rates up to 20–25 L/s/person yields further benefits, but the law of diminishing returns sets in [84].

More recently, Li et al. [42, 44] provided a mechanistic justification for this threshold. Their modeling showed that at a ventilation rate of 10 L/s/person, the concentration decay profile of exhaled aerosols indoors begins to approximate that of an outdoor setting. Essentially, providing 10 L/s/person neutralizes the "indoor penalty," reducing the risk of short-range airborne transmission to levels comparable to being outside [42, 44]. This finding challenges the "room source and people source" theory underlying current standards, arguing instead for higher ventilation rates when interpersonal distances are less than 2 m [42, 44].

4.8.3 Healthcare vs. Non-healthcare Standards

For healthcare facilities, the World Health Organization (WHO) and CDC recommend much higher rates: 6–12 ACH (roughly 60–80 L/s/patient depending on room volume) for airborne precaution rooms [17, 94]. This discrepancy highlights the vulnerability of non-healthcare public spaces. A typical school classroom or office may operate at 2–4 ACH (roughly 5–8 L/s/person). During an airborne pandemic, these spaces become transmission hotspots because their ventilation systems may have been designed for odour control, not pathogen removal [24, 53].

4.9 Monitoring the Invisible: Carbon Dioxide as a Sentinel

Because we cannot measure viruses in the air in real-time, we must rely on proxies. Carbon dioxide (CO_2) has emerged as the most practical, albeit imperfect, sentinel for ventilation performance and infection risk.

4.9.1 The Rebreathed Air Fraction

Humans exhale CO_2 at a predictable rate (approximately 38,000 ppm in exhaled breath). In an indoor space, the elevation of CO_2 above outdoor background levels (approx. 400–420 ppm) is a direct measure of the fraction of air in the room that has been previously exhaled by someone else—the "rebreathed air fraction" [75].

The Rudnick-Milton model utilizes this relationship to estimate the probability of airborne infection. If the indoor CO_2 is 800 ppm, the excess is 400 ppm. Since exhaled breath is ~38,000 ppm above background, the rebreathed fraction is $400 \div 38{,}000 \approx 1\%$. If the CO_2 rises to 2000 ppm, the rebreathed fraction jumps to ~4.2%. For a pathogen like measles or the Delta/Omicron variants of SARS-CoV-2, inhaling 4.2% of other people's breath for hours constitutes a significant exposure event [66, 75].

4.9.2 Establishing CO_2 Limits for Infection Control

Historically, a limit of 1000 ppm CO_2 was suggested by Pettenkofer in the nineteenth century and later adopted by global bodies as a marker for body odour acceptability. However, for infection control, lower targets are now advocated. Other bodies have suggested maintaining CO_2 levels below 800 ppm during pandemics to ensure sufficient dilution [24, 72].

Peng and Jimenez [66] derived analytical expressions showing that the relative risk of infection scales with the excess CO_2 concentration. They argue that CO_2 is the only readily available proxy for quantifying infection risk in real-time. By deploying low-cost NDIR (non-dispersive infrared) CO_2 sensors, building managers can dynamically adjust ventilation rates (demand control ventilation) to keep rebreathed air fractions low [21, 66].

4.9.3 Limitations of the CO_2 Proxy

While valuable, the CO_2 metric has limitations. First, it assumes the room is well-mixed; a sensor on a wall might read 800 ppm while occupants in a crowded corner are breathing 1500 ppm. Second, filtration removes viruses/particles but does not remove CO_2. Therefore, in a room with heavy HEPA filtration, the CO_2 level might be high (indicating low outdoor air exchange), but the viral risk could be low because the filters are cleaning the recirculated air [59]. Relying solely on CO_2 in spaces with air cleaners may lead to a false estimation of risk (but it may still be our best bet due to lack of reliable alternatives). Conversely, in spaces with low occupancy but poor ventilation, CO_2 might be low simply because there are few people generating it, yet if one of them is an infector, the viral concentration could still accumulate [68].

Thus, dilution ventilation, monitored via CO_2 and supplemented by filtration, forms the backbone of engineering defenses. It is a coarse but effective lever. In the next section, we will explore how these principles are applied—and often compromised—in the specific high-risk environments of hospitals, schools, and public transport.

4.10 The Battlefield of Specific Environments: Tailoring Dilution to Risk

While the physics of dilution ventilation—the governing equations of mass balance and decay—remain constant, the *application* of these principles varies radically depending on the built environment. A hospital isolation room, a crowded primary school classroom, and a commuter bus represent distinct aerodynamic domains, each presenting unique challenges to the effective removal of airborne pathogens. The "one size fits all" approach to ventilation rates (e.g., the standard 8–10 L/s/person for offices) crumbles when faced with the high-stakes variability of infectious source strength and occupant density found in these specialized settings.

4.10.1 Hospitals: The Fortress of Negative Pressure

Hospitals represent the apex of ventilation engineering for infection control. Here, the objective shifts from merely maintaining "acceptable" air quality to creating a biological firewall. The gold standard for managing patients with airborne infectious diseases (such as tuberculosis, measles, or SARS-CoV-2) is the airborne infection isolation room (AIIR).

The defining engineering characteristic of an AIIR is not just high dilution (typically 6–12 ACH), but *directional airflow* driven by pressure differentials. By maintaining the room at a negative pressure relative to the corridor (usually a differential of −2.5 Pa or greater), engineers ensure that air flows *into* the room from clean areas, preventing the escape of infectious aerosols into the general hospital population [8, 54].

However, recent research highlights a critical vulnerability in this fortress: the doorway. The simple act of opening a door can induce air exchange volumes that effectively neutralize the pressure differential for short periods, allowing a "bolus" of contaminated air to escape into the corridor—a phenomenon driven by the wake of the person walking through the door and the pumping action of the door itself [35, 86].

This leakage necessitates the use of an *anteroom* (or vestibule). Anterooms act as airlocks or buffer zones. A systematic review by Andalib et al. [8] confirmed that the presence of an anteroom significantly enhances the containment efficiency of isolation units. When a healthcare worker moves from the isolation room to the anteroom, the two-stage pressure gradient (corridor > anteroom > patient room) provides a redundant layer of protection. Furthermore, the anteroom provides a controlled environment for the donning and doffing of personal protective equipment (PPE), a procedure where the reaerosolization of virus particles from contaminated clothing poses a significant risk [8, 32].

Despite these robust designs, outbreaks still occur. A study by Jones and Donskey [34] investigating a SARS-CoV-2 cluster in a hospital administration building found that even with ventilation meeting standard codes (6 ACH), transmission occurred. This suggests that in non-clinical areas of hospitals, where administrative staff congregate without the rigorous PPE protocols of clinical wards, standard ventilation rates may provide a false sense of security against highly transmissible variants [34].

4.10.2 Schools: The Density Dilemma

If hospitals are the fortresses of infection control, schools are the trenches. Classrooms are characterized by high occupant density—often 30 students in a relatively small volume—resulting in rapid accumulation of bioeffluents and potential pathogens. Historically, school ventilation may have been driven by thermal comfort and energy efficiency rather than infection control, leading to a reliance on manual airing (opening windows) which is often erratic and weather-dependent [24].

The "Fresh Air" study and similar interventions have highlighted the stark trade-off in school settings: thermal comfort versus air quality. In colder climates or during winter, teachers are reluctant to open windows due to drafts and heat loss. Consequently, CO_2 levels in classrooms frequently exceed 2000 or even 3000 ppm, indicating extremely low ventilation rates and high fractions of rebreathed air [24, 25].

Recent systematic reviews suggest that to mitigate airborne transmission effectively in schools, ventilation strategies must be decoupled from thermal discomfort. This can be achieved through:

1. *Hybrid Ventilation:* Utilizing mechanical extraction fans to ensure a consistent air change rate regardless of wind pressure, while tempering supply air to avoid cold drafts [24].
2. *Displacement Ventilation (DV):* As discussed in other parts of the book, DV supplies air at floor level. In a classroom, the thermal plumes generated by students (body heat) naturally drive this fresh air upward, carrying respiratory aerosols toward ceiling extraction points. This method is particularly effective in classrooms because it aligns the airflow with the natural buoyancy of body heat, potentially reducing cross-infection risks more effectively than mixing ventilation [24, 70].

However, empirical data on the protective effect of these interventions remains mixed. A study by Varma et al. [87] in New York City schools found that while transmission within schools was lower than in the community, the secondary attack rate was significantly higher when the index case was a teacher rather than a student. This implies that the adult vocalization intensity (lecturing) combined with potential ventilation dead-zones creates a disproportionate risk, necessitating higher ventilation rates or local air cleaning near the teacher's station [87, 88].

4.10.3 Public Transport: The Mobile Vector

Public transportation systems—buses, trains, and subways—present a dynamic and particularly challenging environment for dilution ventilation. The enclosed volume is small, the occupant density fluctuates wildly, and the exposure time is variable.

A critical finding in transport ventilation is the danger of recirculation. To maintain thermal comfort (cooling in summer, heating in winter), vehicle HVAC systems often recirculate a significant fraction (up to 70–80%) of the cabin air. In the absence of high-efficiency filtration (HEPA), this recirculation mechanism effectively homogenizes the viral concentration throughout the bus or train car. A modeling study of a COVID-19 outbreak on a bus in China demonstrated that the air conditioning system facilitated the spread of the virus to passengers sitting seven rows away from the index case—far beyond the range of droplet transmission [1, 64].

Salthammer et al. [77] utilized mobile sensors to track CO_2 levels in buses and trams, revealing a strong correlation between occupancy and CO_2 build-up. They argued that a low CO_2 level (below 1000 ppm) in a moving vehicle is a robust proxy for safety, indicating sufficient intake of fresh air. However, achieving this requires active management of dampers to maximize outdoor air intake, often at the cost of fuel efficiency and thermal comfort [77].

Subway systems introduce another variable: the "piston effect." As trains move through tunnels, they push air ahead of them and draw air behind them. While this contributes to station ventilation, the air quality *inside* the carriage is heavily dependent on the specific HVAC settings. Studies have shown that during rush hours, CO_2 levels in subway cars can spike to dangerous levels, necessitating auxiliary ventilation strategies or reduced occupancy limits [1, 30]. The Delhi Metro Rail Corporation during COVID-19 had come with a time schedule where during cooler morning hours the outdoor air was set at maximum and as the day got hotter, the outdoor supply became lower than the morning, but was still substantial as compared to during pre-COVID-19 days.

4.11 The Variable Source: Occupancy and Activity

The engineering calculations for dilution ventilation often assume a static "source strength." However, humans are dynamic sources. The rate at which an infected individual releases infectious quanta is not constant; it scales exponentially with respiratory activity.

4.11.1 The Super-Spreader Event: The Physics of Vocalization

The concept of *quanta generation rate* (q) is central to the Wells-Riley model. For a resting person breathing nasally, q might be low (e.g., 1–10 quanta/h for SARS-CoV-2). However, vocalization dramatically changes this parameter. Speaking increases aerosol emission by a factor of 10 compared to breathing; shouting or singing can increase it by a factor of 50–100 [16, 53].

This explains the mechanics of "super-spreader" events, such as the Skagit Valley Chorale incident, where a single symptomatic index case infected 52 people during a 2.5-h choir practice. The act of singing not only generated a massive viral load (high "q") but also projected these aerosols deeper into the room. Standard dilution ventilation, designed for sedentary occupancy, is hopelessly overwhelmed by such high-emission events [51].

In the context of the Delta variant outbreak in an auditorium described by Huang et al. [33], the viral emission rate was estimated at 31 quanta/hour even for asymptomatic cases sitting passively (masked audience). This suggests that for highly transmissible variants, the baseline "resting" emission rate is significantly higher, meaning that ventilation rates that were sufficient for ancestral strains may fail to protect against variants like Delta or Omicron [33].

4.11.2 Demand-Controlled Ventilation (DCV): A Pandemic Liability?

In the pursuit of energy efficiency, modern buildings often utilize demand-controlled ventilation (DCV). These systems use CO_2 sensors to estimate occupancy; if the room is sparsely populated (low CO_2), the system throttles down the intake of outdoor air to save energy.

While rational for energy conservation, DCV poses a severe risk during a pandemic. If a single infectious individual enters a room, the DCV system might not detect a significant rise in aggregate CO_2 (especially in a large room) and therefore will not ramp up ventilation. The infected person continues to emit viral aerosols into a stagnant air volume. By the time the CO_2 sensor triggers a response, the viral concentration in the breathing zone may have already reached infectious levels [3, 57].

Consequently, during active pandemic phases, some building codes and operation guidelines explicitly recommend *disabling* DCV features. Ventilation systems should run at nominal speed (design capacity) regardless of partial occupancy, ideally starting 2 h before occupancy and continuing for 2 h after, to purge any lingering aerosols [57, 72]. This operational shift represents a temporary sacrifice of energy efficiency in favor of biological safety—a necessary trade-off in the era of airborne pathogens.

4.12 The Thermodynamic Penalty: Energy Efficiency Versus Infection Control

The widespread implementation of high-volume dilution ventilation faces a formidable adversary: the second law of thermodynamics. Conditioning outdoor air—heating it in winter and cooling or dehumidifying it in summer—represents one of the most energy-intensive processes in the modern built environment. In the latter half of the twentieth century, specifically following the 1973 oil embargo, the philosophy of building design may have shifted radically from "open and breathing" to "tight and sealed." The primary objective became the conservation of thermal energy, often at the direct expense of indoor air quality (IAQ) [80, 84].

4.12.1 The Legacy of the "Tight Building"

To conserve energy, building envelopes were sealed to reduce infiltration, and mechanical ventilation rates were slashed. As also noted above and in other parts of the book, global bodies may have lowered the minimum outdoor air requirement to 2.5 L/s/person in non-smoking areas, a rate now widely recognized as insufficient to dilute human bioeffluents, let alone airborne pathogens [84]. This era gave rise to the phenomenon of "sick building syndrome" (SBS), a constellation of non-specific symptoms—headache, fatigue, mucosal irritation—that afflict occupants of poorly ventilated spaces [19, 46].

While subsequent standards have raised the minimum rates (typically to ~8–10 L/s/person), the tension remains. Increasing ventilation to the levels required for robust infection control (e.g., the 6–12 ACH recommended for hospitals) in a commercial office building may result in higher energy costs and carbon emissions. This creates a moral and engineering dilemma: how to balance the acute risk of pandemic transmission against the chronic existential threat of climate change.

4.12.2 The Outdoor Air Paradox: Pollution vs. Pathogens

The strategy of dilution ventilation relies on the premise that outdoor air is "clean." In many urban centers, this assumption is dangerously flawed. Introducing large volumes of unfiltered outdoor air may dilute indoor viral concentrations but simultaneously introduce high levels of particulate matter ($PM_{2.5}$), nitrogen oxides (NO_x), and ozone (O_3).

Research indicates that exposure to these outdoor pollutants can exacerbate respiratory vulnerability, potentially increasing the severity of viral infections. For instance, chronic exposure to $PM_{2.5}$ leads to airway inflammation, which may facilitate viral entry and replication [48]. Furthermore, ozone is a potent respiratory irritant; ventilation strategies that indiscriminately increase outdoor air intake during high-ozone periods may trade infection risk for chemical injury to the lung parenchyma [80, 93].

Therefore, "dilution" in the modern context cannot simply mean opening dampers. It necessitates a sophisticated approach involving:

1. *Demand-Controlled Filtration:* Cleaning outdoor air of particulates and chemicals before it enters the building.
2. *Economizer Cycles:* Utilizing outdoor air for cooling only when temperature and humidity are favorable (free cooling), but prioritizing recirculation with heavy HEPA filtration when outdoor conditions are hostile (energy-wise or pollution-wise) [10]. But this needs to be localised for conditions which may be low resource where a tuberculosis centre must not wait for hi tech systems when resource constrained and pick up the lowest hanging fruit-simple dilution ventilation.

But a caveat to this is settings in low resource settings where filtration, if available, may not be maintained, filters not replaced, and these may become breeding grounds for harm than good.

4.13 The Physics of Failure: Why General Dilution Sometimes Fails

Despite adherence to ventilation standards, outbreaks continue to occur in "compliant" buildings. This suggests that the simplified "well-mixed" box models used to calculate ventilation rates often fail to capture the complex reality of airflow dynamics.

4.13.1 The ZADIR Model and the Auditorium Outbreak

A profound illustration of the limitations of general dilution was provided by the analysis of a COVID-19 Delta variant outbreak in an auditorium, detailed by Huang et al. [33]. In this event, three index cases infected a secondary case seated in a different row, despite the facility operating with a mechanical ventilation system.

To understand this transmission, researchers utilized a novel modeling approach: *zonal airflow and dynamically integrated risk (ZADIR).* Unlike standard computational fluid dynamics (CFD) which can be computationally prohibitive for long durations, or simple box models which ignore spatial heterogeneity, ZADIR divides the indoor space into thousands of interconnected zones (e.g.,

2951 zones for the auditorium, matching the dimensions of individual seats). It simulates the mass balance of viral aerosols, heat, and airflow between these micro-zones [33].

The simulation revealed that the "dilution" air did not mix uniformly. Instead, the thermal plumes from the audience and the momentum of the supply air created a specific, directional "viral plume" that travelled from the index cases, moving upwards and backwards toward the ceiling exhaust vents. The secondary case was located precisely in the wake of this plume. The study demonstrated that even with active ventilation, local concentrations of infectious quanta can remain dangerously high in specific streamlines—a phenomenon termed "short-range airborne transmission" extended over distance [33].

This finding is critical: Dilution ventilation reduces the *average* concentration in a room, but may not always necessarily disrupt the high-concentration *plumes* that connect an infector to a susceptible host. The airflow pattern (the path of the air) is as important as the air change rate (the amount of air).

4.13.2 Stratification and "Lock-Up"

Another failure mode occurs in displacement ventilation systems (as introduced above and in other parts of the book). While generally superior for removing bioeffluents, these systems rely on a stable vertical temperature gradient. If the supply air velocity is too high, or if the heat load in the room is insufficient to drive the thermal plumes to the ceiling, a layer of contaminated air can become trapped or "locked up" in the breathing zone. In such scenarios, the "old" air recirculates locally rather than being exhausted, leading to a rapid accumulation of viral quanta despite the system theoretically providing adequate fresh air volume [43, 70].

4.14 Empirical Evidence: Carbon Dioxide and Tuberculosis

While fluid dynamics models provide theoretical insight, empirical evidence links ventilation deficits directly to biological outcomes. The most compelling data often comes from tuberculosis (TB) wards, where the pathogen is unequivocally airborne and measuring infection (via skin tests or blood assays) is standardized.

4.14.1 The CO_2-TB Correlation

A study by Nathavitharana et al. [61] provided a stark demonstration of the relationship between ventilation, carbon dioxide (CO_2) levels, and infection risk. The researchers monitored CO_2 levels in healthcare settings and correlated them with the incidence of latent TB infection (measured by interferon gamma release assay, IGRA) among healthcare workers (HCWs).

The results showed a statistically significant association: HCWs who converted to a positive IGRA (indicating new infection) worked in areas with significantly higher average CO_2 concentrations compared to those who remained uninfected. Specifically, a box plot analysis revealed that IGRA converters were exposed to median CO_2 levels that were consistently elevated, indicating lower ventilation rates and higher fractions of rebreathed air [61].

This study validates the use of CO_2 as a biological proxy. It confirms that the "rebreathed air fraction" calculated by the Rudnick-Milton equation is not just a theoretical construct but a predictor of actual biological transmission. When CO_2 rises, indicating that the ventilation system is failing to dilute human exhalations faster than they are produced, the risk of inhaling an infectious dose of *Mycobacterium tuberculosis* (or SARS-CoV-2) rises commensurately [61, 75].

4.15 Beyond the Building: Wastewater Surveillance as a Macro-indicator

While dilution ventilation manages risk at the building level, assessing the need for such interventions requires monitoring at the community level. If the prevalence of a pathogen in the community is zero, the ventilation rate in a school is irrelevant to infection control (though still relevant for general health). Conversely, during a surge, even high ventilation rates may be insufficient.

4.15.1 The Sewer as a Sentinel

Wastewater-based epidemiology (WBE) has emerged as a powerful tool to gauge community infection loads, serving as a macro-scale "smoke detector" for public health. SARS-CoV-2 is shed in the feces of infected individuals, often days before symptoms appear [41, 96]. By quantifying the concentration of viral RNA in sewage, public health officials can estimate the prevalence of COVID-19 in a catchment area [41].

However, translating sewage RNA concentrations $C_{(RNA)}$ back to the number of infected individuals is complex. It depends on the "shedding profile" of the virus (how much virus is excreted per gram of feces) and the hydraulic retention time (HRT) in the sewer system. Li et al. [41] utilized Monte Carlo simulations to model these variables, revealing that faecal shedding alone often underestimated the viral load found in wastewater. They proposed that *sputum* (respiratory mucus swallowed or spit into sinks/toilets) contributes significantly to the viral load in sewage, especially given the high viral titers found in the upper respiratory tract.

This finding connects WBE back to building hygiene. The same sputum and respiratory fluids that generate airborne aerosols also enter the wastewater stream.

A spike in wastewater viral load acts as an early warning signal, triggering the need for enhanced dilution ventilation and mask mandates in the buildings within that sewer shed, effectively linking environmental engineering with epidemiological surveillance [29, 41].

4.16 The Chronic Cost of Poor Ventilation: Sick Building Syndrome

Finally, it is crucial to recognize that the failure of dilution ventilation has consequences beyond infectious disease. The "sick building syndrome" (SBS) represents a chronic failure of the indoor environment [83].

4.16.1 Neurogenic Switching and Inflammation

The mechanism of SBS may share pathways with the body's response to pathogens. Meggs [49, 50] proposed the hypothesis of "neurogenic switching," where chemical irritants (accumulated due to poor ventilation) stimulate sensory nerves in the airways. This stimulation can trigger an inflammatory response at a distant site (e.g., headache, skin rash) via the central nervous system. This model explains why occupants of poorly ventilated buildings report diverse systemic symptoms—fatigue, difficulty concentrating, skin irritation—that resolve upon leaving the building [49, 50].

Furthermore, exposure to dampness and molds (like *Stachybotrys chartarum*) in poorly ventilated, water-damaged buildings can produce mycotoxins (e.g., trichothecenes) that inhibit protein synthesis and impair immune function [47]. Occupants in such environments not only suffer from SBS but may also be more susceptible to respiratory infections due to compromised mucosal immunity.

4.16.2 Ventilation Rates and SBS Prevalence

Epidemiological reviews consistently show a dose-response relationship between ventilation rates and SBS symptoms. Seppänen et al. [81] analyzed over 20 studies and found that relative risk of SBS symptoms decreased significantly as ventilation rates increased up to 10 L/s/person, with some studies showing benefits up to 20–25 L/s/person [81].

This convergence of evidence highlights that dilution ventilation is a dual-use technology. The same engineering controls required to dilute the viral Aerosols of a pandemic are required to flush the chemical irritants and bioeffluents that cause chronic SBS. The "cost" of ventilation, therefore, should be weighed not just against the probability of a rare pandemic event, but against the daily, tangible loss of productivity and health associated with "sick" buildings.

4.17 The Economic Calculus: The Cost of Clean Air Versus the Cost of Infection

The most formidable barrier to the implementation of robust dilution ventilation is not technological but economic. In the lexicon of building management, ventilation is often viewed exclusively as a cost center—a thermal load that inflates utility bills. This perspective, however, represents a fundamental accounting error that ignores the human occupants who constitute the primary value proposition of any building. To understand the true value of dilution ventilation, we must shift our calculus from the cost of energy to the cost of health and productivity.

4.17.1 The 1-9-90 Rule and the Productivity Multiplier

A commonly cited heuristic in commercial real estate is the "1-9-90" rule: approximately 1% of operating costs are energy, 9% are rent and operations, and 90% are salaries and benefits [15, 27]. Consequently, a marginal increase in energy costs (the 1%) required to improve ventilation is negligible if it yields even a fractional improvement in human health or productivity (the 90%).

Historical data establishes a compelling link between low ventilation rates and "sick building syndrome" (SBS) symptoms, which in turn correlate with reduced productivity and increased absenteeism. In a landmark analysis, Fisk and Rosenfeld (1997) estimated that improving indoor environmental quality (IEQ) in the United States could result in annual savings of \$6–\$14 billion from reduced respiratory infections, \$1–\$4 billion from reduced allergies and asthma, and \$20 to \$160 billion from direct productivity gains (Fisk and Rosenfeld 1997; [82]).

Specifically regarding infectious disease, the economic argument becomes starker. The cost of a single viral outbreak—measured in sick leave, temporary closures, and long-term disability (Long COVID)—dwarfs the incremental cost of running fans at a higher setting or installing heat recovery systems. As noted by Seppänen and Fisk [82], the cost of ventilation is often repaid if the rate of sick leave decreases by as little as 1% [82]. In the post-COVID-19 era, "business continuity" has replaced "energy savings" as the dominant metric for high-performance buildings; a building that cannot remain open because it is a vector for transmission is a stranded asset.

4.17.2 Energy Efficiency and Infection Control: Resolving the Tension

Critics of high-volume dilution ventilation point to its carbon footprint. How can we advocate for 6–12 air changes per hour (ACH) in a climate crisis? The resolution lies in the decoupling of *ventilation* from *thermal conditioning*. Technologies such as dedicated outdoor air systems (DOAS) with high-efficiency energy recovery ventilators (ERVs) allow for the transfer of heat (and moisture) from the exhaust air stream to the incoming fresh air stream without cross-contamination of air, recovering 60–80% of the energy [59, 98].

Furthermore, the "hybrid" approach—using natural ventilation when weather permits and mechanical systems only when necessary—offers a sustainable path forward. As demonstrated by the joint committee meetings of the Central Pollution Control Board (CPCB), developing nations are increasingly looking toward "mixed-mode" buildings that leverage climate-responsive architecture to achieve dilution targets without prohibitive energy costs [20].

4.18 Implementing Dilution: A Practical Framework for Building Managers

Moving from theory to practice requires actionable protocols. Based on the consensus of global bodies and recent governmental task forces [20, 95], a practical framework for implementing dilution ventilation for infection control involves four key operational shifts:

1. *Disable Demand-Controlled Ventilation (DCV):* As discussed in other parts of the book, DCV systems save energy by reducing fresh air intake when occupancy (CO_2) is low. During a pandemic, this logic is dangerous. A single infectious individual in a sparsely occupied room requires *more* dilution, not less. Systems should be locked to supply nominal airflow regardless of occupancy sensors [20, 72].
2. *Extended Operation Times (Flush-Out):* Ventilation systems should not be coupled strictly to working hours. Best practice dictates starting systems at nominal speed at least 2 h before occupancy and continuing for 2 h after occupancy to "flush out" any viral aerosols accumulated during the day or settled on surfaces [72].
3. *Filtration of Recirculated Air:* In systems where 100% outdoor air is not feasible due to thermal capacity, the recirculated portion must be treated as if it were contaminated. It should pass through a filter with a minimum efficiency reporting value (MERV) of 13 or higher (or ISO ePM1 >50%) to ensure that the "dilution" provided by recirculation is effectively removing pathogen-laden droplet nuclei [10, 20].
4. *Strategic Monitoring:* Monitoring should move beyond the central plant. Installing CO_2 sensors in "critical zones"—high-density areas like meeting rooms, cafeterias, and waiting areas—provides a real-time proxy for ventilation effectiveness. If CO_2 exceeds 800–1000 ppm, it triggers a visual alarm for occupants to open windows or vacate the space [20, 66].

4.19 The Limits of Dilution: The Law of Diminishing Returns

It is imperative to recognize that dilution ventilation is not a panacea. It is subject to the law of diminishing returns. The relationship between infection risk and ventilation rate is non-linear; the first few air changes provide the most dramatic risk reduction. Increasing ventilation from 1 to 3 ACH significantly reduces the steady-state concentration of droplet nuclei. However, increasing from 12 to 15 ACH yields a negligible reduction in risk while imposing a severe energy penalty [43, 59].

Furthermore, dilution ventilation has a fundamental physical limitation: it cannot prevent transmission in the "near-field" (within 1–2 m). If a susceptible person is standing in the direct exhalation plume of an infected individual, no amount of room-level air change will prevent exposure. The concentration of the virus in the direct plume is orders of magnitude higher than the room average. This reality necessitates the "layered" defense strategy: masks to contain the source plume, distancing to avoid the near-field, and dilution ventilation to clear the far-field accumulation [42, 44, 83].

When the required dilution rate to achieve safety exceeds the mechanical or economic capacity of the building (e.g., requiring >12 ACH in an old school building), engineers must pivot to "equivalent" dilution technologies. This is where air cleaning—specifically upper-room ultraviolet germicidal irradiation (UVGI)—becomes superior. As Nardell [59] argues, UVGI can generate an "equivalent" 24 ACH in the breathing zone for a fraction of the energy cost of moving that volume of air, effectively breaking the ceiling of what mechanical ventilation can achieve.

4.20 Future Paradigms: Toward Infection-Resilient Environments

The COVID-19 pandemic has precipitated a paradigm shift in building standards, analogous to the sanitation revolution of the nineteenth century. Just as we no longer accept water contaminated with cholera in our taps, we can no longer accept air contaminated with respiratory pathogens in our buildings.

The Royal Academy of Engineering [74] has proposed a framework for "Infection-Resilient Environments," advocating that infection control be elevated to a core building performance metric alongside structural stability and fire safety. This framework envisions buildings that are:

- *Adaptable:* Capable of switching from "energy save" mode to "pandemic mode" (high ventilation/filtration) at the flick of a switch.
- *Visible:* Displaying real-time air quality metrics to occupants to build trust and agency.
- *Regulated:* Subject to rigorous, legally enforceable indoor air quality (IAQ) standards rather than voluntary guidelines.

This shift will require a multidisciplinary convergence of engineering, microbiology, and public health policy. It demands that we stop designing buildings merely to shelter us from the elements and start designing them to protect us from each other.

4.21 Conclusion: The Invisible Shield

Dilution ventilation is the lung of the built environment. It is the primary physiological process by which a building expels metabolic and pathogenic waste. Throughout this chapter, we have explored the physics of this mechanism—from the Wells-Riley equation to the behavior of turbulent gas clouds. We have compared it to filtration and UVGI, noting that while it may not always be the most energy-efficient method for pathogen removal, it remains the only method that broadly controls all gaseous and aerosol contaminants simultaneously.

We have seen that the "solutions" to airborne infection are not singular but systemic. Natural ventilation offers immense capacity but lacks reliability; mechanical ventilation offers control but faces thermodynamic limits. The future lies in hybrid systems that are intelligent, responsive, and human-centric.

Ultimately, dilution ventilation is an invisible shield. When it works, nobody notices. The air simply feels "fresh," and the headache or the viral infection that *didn't* happen remains unrecorded. But as we move forward into an era of increasing biosecurity threats, making this invisible shield visible, measurable, and robust is one of the defining engineering challenges of our time.

Acknowledgments Many thanks to Abha Durgesh. The authors acknowledge the support provided by the institutions including School of Planning and Architecture, New Delhi, All India Institute of Medical Sciences, New Delhi, and Drexel University. Special thanks to Rajshekhar Pullabhatla and Group Captain P Aanand Naidu of ISAC Centre for Built Environment Policy and Tathatara Foundation. Many thanks to Dr Arthur L Frank, MD. Many thanks to all the people who supported this work in many ways.

Declarations The authors Raja Singh, Nirupam Madaan, and Anil Dewan declare no conflict of interests or competing interests in this work. There is no involvement of human participants, animals, human or animal tissue. All authors declare that there was no specific financial support received from any organization for the submitted work. All authors declare that they have no financial relationships at present or within the previous 3 years with any organizations that might have an interest in the submitted work. While all care has been taken in ensuring the accuracy of this work, any inadvertent error may be reported at the earliest. The authors acknowledge the use of supervised language learning models/large language models for enhancement of the work, with responsibility lying with the authors. For more information, the corresponding author may be contacted at email rajaresearch@proton.me.

CRediT Statement The following is the CRediT statement which declares the author credits for this chapter:

Raja Singh: Conceptualization, Methodology, Formal Analysis, Investigation, Data Curation, Writing-Original Draft, Writing-Review & Editing, Visualization, Project Administration.
Nirupam Madaan: Conceptualization, Resources, Validation, Supervision, Project Administration.
Anil Dewan: Resources, Validation Supervision.

References

1. Abduljabbar RL, Liyanage S, Dia H. The role of urban transport in the spread of COVID-19: a systematic review. Transport Res Interdiscip Perspect. 2022;15:100653.
2. Adams NJ, Johnson DL, Lynch RA. The effect of pressure differential and care provider movement on airborne infectious isolation room containment effectiveness. Am J Infect Control. 2011;39(2):91–7.
3. Afshari A, Hultmark G, Nielsen PV, Maccarini A. Ventilation system design and the coronavirus (COVID-19). Front Built Environ. 2021;7:662489.
4. Agarwal N, Meena CS, Raj BP, Saini L, Kumar A, Gopalakrishnan N, et al. Indoor air quality improvement in COVID-19 pandemic: review. Sustain Cities Soc. 2021;70:102942.
5. Alameddine M, Tamim H, Hitti E. Resilience of the healthcare system: the impact of COVID-19. Front Public Health. 2021;9:642.
6. Allen JG, MacNaughton P, Satish U, Santanam S, Vallarino J, Spengler JD. Associations of cognitive function scores with carbon dioxide, ventilation, and volatile organic compound exposures in office workers: a controlled exposure study of green and conventional office environments. Environ Health Perspect. 2016;124(6):805–12.
7. Amoatey P, Omidvarborna H, Baawain MS, Al-Mamun A. Impact of building ventilation systems and habitual indoor incense burning on SARS-CoV-2 virus transmissions in Middle Eastern countries. Sci Total Environ. 2020;733:139356.
8. Andalib D, Sheibani K, Vahabi S. The effectiveness of the anteroom on hospital infection control: a systematic review. Front Public Health. 2022;10:828845.
9. ASHRAE. Standard 62.1-2019, ventilation for acceptable indoor air quality. American Society of Heating, Refrigerating and Air-Conditioning Engineers; 2019.
10. Azimi P, Stephens B. HVAC filtration for controlling infectious airborne disease transmission in indoor environments: predicting risk reductions and operational costs. Build Environ. 2013;70:150–60.
11. Beggs CB, Kerr KG, Noakes CJ, Hathway EA, Sleigh PA. The ventilation of multiple-bed hospital wards: review and analysis. Am J Infect Control. 2003;31(5):280–9.
12. Bhagat RK, Davies Wykes MS, Dalziel SB, Linden PF. Effects of ventilation on the indoor spread of COVID-19. J Fluid Mech. 2020;903:F1.
13. Bourouiba L. Turbulent gas clouds and respiratory pathogen emissions: potential implications for reducing transmission of COVID-19. JAMA. 2020;323(18):1837–8.
14. Brickner PW, Vincent RL, First M, Nardell E, Murray M, Kaufman W. The application of ultraviolet germicidal irradiation to control transmission of airborne disease: bioterrorism countermeasure. Public Health Rep. 2003;118(2):99–114.
15. Britigan N, Alshawa A, Nizkorodov SA. Quantification of ozone formation in indoor air due to corona discharges. Environ Sci Technol. 2006;40(12):3963–8.
16. Buonanno G, Stabile L, Morawska L. Estimation of airborne viral emission: quanta emission rate of SARS-CoV-2 for infection risk assessment. Environ Int. 2020;141:105794.
17. Centres for Disease Control and Prevention (CDC). Guidelines for preventing the transmission of Mycobacterium tuberculosis in health-care settings, 2005. MMWR Recomm Rep. 2005;54(RR-17):1–141.
18. Chenari B, Dias Carrilho J, Gameiro Da Silva M. Towards sustainable, energy-efficient and healthy ventilation strategies in buildings: a review. Renew Sust Energ Rev. 2016;59:1426–47.

19. Chester AC. Sick-building syndrome fatigue as a possible predation defence. Integr Physiol Behav Sci. 1999;34(1):71–83.
20. CPCB (Central Pollution Control Board). Report of the Joint committee on indoor air quality management. Ministry of Environment, Forest & Climate Change, Government of India; 2022.
21. Dinh TV, Lee JY, Ahn JW, Kim JC. Development of a wide-range non-dispersive infrared analyser for the continuous measurement of CO_2 in indoor environments. Atmosphere. 2020;11(10):1024.
22. Du CR, Wang SC, Yu MC, Chiu TF, Wang JY, Chuang PC, et al. Effect of ventilation improvement during a tuberculosis outbreak in under ventilated university buildings. Indoor Air. 2019;30(3):422–32.
23. Escombe AR, Oeser CC, Gilman RH, Navincopa M, Ticona E, Pan W, et al. Natural ventilation for the prevention of airborne contagion. PLoS Med. 2007;4(2):e68.
24. Ferrari S, Blázquez T, Cardelli R, Puglisi G, Suárez R, Mazzarella L. Ventilation strategies to reduce airborne transmission of viruses in classrooms: a systematic review of scientific literature. Build Environ. 2022;222:109366.
25. Ferreira de Oliveira A, Urrutia-Pereira M, Solé D. School environment and children's health: a systematic review. Int J Environ Res Public Health. 2023;20(3):1746.
26. First MW, Weker RA, Yasui S, Nardell EA. Monitoring human exposures to upper-room germicidal ultraviolet irradiation. J Occup Environ Hyg. 2005;2(5):285–92.
27. Fisk, WJ, Rosenfeld AH. Estimates of improved productivity and health from better indoor environments. Indoor Air. 1997;7:158–72. https://doi.org/10.1111/j.1600-0668.1997.t01-1-00002.x.
28. Gilkeson C, Camargo-Valero M, Pickin L, Noakes C. Measurement of ventilation and airborne infection risk in large naturally ventilated hospital wards. Build Environ. 2013;65:35–48.
29. Graham KE, Loeb SK, Wolfe MK, Catoe D, Sinnott-Armstrong N, Kim S, et al. SARS-CoV-2 RNA in wastewater settled solids is associated with COVID-19 cases in a large urban sewershed. Environ Sci Technol. 2021;55(1):488–98.
30. Hamidi S, Hamidi I. Subway ridership, crowding, or population density: determinants of COVID-19 infection rates in New York City. Am J Prev Med. 2021;60(5):614–20.
31. Hammond A, Khalid T, Thornton HV, Woodall CA, Hay AD. Should homes and workplaces purchase portable air filters to reduce the transmission of SARS-CoV-2 and other respiratory infections? A systematic review. PLoS ONE. 2021;16(4):e0251049.
32. Herlihey TA, Gelmi S, Flewwelling CJ, Hall TN, Bañez C, Morita PP, et al. Personal protective equipment for infectious disease preparedness: a human factors evaluation. Infect Control Hosp Epidemiol. 2016;37(9):1022–8.
33. Huang J, Hao T, Liu X, Jones P, Ou C, Liang W, Liu F. Airborne transmission of the Delta variant of SARS-CoV-2 in an auditorium. Build Environ. 2022;219:109212.
34. Jones LD, Donskey CJ. Investigation of a cluster of severe acute respiratory syndrome coronavirus 2 (SARS-CoV-2) infections in a hospital administration building. Infect Control Hosp Epidemiol. 2023;44:277–83.
35. Kalliomäki P, Saarinen P, Tang JW, Koskela H. Airflow patterns through single hinged and sliding doors in hospital isolation rooms. Int J Vent. 2015;14(2):111–26.
36. Knibbs LD, Morawska L, Bell SC. The risk of airborne influenza transmission in passenger cars. Epidemiol Infect. 2011;140(3):474–8.
37. Kowalski W. Ultraviolet germicidal irradiation handbook: UVGI for air and surface disinfection. Springer Science & Business Media; 2009.
38. Kujundzic E, Hernandez M, Miller SL. Ultraviolet germicidal irradiation inactivation of airborne fungal spores and bacteria in upper-room air and HVAC in-duct configurations. J Environ Eng Sci. 2007;6(1):1–9.
39. Kurnitski J. Ventilation rate and room size effects on infection risk of COVID-19. REHVA J. 2020;57(3):26–31.
40. Ledo Gomis L, Fiorentini M, Daly D. Potential and practical management of hybrid ventilation in buildings. Energy Build. 2021;231:110597.

41. Li X, Zhang S, Liu W, Chen C, Ho SH, Li F. Potential role of sputum in the detection of SARS-CoV-2 RNA in wastewater. J Hazard Mater. 2022;432:128667.
42. Li Y, Cheng P, Jia W. Poor ventilation worsens short-range airborne transmission of respiratory infection. Indoor Air. 2021a;32:e12946.
43. Li Y, Leung GM, Tang JW, Yang X, Chao CYH, Lin JZ, et al. Role of ventilation in airborne transmission of infectious agents in the built environment—a multidisciplinary systematic review. Indoor Air. 2007;17(1):2–18.
44. Li Y, Qian H, Hang J, Chen X, Hong L, Liang P, et al. Probable airborne transmission of SARS-CoV-2 in a poorly ventilated restaurant. Build Environ. 2021b;196:107788.
45. Lu J, Gu J, Li K, Xu C, Su W, Lai Z, et al. COVID-19 outbreak associated with air conditioning in restaurant, Guangzhou, China, 2020. Emerg Infect Dis. 2020;26(7):1628.
46. Lyles WB, Greve KW, Bauer RM, Ware MR. Sick building syndrome. South Med J. 1991;84(1):65–75.
47. Mahmoudi M, Gershwin ME. Sick building syndrome. III. Stachybotrys chartarum. J Asthma. 2000;37(3):191–8.
48. Mao N, An CK, Guo LY, Wang M, Guo L, Guo SR, Long ES. Transmission risk of infectious droplets in physical spreading process at different times: a review. Build Environ. 2020;185:107307.
49. Meggs WJ. Neurogenic switching: a hypothesis for a mechanism for shifting the site of inflammation in allergy and chemical sensitivity. Environ Health Perspect. 1995;103(1):54–6.
50. Meggs WJ. Pathology of chemical sensitivity. Environ Health Perspect. 1997;105(Suppl 2):473–8.
51. Miller SL, Nazaroff WW, Jimenez JL, Boerstra A, Buonanno G, Dancer SJ, et al. Transmission of SARS-CoV-2 by inhalation of respiratory aerosol in the Skagit Valley Chorale superspreading event. Indoor Air. 2021;31(2):314–23.
52. Morawska L, Milton DK. It is time to address airborne transmission of coronavirus disease 2019 (COVID-19). Clin Infect Dis. 2020;71(9):2311–3.
53. Morawska L, Tang JW, Bahnfleth W, Bluyssen PM, Boerstra A, Buonanno G, et al. How can airborne transmission of COVID-19 indoors be minimised? Environ Int. 2020;142:105832.
54. Mousavi ES, Grosskopf KR. Airflow patterns due to door motion and pressurization in hospital isolation rooms. Sci Technol Built Environ. 2016;22(3):379–84.
55. Mousavi ES, Kananizadeh N, Martinello RA, Sherman JD. COVID-19 outbreak and hospital air quality: a systematic review of evidence on air filtration and recirculation. Environ Sci Technol. 2021;55(7):4134–47.
56. Mphaphlele M, Dharmadhikari AS, Jensen PA, Rudnick SN, van Reenen TH, Pagano MA, et al. Institutional tuberculosis transmission. Controlled trial of upper room ultraviolet air disinfection: a basis for new dosing guidelines. Am J Respir Crit Care Med. 2015;192(4):477–84.
57. Nair AN, Anand P, George A, Mondal N. A review of strategies and their effectiveness in reducing indoor airborne transmission of COVID-19. Environ Res. 2022;213:113579.
58. Nardell EA. Indoor environmental control of tuberculosis and other airborne infections. Indoor Air. 2016;26(1):79–87.
59. Nardell EA. Air disinfection for airborne infection control with a focus on COVID-19: why germicidal UV is essential. Photochem Photobiol. 2021;97(3):493–7.
60. Nardell EA, Bucher SJ, Brickner PW, Wang C, Vincent RL, Becan-McBride K, et al. Safety of upper-room ultraviolet germicidal air disinfection for room occupants: results from the Tuberculosis Ultraviolet Shelter Study. Public Health Rep. 2008;123(1):52–60.
61. Nathavitharana RR, Rylance J, Nardell E, Lederer P. CO_2 levels may predict TB infection risk. Clin Infect Dis. 2022;75(8):1297–306.
62. Nazarenko Y. Air filtration and SARS-CoV-2. Epidemiol Health. 2021;42:e2020049.
63. Noakes CJ, Beggs CB, Sleigh PA. Modelling the performance of upper room ultraviolet germicidal irradiation devices in ventilated rooms: comparison of analytical and CFD methods. Indoor Built Environ. 2004;13(6):477–88.

64. Ou C, Hu S, Luo K, Yang H, Hang J, Cheng P, et al. Insufficient ventilation led to a probable long-range airborne transmission of SARS-CoV-2 on two buses. Build Environ. 2022;207:108414.
65. Pantelic J, Sze-To GN, Tham KW, Chao CY, Khoo YCM. Personalized ventilation as a control measure for airborne transmissible disease spread. J R Soc Interface. 2009;6(Suppl 6):S715–26.
66. Peng Z, Jimenez JL. Exhaled CO_2 as a COVID-19 infection risk proxy for different indoor environments and activities. Environ Sci Technol Lett. 2021;8(5):392–7.
67. Persily A. Challenges in developing ventilation and indoor air quality standards: the story of ASHRAE Standard 62. Build Environ. 2015;91:61–9.
68. Persily A, de Jonge L. Carbon dioxide generation rates for building occupants. Indoor Air. 2017;27(5):868–79.
69. Qian H, Zheng X. Ventilation control for airborne transmission of human exhaled bio-aerosols in buildings. J Thoracic Dis. 2018;10(Suppl 19):S2295.
70. Qian H, Li Y, Nielsen PV, Hyldgaard CE, Wong TW, Chwang AT. Dispersion of exhaled droplet nuclei in a two-bed hospital ward with three different ventilation systems. Indoor Air. 2006;16(2):111–28.
71. Qian H, Li Y, Seto WH, Ching P, Ching WH, Sun HQ. Natural ventilation for reducing airborne infection in hospitals. Build Environ. 2010;45(3):559–65.
72. REHVA. REHVA COVID-19 guidance document: how to operate and use building services in order to prevent the spread of the coronavirus disease (COVID-19) in workplaces. Federation of European Heating, Ventilation and Air Conditioning Associations; 2020.
73. Riley EC, Murphy G, Riley RL. Airborne spread of measles in a suburban elementary school. Am J Epidemiol. 1978;107(5):421–32.
74. Royal Academy of Engineering. Infection resilient environments: time for a major upgrade. National Engineering Policy Centre; 2022.
75. Rudnick SN, Milton DK. Risk of indoor airborne infection transmission estimated from carbon dioxide concentration. Indoor Air. 2003;13(3):237–45.
76. Salonen H, Salthammer T, Morawska L. Human exposure to ozone in school and office indoor environments. Environ Int. 2018;119:503–14.
77. Salthammer T, Fauck C, Omelan A, Wientzek S, Uhde E. Time and spatially resolved tracking of the air quality in local public transport. Sci Rep. 2022;12(1):1–11.
78. Satish U, Mendell MJ, Shekhar K, Hotchi T, Sullivan D, Streufert S, Fisk WJ. Is CO_2 an indoor pollutant? Direct effects of low-to-moderate CO_2 concentrations on human decision-making performance. Environ Health Perspect. 2012;120(12):1671–7.
79. Seppänen OA, Fisk WJ. Association of ventilation system type with SBS symptoms in office workers. Indoor Air. 2002;12(2):98–112.
80. Seppänen OA, Fisk WJ. Summary of human responses to ventilation. Indoor Air. 2004;14(Suppl 7):102–18.
81. Seppänen OA, Fisk WJ, Mendell MJ. Association of ventilation rates and CO_2 concentrations with health and other responses in commercial and institutional buildings. Indoor Air. 1999;9(4):226–52.
82. Seppänen OA, Fisk WJ. Some quantitative relations between indoor environmental quality and work performance or health. HVACR Res. 2006;12(4):957–73.
83. Stephens B, Azimi P, Thoemmes MS, Heidarinejad M, Allen JG, Gilbert JA. Microbial exchange via fomites and implications for human health. Curr Pollut Rep. 2013;5:198–213.
84. Sundell J, Levin H, Nazaroff WW, Cain WS, Fisk WJ, Grimsrud DT, et al. Ventilation rates and health: multidisciplinary review of the scientific literature. Indoor Air. 2011;21(3):191–204.
85. Tang JW, Bahnfleth WP, Bluyssen PM, Buonanno G, Jimenez JL, Kurnitski J, et al. Dismantling myths on the airborne transmission of severe acute respiratory syndrome coronavirus-2 (SARS-CoV-2). J Hosp Infect. 2021;110:89–96.
86. Tang JW, Eames I, Li Y, Taha Y, Wilson P, Bellingan G, et al. Door-opening motion can potentially lead to a transient breakdown in negative-pressure isolation conditions: the importance of vorticity and buoyancy airflows. J Hosp Infect. 2005;61(4):283–6.

87. Varma JK, Thamkittikasem J, Whittemore K, Alexander M, Stephens DH, Arslanian K, et al. COVID-19 infections among students and staff in New York City public schools. Pediatrics. 2021;147(5):e2021050605.
88. Viner RM, Waddington C, Mytton OT, Booy R, Ho ZJ, Kinra S. Transmission of SARS-CoV-2 by children and young people in households and schools: a meta-analysis of population-based and contact-tracing studies. J Infect. 2022;84(3):361–82.
89. Waring MS, Siegel JA. Indoor air quality implications of using ozone-based air cleaners. Indoor Air. 2011;21:266–7.
90. Wargocki P, Sundell J, Bischof W, Brundrett G, Fanger PO, Gyntelberg F, et al. Ventilation and health in non-industrial indoor environments: report from a European Multidisciplinary Scientific Consensus Meeting (EUROVEN). Indoor Air. 2002;12(2):113–28.
91. Welch D, Buonanno M, Grilj V, Shuryak I, Crickmore C, Bigelow AW, et al. Far-UVC light: A new tool to control the spread of airborne-mediated microbial diseases. Sci Rep. 2018;8(1):1–7.
92. Wells WF. Airborne contagion and air hygiene. An ecological study of droplet infections. Harvard University Press; 1955.
93. Weschler CJ. Ozone's impact on public health: contributions from indoor exposures to ozone and products of ozone-initiated chemistry. Environ Health Perspect. 2006;114(10):1489–96.
94. WHO. Natural ventilation for infection control in health-care settings. World Health Organization; 2009.
95. WHO. Roadmap to improve and ensure good indoor ventilation in the context of COVID-19. World Health Organization; 2021.
96. Wu Y, Guo C, Tang L, Hong Z, Zhou J, Dong X, et al. Prolonged presence of SARS-CoV-2 viral RNA in faecal samples. Lancet Gastroenterol Hepatol. 2020;5(5):434–5.
97. Zeng Y, Manwatkar P, Laguerre A, Boreson M, Stephan C. Evaluating a commercially available in-duct bipolar ionization device for pollutant removal and potential byproduct formation. Build Environ. 2021;195:107750.
98. Zhang J, Huntley D, Fox A, Gerhardt B, Vatine A, Cherne J. Study of viral filtration performance of residential HVAC filters. ASHRAE J. 2022;63(8).

Surrogate for Ventilation for Infection Control: Using Carbon Dioxide Biomarker

5

Raja Singh, Nirupam Madaan, and Anil Dewan

5.1 The Invisible Tracer: Breathing in the Anthropocene

In the realm of indoor environmental quality and infection control, we are often tasked with measuring the invisible to prevent the intangible. Unlike a puddle of water on the floor or a visible cloud of smoke, the biological hazards of the indoor environment—viruses like SARS-CoV-2, bacteria like *Mycobacterium tuberculosis*, and various fungal spores—are imperceptible to the human senses until the onset of pathology. We cannot see the viral plume emitted by an asymptomatic carrier speaking across a conference table, nor can we taste the lingering aerosols of a previous occupant in a poorly ventilated elevator. To manage these invisible risks, building scientists and public health officials rely on proxies—measurable indicators that reveal the hidden dynamics of air movement and contaminant accumulation. Among these, carbon dioxide (CO_2) stands as the preeminent, albeit complex, sentinel of the indoor environment.

For over a century, CO_2 has served as the fundamental metric for ventilation standards, primarily driven by the need to control human bioeffluents (body odors). However, the twenty-first century has necessitated a paradigm shift. We have moved from viewing CO_2 merely as a marker of "stuffiness" or comfort to recognizing it as a critical biomarker for the "rebreathed air fraction"—a direct quantitative link to

R. Singh
Founder/Researcher, The Built, New Delhi, Delhi, India

Former Post Doctoral Fellow, Department of Environmental and Occupational Health, Dornsife School of Public Health, Drexel University, Philadelphia, Pennsylvania, USA

N. Madaan
Department of Hospital Administration, All India Institute of Medical Sciences, New Delhi, Delhi, India

A. Dewan
Department of Architecture, School of Planning and Architecture, New Delhi, Delhi, India

R. Singh et al., *Infection Control in the Everyday Built Environment*,
https://doi.org/10.1007/978-981-95-8624-0_5

the probability of airborne infection transmission [36, 44]. Every time humans exhale, they release a plume of warm, moist air containing approximately 38,000–40,000 parts per million (ppm) of CO_2, roughly 100 times the concentration found in the ambient outdoor atmosphere [38, 44]. If this exhalation occurs in a sealed room, the CO_2 concentration rises inexorably, mirroring the accumulation of potentially infectious aerosols emitted alongside it.

This chapter explores the physics, physiology, and utility of using CO_2 as a surrogate for ventilation and infection control. We will dissect the historical evolution of CO_2 standards, the mathematical derivation of the "rebreathed fraction," and the nuances of monitoring in diverse built environments. Crucially, we must also confront the limitations of this proxy: while high CO_2 almost always indicates a risk of airborne transmission, low CO_2 does not guarantee safety, particularly in the era of high-efficiency particulate air (HEPA) filtration which cleans the air of pathogens without altering gas concentrations [19, 31].

5.2 The Physiology of the Source: Humans as Carbon Engines

To utilize CO_2 effectively as a tracer for infection risk, one must first understand the emission source. Unlike volatile organic compounds (VOCs) which may off-gas from furniture or paints, or particulate matter ($PM_{2.5}$) which may infiltrate from traffic pollution or cooking, the primary source of indoor CO_2 in non-industrial settings is human metabolism [38, 51]. The human body is a combustion engine, consuming oxygen and producing carbon dioxide as a byproduct of cellular respiration.

The rate of CO_2 generation G_{CO2} is not a static constant; it is a dynamic variable dependent on body surface area (a function of age, sex, and height) and, most critically, physical activity level (metabolic rate). A resting adult might generate approximately 0.004–0.005 L/s of CO_2, while the same individual engaged in light office work produces roughly 30% more, and heavy exercise can increase this rate by a factor of 5–10 [7, 38].

This variability is critical for infection control modeling. A classroom of sedentary 6-year-olds generates significantly less CO_2 than a gym full of adults exercising, yet the children may be more susceptible to certain infections due to differing immune profiles and social behaviors. Persily and de Jonge [38] revised the standard generation rates used in building codes, noting that historically cited values often overestimated generation rates for women and children while underestimating them for larger modern adult body types. Accurate estimation of G_{CO2} is the foundational variable in the mass balance equations used to determine ventilation rates from observed concentrations [5, 38].

Furthermore, the emission of CO_2 correlates temporally with the emission of bioaerosols. Activities that increase metabolic demand and CO_2 production—such as singing, shouting, or heavy breathing during exercise—also increase the atomization of respiratory fluids from the bronchioles and larynx [4, 27]. Consequently, a spike in indoor CO_2 is often a dual signal: it indicates both a failure of dilution ventilation and a likely period of high-intensity aerosol generation, compounding the risk of viral transmission [9, 26].

5.3 The Historical Trajectory: From Odour to Pathogen

The use of CO_2 as a ventilation metric is rooted in the nineteenth-century hygiene movement. Max von Pettenkofer, a German hygienist, was among the first to propose that while CO_2 itself was not toxic at typical indoor levels, it served as a reliable measuring stick for other, more noxious human emanations. In 1858, Pettenkofer proposed a limit of 1000 ppm (parts per million) for indoor spaces, not because 1000 ppm of CO_2 was dangerous, but because his empirical observations suggested that above this level, the air became perceived as "stuffy" and malodorous to occupants [39, 50].

This "Pettenkofer number" of 1000 ppm remained the de facto standard for nearly a century. In the 1930s, Yaglou and colleagues at Harvard University conducted seminal chamber studies to quantify the ventilation required to dilute body odors to an acceptable level. They determined that approximately 7.5 L/s (15 cubic feet per minute) per person of outdoor air was necessary to satisfy the olfactory comfort of visitors entering a room [50, 56]. This roughly correlates to maintaining steady-state CO_2 levels around 1000 ppm, assuming standard adult metabolism.

However, the energy crisis of the 1970s disrupted this consensus. In a bid to conserve thermal energy, the globally used standards lowered the minimum ventilation rate to 2.5 L/s (5 cfm) per person in non-smoking areas. This reduction led to a widespread accumulation of indoor pollutants and the emergence of "Sick Building Syndrome" (SBS), characterized by non-specific symptoms such as headaches, fatigue, and mucosal irritation [47, 50]. Empirical studies during this era repeatedly showed that as ventilation rates dropped and CO_2 levels rose, the prevalence of SBS symptoms increased significantly [3, 47].

It was not until the resurgence of tuberculosis in the late 1980s and the subsequent SARS-CoV-1 outbreak in 2003 that the focus shifted from odour and comfort back to infection control. Epidemiological investigations, such as those analyzing the tuberculosis outbreak in a Harvard office building [32] or the spread of measles in schools [43], utilized CO_2 not as a smell proxy, but as a tracer gas to calculate the fraction of air that had been previously exhaled by an infector. This marked the transition of CO_2 monitoring from an amenity metric to a "biosecurity" tool [30, 44].

5.4 The Rudnick-Milton Concept: The Rebreathed Air Fraction

The theoretical bridge between CO_2 concentration and infection risk is the concept of the "rebreathed air fraction" (f). In any enclosed space where people are present, the air is a mixture of fresh air (from outdoors or filtered supply) and air that has recently exited the lungs of the occupants. For airborne pathogens like

SARS-CoV-2, measles, and tuberculosis, the risk of infection is directly proportional to the volume of this rebreathed air inhaled by a susceptible person [36, 44].

Rudnick and Milton [44] derived a modification of the classic Wells-Riley equation, replacing the difficult-to-measure ventilation rate (Q) with the readily measurable CO_2 concentration. The fraction of air that is exhaled breath (f) can be approximated as:

$$f = \frac{C_{\text{indoor}} - C_{\text{outdoor}}}{C_{\text{exhaled}}}$$

where:

- C_{indoor} is the measured indoor CO_2 concentration (ppm).
- C_{outdoor} is the outdoor background CO_2 concentration (typically 400–420 ppm or more).
- C_{exhaled} is the CO_2 concentration in exhaled breath (approximately 38,000 ppm).

For example, if a classroom measures 800 ppm of CO_2, the excess CO_2 produced by occupants is

$$800 - 400 = 400\,\text{ppm}.$$

The fraction of rebreathed air is therefore

$$400 \div 38{,}000 \approx 0.01, \text{which is } 1\%.$$

This means that for every breath a student takes, 1% of the volume consists of air that was recently inside someone else's lungs. If the CO_2 level rises to 2400 ppm (an excess of 2000 ppm), the rebreathed fraction rises to [36, 44]

$$\frac{2000}{38{,}000} \approx 5.2\%.$$

This mathematical relationship transforms the abstract concept of "ventilation" into a tangible biological risk metric. While 1% rebreathed air might seem low, over an 8-h workday or school day, the cumulative volume of rebreathed air can be substantial—enough to inhale an infectious dose (a "quantum") if an infector is present. Studies have shown that maintaining CO_2 below specific thresholds (often 800 or 1000 ppm) may significantly reduce the reproduction number (R_0) of airborne events [14, 23].

5.5 Quantifying the Association: CO_2 and Health Outcomes

The utility of CO_2 as a biomarker is supported by a robust body of epidemiological evidence linking elevated concentrations to adverse health outcomes. These outcomes range from the non-specific symptoms of sick building syndrome (SBS) to confirmed transmission of infectious diseases.

5.5.1 Sick Building Syndrome (SBS) and Cognitive Function

A seminal review by Seppänen et al. [47] analyzed over 20 studies involving 30,000 subjects and found a consistent association: ventilation rates below 10 L/s/person (often corresponding to CO_2 levels above ~1000 ppm) were associated with a statistically significant worsening of health outcomes. Specifically, the relative risk of SBS symptoms was 1.1–6 times higher in low ventilation environments compared to high ventilation ones [47].

Furthermore, recent research has suggested that CO_2 may have direct physiological effects independent of its role as a proxy for other contaminants. Satish et al. [45] and Allen et al. [2] demonstrated that at CO_2 concentrations of 2500 ppm—levels occasionally seen in crowded meeting rooms and classrooms—measures of human decision-making performance declined significantly. While the mechanism for this direct toxicity is debated, the correlation reinforces the value of CO_2 monitoring for productivity and general health, beyond infection control [2, 45].

5.5.2 Infectious Disease Transmission

In the specific context of infectious disease, the correlation between CO_2 and transmission is even more direct. In a landmark study of tuberculosis transmission in South African hospitals, Nathavitharana et al. [33] used personal CO_2 monitors worn by healthcare workers. They found that workers who converted to a positive tuberculosis test (IGRA conversion) had been exposed to significantly higher median CO_2 levels than those who did not convert. This provided empirical validation that the "rebreathed air fraction," as measured by CO_2, is a predictor of biological infection risk in real-world clinical settings, or more accurately demonstrates a statistically significant association between elevated CO_2 exposure and TB infection risk [33].

Similarly, during the COVID-19 pandemic, outbreaks in high-density environments like schools and buses were frequently associated with poor ventilation. A study of a COVID-19 outbreak on a bus in China revealed that the air recirculation system, which offered minimal fresh air supply, likely facilitated transmission to passengers seated far from the index case. While CO_2 was not measured in real-time during the ride, subsequent modeling of the bus environment indicated that low air exchange rates (which correlate with high CO_2) were the critical failure point [35, 48].

5.6 The Steady-State Assumption and Its Pitfalls

A critical nuance in using CO_2 as a ventilation surrogate is the concept of "steady state." The standard mass balance equations (like the one used to derive 15 cfm from 1000 ppm) assume that the concentration of CO_2 in the room has stabilized—that the rate of generation equals the rate of removal. However, in many real-world scenarios, equilibrium is never reached.

Consider a school classroom that starts empty at 400 ppm. When 30 students enter at 8:00 AM, CO_2 levels begin to rise. Depending on the ventilation rate and room volume, it may take 30 min to 2 h to reach a steady state. If the class duration is only 45 min, a single point measurement taken at the end of the class might read 1200 ppm, but the average exposure during the period was much lower. Conversely, if ventilation fails mid-day, levels might climb continuously [7, 37].

Therefore, relying on "spot checks" of CO_2 can be misleading. A low reading might simply mean the room was recently vacated or the door was briefly opened, not that the ventilation system is adequate. For infection control, continuous monitoring or "time-weighted averages" are far more reliable indicators of cumulative risk [21, 36].

5.7 The Dynamics of Accumulation: Steady-State vs. The Transient Reality

While the Rudnick-Milton model and the Wells-Riley equation provide elegant mathematical frameworks for linking carbon dioxide (CO_2) to infection risk, they rely heavily on the assumption of a "steady-state" environment. This assumption posits that the rate of CO_2 generation by occupants is perfectly balanced by the rate of removal via ventilation, resulting in a constant indoor concentration. However, the built environment is rarely a static system; it is a dynamic theatre of fluctuating occupancy, variable metabolic rates, and intermittent ventilation operation. Understanding the physics of transient conditions is essential for interpreting CO_2 data correctly and avoiding dangerous false assurances.

5.7.1 The Lag Time of Detectability

When a group of people enters a room, CO_2 levels do not rise instantaneously to their maximum value. Instead, they follow a logarithmic growth curve, asymptotically approaching the steady-state concentration determined by the ventilation rate. The speed of this rise is governed by the room's air change rate (ACH). In a poorly ventilated room (low ACH), the air is "sluggish"; it takes a long time for the concentration to stabilize. Conversely, in a highly ventilated room (high ACH), the air volume is flushed rapidly, and steady state is reached quickly [7].

This physical reality introduces a critical "lag time" in risk assessment. Consider a 45-min school lesson in a poorly ventilated classroom. The class begins with CO_2 at background levels (400 ppm). Thirty students enter. Due to the low ventilation, the CO_2 accumulates slowly. By the end of the 45-min period, the concentration might only reach 1200 ppm, even though the steady-state concentration (if they stayed for 4 h) would be 3000 ppm. An observer glancing at a sensor reading of 1000 ppm halfway through the lesson might erroneously conclude that the ventilation is adequate (meeting the 1000 ppm standard), when in fact, the system is grossly insufficient to handle the bio-load [7, 37]. The sensor is reading the *history* of the air, not just its current quality.

This transient behavior is particularly treacherous in high-density, short-duration settings such as public transport or waiting rooms. A study on bus transmission showed that even short trips could facilitate infection if air recirculation is high and fresh air intake is low, yet a CO_2 monitor might not alarm until the journey is nearly over [35]. Therefore, for infection control, the *rate of rise* in CO_2 is often as diagnostically valuable as the absolute value. A rapid climb in CO_2 indicates a severe ventilation deficit relative to the occupancy load, signaling an urgent need for intervention before the "rebreathed air fraction" reaches critical levels [36].

5.7.2 The Decay Curve and "Flush Out"

The dynamic relationship works in reverse when occupants leave. The "decay" of CO_2 levels back to baseline is a direct measure of the room's effective air change rate. This principle is utilized in the "concentration decay method" for measuring ventilation: researchers release a tracer gas (or use occupant-generated CO_2), stop the source (occupants leave), and measure the slope of the decline [7].

In the context of pandemic management, this decay profile dictates the necessary "flush-out" time between occupancies. If a meeting room is used by different groups, how long must it stand empty for the potentially infectious aerosols from Group A to be removed before Group B enters? In a room with 6 ACH, 99% of airborne contaminants are removed in roughly 46 min. In a poorly ventilated room with 1 ACH, this same clearance takes over 4 h [10]. Real-time CO_2 monitoring can visualize this purge process. If the CO_2 level remains elevated long after occupants have departed, it is a definitive marker of stagnant air and a high risk of cross-infection between temporally separated groups—a phenomenon documented in the transmission of measles and tuberculosis in medical waiting areas [30].

5.8 The Technology of Detection: Sensors and Deployment

To use CO_2 as a proxy for biological safety, we rely on the fidelity of the measurement technology. The proliferation of low-cost sensors has democratized air quality monitoring, but it has also introduced significant variability in data quality. Understanding the mechanism of detection is requisite for interpreting the data.

5.8.1 NDIR: The Gold Standard

The most reliable technology for indoor CO_2 monitoring is non-dispersive infrared (NDIR) detection. CO_2 molecules absorb infrared light at a specific wavelength (4.26 microns). An NDIR sensor consists of an infrared source, a sample chamber (tube), and a detector. The gas is pumped or diffuses into the chamber, and the reduction in light intensity reaching the detector is proportional to the concentration of CO_2 according to the Beer-Lambert law [53, 54].

Recent advancements have led to the miniaturization of these components using micro-electro-mechanical systems (MEMS). For instance, ScAlN-based pyroelectric detectors have been developed to create CMOS-compatible NDIR sensors that are smaller, cheaper, and consume less power, making them suitable for widespread deployment in schools and offices [34, 53, 54]. These sensors generally offer good specificity to CO_2, resisting interference from other common indoor gases, although they can be sensitive to temperature and humidity variations which must be compensated for by the device firmware [53, 54].

5.8.2 The Pitfall of Electrochemical Sensors (eCO_2)

A critical distinction must be made between "true" CO_2 sensors (NDIR) and "equivalent" CO_2 sensors (eCO_2). Many cheap consumer-grade air quality monitors use metal-oxide semiconductor (MOS) sensors to detect volatile organic compounds (VOCs) and then use an algorithm to *estimate* a CO_2 value. These devices do not detect CO_2 molecules directly. Instead, they assume that because humans emit both VOCs and CO_2, the two will correlate. This assumption fails catastrophically in the context of infection control. For example, the use of hand sanitizers (alcohol) or cleaning products can cause a massive spike in VOC readings, causing an eCO_2 sensor to report dangerously high "CO_2" levels when the actual ventilation is adequate. Conversely, a room full of people wearing masks (which might trap some breath VOCs) or simply breathing without generating other odors might register low on an eCO_2 sensor while actual CO_2 and viral aerosols accumulate to unsafe levels [7, 53, 54]. For biosecurity purposes, eCO_2 sensors are prone to error and should be avoided.

5.8.3 Strategic Sensor Placement

The placement of the sensor is as important as the technology. The assumption of a "well-mixed" room is a mathematical convenience, not a physical reality. CO_2 concentrations can vary significantly within a single space due to thermal plumes, ventilation short-circuiting, and proximity to sources (people).

- *Breathing Zone vs. Exhaust:* Ideally, monitoring should reflect the air being inhaled by occupants. Placing sensors at the "breathing height" (approx. 1.2–1.5 m for seated adults) is standard practice. However, placing a sensor too close to an occupant (e.g., on a desk right next to someone) results in measuring their direct exhalation plume rather than the mixed room air, leading to artificially high readings [53, 54].

- *Dead Zones:* Sensors should be placed in areas likely to have the poorest ventilation effectiveness, such as corners away from supply diffusers or areas with high occupant density.
- *Avoidance of Fresh Air:* Sensors must not be placed near windows, doors, or supply vents, where they will measure fresh air rather than the mixed room air, leading to a false sense of security [53, 54].

5.9 Carbon Dioxide and the "Indoor Penalty"

The most profound application of CO_2 monitoring is its ability to quantify the "indoor penalty"—the inherent increase in transmission risk associated with moving social interactions from outdoors to indoors.

5.9.1 Quantifying the Outdoor Reference

Outdoor air generally has a CO_2 concentration typically 410–430 ppm globally, often higher in urban environments (450–500+ ppm). In an outdoor setting, the infinite reservoir of fresh air and natural air currents (wind) dilute exhaled breath so rapidly that the "rebreathed fraction" is essentially zero, barring immediate close-range interactions [22]. This establishes the baseline for safety. When we move indoors, we restrict the volume of dilution air. The rise in CO_2 above the 400–420 ppm baseline is a direct metric of how much we have compromised that safety.

5.9.2 Ventilation and Short-Range Transmission

Traditionally, it was believed that general ventilation (and thus room-level CO_2) only mitigated "long-range" airborne transmission (infection across the room), while "short-range" transmission (droplets/aerosols within 1–2 m) was governed solely by distance and was impervious to ventilation rates. Recent mechanistic modelling by Li et al. [22] has dismantled this dichotomy.

Li et al. [22] demonstrated that the concentration of pathogens in the short-range "jet" of exhaled breath is determined not only by the source strength but by the entrainment of the surrounding background air. If the background air is stale (high CO_2, high viral load), the jet entrains contaminated air, maintaining a higher viral concentration even as it dilutes. Conversely, if the background air is clean (low CO_2, high ventilation), the jet entrains clean air, accelerating the dilution of the viral plume before it reaches the face of a susceptible person nearby. The study showed that a ventilation rate of *10 L/s per person* (roughly corresponding to maintaining CO_2 below 800–900 ppm) creates a concentration decay profile for exhaled aerosols that begins to approximate outdoor conditions. When ventilation is poor (e.g., 1 L/s/

person, leading to high CO_2), the risk of infection increases for *both* long-range and short-range exposures. This finding elevates CO_2 monitoring from a tool for managing "room air" to a tool for mitigating close-contact risk [22]. It implies that maintaining low CO_2 is a protective layer even for people standing in conversation, reducing the "indoor penalty" imposed by the enclosure.

5.9.3 The 1000 ppm Threshold: History vs. Virology

The benchmark of 1000 ppm CO_2 has been a cornerstone of indoor air quality standards for over a century, tracing back to Pettenkofer's work on body odor perception [50]. However, the validity of this threshold for *viral* infection control is context-dependent.

- *Odor vs. Infection:* The 1000 ppm limit (roughly 7.5 L/s/person) was designed to keep bioeffluents (odors) below the threshold of annoyance for 80% of visitors [50]. Viruses do not follow olfactory thresholds. A highly infectious pathogen like the measles virus or the Omicron variant of SARS-CoV-2 can spread at concentrations well below those that cause noticeable odor or "stuffiness."
- *The Re-evaluation:* While 1000 ppm indicates "acceptable" ventilation for comfort, for infection control—especially in high-risk settings like hospitals or during pandemic surges—a target of *800 ppm* or even lower is increasingly advocated [22, 36]. Maintaining levels closer to outdoor background (e.g., 600 ppm) provides a significantly higher safety margin, reducing the rebreathed fraction to below 0.5% [44].

In summary, CO_2 is a powerful, albeit nuanced, biomarker. It captures the complex interplay of occupancy, ventilation, and room volume into a single, actionable number. However, relying on it requires an understanding of its temporal dynamics and the technology used to measure it. A "green" light on a sensor does not guarantee sterility, but a "red" light is a definitive warning of a failure in the biological "firewall" of the building.

5.10 From Comfort to Biosecurity: Evolving Standards and Guidelines

The transition of carbon dioxide (CO_2) from a metric of olfactory comfort to a sentinel of biosecurity has necessitated a rigorous re-evaluation of global building standards. For decades, the dominant paradigm in heating, ventilation, and air conditioning (HVAC) engineering was governed by the metabolic demands of occupants and the dilution of body odors, codified in standards. However, the exigencies of the COVID-19 pandemic and the persistent threat of tuberculosis have forced a regulatory decoupling: "acceptable" air quality for comfort is no longer synonymous with "safe" air quality for infection prevention.

5.10.1 The Legacy Standard: The Pettenkofer Limit and ASHRAE

As established earlier, the historical benchmark for indoor CO_2 has been 1000 ppm. This limit, derived from Max von Pettenkofer's nineteenth-century observations and formalized by Yaglou's chamber studies in the 1930s, was predicated on the threshold at which body odors became perceptible to 80% of unadapted visitors entering a space [50, 56]. In engineering terms, maintaining CO_2 below 1000 ppm generally requires a ventilation rate of approximately 7.5–8 L/s per person, assuming standard adult metabolic activity [37].

While this rate is sufficient to control bioeffluents, it does not account for the probabilistic nature of viral transmission. Pathogens do not follow the same psychophysical laws as odors. A highly infectious agent, such as the measles virus or the Delta variant of SARS-CoV-2, possesses a low infectious dose (ID_{50}), meaning that infection can occur even at ventilation rates that successfully dilute odors. Conversely, less transmissible pathogens might be controlled adequately at the odor threshold. Therefore, the 1000 ppm standard represents a *minimum hygiene* level, not a sterile safety limit [22, 28]. For context, occupational exposure limits historically treat CO_2 primarily as a bulk asphyxiant rather than a pathogen proxy; Some older hygiene/occupational standards for CO_2 has long been set at 5000 ppm (with a short-term exposure limit), a level far above comfort and infection-control targets [1].

5.10.2 The Pandemic Paradigm Shift: Targeting 800 ppm

During the COVID-19 crisis, public health agencies and engineering bodies (including REHVA, ASHRAE, and the CDC) issued guidance recommending enhanced ventilation. A converging consensus emerged around a lower threshold for high-occupancy spaces: *800 ppm*. This target is not arbitrary; it is rooted in the non-linear relationship between the rebreathed air fraction and infection risk described by the Wells-Riley equation.

Lowering the limit from 1000 ppm (an excess of ~600 ppm above background) to 800 ppm (an excess of ~400 ppm) represents a 33% reduction in the rebreathed air fraction. Because the probability of infection scales exponentially with the dose of inhaled quanta, this reduction can have a disproportionate impact on the reproduction number (R_0) of an outbreak event. For example, Li et al. [22] demonstrated through continuum modelling that a ventilation rate of 10 L/s per person—which roughly corresponds to maintaining steady-state CO_2 below 800–900 ppm—is the inflection point where the "indoor penalty" of transmission likely begins to approximate outdoor risk levels.

Consequently, recent interim guidelines for indoor air quality management in public places, such as those deliberated by the Central Pollution Control Board (CPCB) in India, have explicitly included CO_2 as a critical parameter for monitoring, recognizing its utility in gauging ventilation adequacy in real-time [11, 12]. These guidelines emphasize that while CO_2 is not a direct measure of viral load, it is the most viable proxy for the *potential* accumulation of airborne pathogens in spaces like malls, auditoriums, and offices.

5.10.3 The "Traffic Light" System

To operationalize these standards for laypersons (teachers, office managers), many jurisdictions have adopted a "traffic light" visualization for CO_2 monitors:

- *Green (<800 ppm):* Ventilation is likely adequate. Risk of long-range airborne transmission is reduced. Ideally, it should be 500 ppm and below.
- *Amber (800–1500 ppm):* Ventilation is suboptimal. Measures such as opening windows or reducing occupancy should be taken.
- *Red (>1500 ppm):* Ventilation is critically insufficient. The rebreathed air fraction is high (>3–4%), indicating a significant risk of pathogen accumulation. Immediate remediation is required [36, 41].

It is crucial to note that these thresholds assume a steady state and standard occupancy. In dynamic environments, a rapid rise from 400 to 800 ppm in a short period (e.g., 15 min) is a "Red" signal regarding the ventilation rate's capacity to handle the load, even if the absolute value is still "Green" or "Amber" [7].

5.11 The Decoupling Effect: The Limits of CO_2 as a Proxy

While CO_2 is an invaluable tool, it is not a perfect "crystal ball". The fundamental limitation of CO_2 monitoring in the modern era of infection control is the phenomenon of *decoupling*. The relationship between CO_2 and airborne pathogens relies on the premise that both are removed by the same mechanism: ventilation (exchange with outdoor air). However, modern air cleaning technologies can break this link.

5.11.1 The Filtration Paradox

High-efficiency particulate air (HEPA) filters and minimum efficiency reporting value (MERV-13+) filters are highly effective at capturing respiratory aerosols and droplet nuclei carrying viruses [6]. However, fibrous filters are completely transparent to gas molecules like carbon dioxide (CO_2 is ~0.3 nm, while viruses are ~100 nm and droplets >1000 nm).

Consider a sealed room with a high-capacity portable HEPA air cleaner running at 6 air changes per hour (ACH). The HEPA filter will rapidly strip the air of viral particles, significantly lowering the risk of infection. However, the HEPA filter will *not* remove the occupant-generated CO_2. Consequently, the CO_2 meter might read 2000 ppm (indicating "danger"), while the actual viral concentration is negligible due to filtration. In this scenario, CO_2 monitoring yields a *false positive* for probable infection risk [19, 31].

This paradox necessitates a modification of how we interpret CO_2 data in spaces with air cleaning. The "effective ventilation rate" (Q_{eff}) for pathogen removal is the sum of outdoor air ventilation (Q_{vent}) and the clean air delivery rate of the filtration system (Q_{filter}). CO_2 only measures Q_{vent}. Therefore, in spaces with aggressive filtration, CO_2 remains a valid indicator of *ventilation* (and bioeffluent control) but may become a conservative overestimate of *infection risk*. This distinction is vital for facility managers to avoid unnecessary panic or energy waste [31]. Yet, even in these situations, the indication of low ventilation may still serve as a warning for high odours or general stuffiness in the room.

5.11.2 The Influence of Non-human Sources

The utility of CO_2 as a tracer assumes that humans are the sole source. In environments with indoor combustion—such as kitchens with gas stoves, laboratories with Bunsen burners, or spaces with unvented gas heaters—CO_2 levels can be elevated by non-biological sources [51]. In these settings, a reading of 1500 ppm does not imply that 3% of the air is rebreathed; it implies that the air is polluted with combustion byproducts (which pose their own respiratory risks, such as NO_2 and PM). Similarly, in highly polluted urban centers, the outdoor background CO_2 can fluctuate significantly above 400 ppm due to traffic density, requiring local calibration of the baseline [11, 12].

5.11.3 Variability in Generation Rates

The rate of CO_2 generation is metabolically driven. A gym class will generate significantly more CO_2 per person than a library reading room. Crucially, the emission of viral aerosols also scales with respiratory activity—shouting and heavy breathing generate exponentially more aerosols than tidal breathing [4, 27]. While CO_2 generation and aerosol generation correlate, the relationship is not perfectly linear across all vocalization activities. For instance, "super-emitters" of aerosols may not necessarily be "super-emitters" of CO_2. Thus, a room with low CO_2 could still harbor a risk if a specific activity (like singing) is generating a disproportionately high viral load compared to the metabolic output [26].

5.12 Interpreting the Signal: Mathematical Adjustments

To address the filtration paradox, researchers have proposed modified equations that adjust the CO_2-derived risk assessment based on the clean air delivery rate (CADR) of air cleaners.

The standard Rudnick-Milton approach estimates the fraction of rebreathed air (f). When filtration is present, the concentration of virus (C_y) decays faster than the concentration of CO_2. The equivalent ventilation rate for virus removal (Q_{virus}) is:

$$Q_{\text{virus}} = Q_{\text{vent}} + Q_{\text{filter}} + Q_{\text{deposition}} + Q_{\text{inactivation}}$$

While the ventilation rate measured by CO_2 (Q_{CO2}) is simply:

$$Q_{\text{CO2}} \approx Q_{\text{vent}}$$

Therefore, to use CO_2 as a proxy in a filtered room, one must apply a correction factor. If the filtration system provides an additional 4 ACH on top of the 2 ACH from ventilation, the total removal rate for the virus is 6 ACH. The CO_2 sensor will only "see" the 2 ACH. The actual risk is roughly one-third of what the CO_2 level suggests (assuming perfect mixing). Building operators must maintain a "logbook" of filtration efficacy to interpret sensor data correctly: high CO_2 is acceptable *only if* confirmed, high-efficiency filtration is active [16, 31]. Yet, it is a warning sign for stuffiness and hygiene issues like possible odours.

5.13 Case Studies in CO_2 Monitoring

The theoretical framework of CO_2 monitoring has been validated—and its limitations exposed—in numerous field studies across diverse environments.

5.13.1 The Educational Sector: Schools as Crucibles of Transmission

Schools represent a primary use-case for CO_2 monitoring due to high occupant density and historically poor ventilation. A study by Richardson et al. [42] in South African schools highlighted the critical role of ventilation in tuberculosis (TB) transmission. They monitored CO_2 in naturally ventilated classrooms and found that levels frequently exceeded 1000 ppm, often reaching 3000–4000 ppm in winter when windows were closed. Using the rebreathed air fraction model, they calculated that the cumulative risk of TB transmission was high. The study concluded that achieving a target of 1000 ppm (approximately 12 ACH in their model context) could significantly reduce the effective contact number for TB. This demonstrated that simple CO_2 monitoring could identify "hotspot" classrooms requiring structural intervention [42].

Similarly, during the COVID-19 pandemic, data from European schools showed that classrooms relying on manual airing (opening windows) often failed to maintain safe levels during cold weather. A study reviewing ventilation strategies in schools (Ferrari et al. 2022) noted that while mechanical systems could maintain lower CO_2, naturally ventilated rooms exhibited "sawtooth" profiles—rapid drops when windows opened during breaks, followed by steep rises during lessons. This intermittent exposure suggests that continuous logging, rather than spot checks, is essential for accurate risk profiling in schools.

5.13.2 Public Transportation: The Mobile Enclosure

Public transport vehicles are unique microenvironments characterized by small volumes and variable occupancy. A study investigating a COVID-19 outbreak on a bus in Eastern China [48] indicated that the recirculation of air (to save energy on cooling) likely facilitated transmission. While real-time CO_2 data was not available during the outbreak, subsequent modeling suggests that CO_2 would have risen rapidly.

Conversely, a study on trams [46] demonstrated the rapid decay of pollutants when doors open. They measured particulate matter and CO_2 decay rates, finding that the frequent opening of doors at stops acted as a powerful "pulse" ventilation mechanism, with decay constants explaining the rapid clearance of airborne contaminants. However, if doors remained closed (e.g., between distant stops), concentrations climbed. This suggests that CO_2 sensors in transport should be linked to automated damper controls—increasing fresh air intake when the vehicle is in motion and occupancy is detected [46].

5.13.3 Healthcare Settings: Validating the Biological Link

Perhaps the most compelling validation comes from the clinical setting. The study by Nathavitharana et al. [33] deserves detailed scrutiny here. In this study, personal CO_2 monitors were worn by healthcare workers in TB wards. The study found a statistically significant association between the *average* CO_2 exposure and the likelihood of converting to a positive interferon-gamma release assay (IGRA), which indicates latent TB infection. Specifically, workers who became infected had higher median CO_2 exposure levels compared to those who did not. This study effectively closed the loop between the physics of ventilation (measured by CO_2) and the biology of transmission (measured by immune response). It provides the empirical justification for using CO_2 targets (e.g., <800 ppm) not just as comfort goals, but as occupational safety limits for airborne pathogens [33].

5.14 The Future of Monitoring: From Passive Sensors to Active Control

The integration of CO_2 sensors into the "Internet of Things" (IoT) allows for a shift from passive monitoring to active control. Demand-controlled ventilation (DCV) systems traditionally use CO_2 to *lower* ventilation during low occupancy to save energy. In the post-pandemic era, the logic must be inverted or at least modified. "Infection-mode" DCV would use CO_2 data to *maximize* ventilation when occupancy rises, prioritizing health over energy savings. Furthermore, integrating CO_2 sensors with automated window openers in naturally ventilated schools could remove the human error of forgetting to air out classrooms (Ferrari et al. 2022; [11, 12]).

The emerging field of "smart" building management envisions sensors that not only track CO_2 but correlate it with real-time occupancy counts and particulate matter levels to generate dynamic "Air Quality Indexes" displayed on public screens. This transparency empowers occupants to make informed decisions—such as leaving a crowded, stuffy room—effectively using CO_2 data as a tool for behavioral adaptation [55].

5.15 The Cognitive Cost: Carbon Dioxide as a Direct Pollutant

For decades, the prevailing dogma in building science and industrial hygiene was that carbon dioxide (CO_2) at indoor concentrations (typically 400–3000 ppm) was biologically inert—a benign asphyxiant relevant only insofar as it displaced oxygen or indicated the presence of other bioeffluents. This assumption relegated CO_2 to the status of a mere proxy, a "canary in the coal mine" for body odours and, more recently, for airborne pathogens [37]. However, a growing body of toxicological and epidemiological evidence challenges this view, suggesting that CO_2 may be a direct pollutant with significant impacts on human cognitive function and decision-making capabilities. This paradigm shift has profound implications for infection control strategies, particularly those relying heavily on air cleaning (filtration) which removes pathogens but leaves CO_2 accumulation unchecked.

5.15.1 The Satish and Allen Studies: A Wake-Up Call

The reassessment of CO_2 toxicity was catalyzed by controlled exposure studies that isolated CO_2 from other indoor pollutants. In a landmark study, Satish et al. [45] exposed participants to CO_2 concentrations of 600, 1000, and 2500 ppm in an environmental chamber while measuring decision-making performance using the strategic management simulation (SMS). The results were startling: at 1000 ppm—a level considered "acceptable" by ASHRAE standards and ubiquitous in schools and offices—moderate decrements were observed in six of nine scales of decision-making performance. At 2500 ppm, a level frequently reached in crowded meeting rooms and classrooms, large and statistically significant reductions occurred in seven scales, with some performance metrics dropping to "dysfunctional" levels [45].

These findings were corroborated and expanded upon by Allen et al. [2] in a study of office workers. They found that cognitive function scores were 15% lower for a day with moderate CO_2 (~945 ppm) and 50% lower for a day with high CO_2 (~1400 ppm) compared to days with low CO_2 (~550 ppm). Critically, this effect was independent of ventilation rate; when the ventilation rate was held constant but pure CO_2 was injected into the space, cognitive scores still declined. This suggests that the impairment is driven by the CO_2 molecule itself, not just by the other bioeffluents that usually accompany it [2].

5.15.2 Mechanisms of Action and Physiological Implications

The biological mechanism by which moderately elevated CO_2 impairs cognition remains an area of active investigation. Hypotheses include subtle changes in blood pH (respiratory acidosis) leading to alterations in cerebral blood flow or direct neuronal inhibition. While healthy humans possess robust buffering systems to maintain blood pH, even minor shifts in the acid-base balance within the central nervous system can modulate neuronal excitability [45].

In the context of infection control, these findings create a "double-bind." Strategies that rely solely on filtration (e.g., HEPA purifiers) to mitigate SARS-CoV-2 risk may successfully reduce the viral load (quanta per cubic meter) but fail to remove the metabolically generated CO_2. If a classroom is sealed to conserve energy and outfitted with HEPA units, the air may be "virus-free" but "carbon-rich." Students might be safe from infection but suffer from reduced concentration, fatigue, and impaired learning ability due to CO_2 levels exceeding 2000 ppm—a scenario often observed in schools during winter months [7, 15].

Therefore, the "traffic light" indicators on CO_2 monitors serve a dual purpose. A "red" light (>1500 ppm) warns of two distinct hazards: a high probability of inhaling rebreathed, potentially infectious air (if filtration is absent), and a high probability of cognitive impairment (regardless of filtration). This convergence reinforces the primacy of *dilution*(bringing in fresh air) over *cleaning* (recirculating filtered air) whenever feasible.

5.16 The Illusion of Homogeneity: Spatial Variability and the "Breath Cloud"

The standard models used to estimate infection risk from CO_2 data, such as the Rudnick-Milton equation, rely on the "well-mixed" assumption. They posit that the air in a room is a homogeneous mixture, where the concentration of CO_2 (and by extension, viral aerosols) measured at the sensor on the wall represents the concentration inhaled by every occupant. In reality, the indoor environment is a turbulent seascape of thermal plumes, convective currents, and stagnant zones.

5.16.1 The Short-Range "Bubble"

Recent research has highlighted the danger of the "short-range" zone (within 1.5–2 m of an infector). Li et al. [22] demonstrated that when two people converse, the susceptible person is exposed to a concentrated "jet" of exhaled breath from the infector. This jet contains levels of CO_2 and viral quanta significantly higher than the room average.

If the background ventilation is poor (low air change rate), the jet entrains stagnant, contaminated air, preserving its high concentration over a longer distance. If the background ventilation is high, the jet entrains clean air, diluting the plume more rapidly [22]. A wall-mounted CO_2 sensor reading 800 ppm might suggest a safe environment, but two colleagues talking face-to-face could be exchanging air with a local effective CO_2 concentration of 2000 ppm or higher within their micro-environment. This "proximity penalty" means that global CO_2 metrics underestimate the risk for close-contact interactions.

5.16.2 Stratification and Sensor Placement

Thermal stratification poses another challenge. In rooms with high ceilings or displacement ventilation (where cool air is supplied at the floor and warm air rises), CO_2 and bioaerosols can accumulate in a stratified layer near the ceiling or in the "breathing zone" of standing occupants. Ideally, sensors should be placed within the breathing zone (height of 1.1–1.7 m), away from doors, windows, and supply vents which can artificially lower readings [5, 7].

A common error is placing sensors too close to occupants. A sensor on a teacher's desk, directly in the path of their exhaled breath, will record spikes that reflect the teacher's immediate exhalation rather than the mixed room air. Conversely, a sensor placed near an open window or a supply diffuser will read near-ambient levels (400–450 ppm), masking the accumulation of contaminants in the center of the room. This spatial heterogeneity necessitates a strategic approach to monitoring: in large spaces, multiple sensors may be required to map the "ventilation dead zones" where risk is highest [8].

5.17 The Calibration Conundrum: Ensuring Data Integrity

The utility of CO_2 as a biomarker is entirely dependent on the accuracy of the sensors employed. The rapid proliferation of low-cost monitoring devices during the COVID-19 pandemic has introduced significant data quality issues.

5.17.1 The Drift Problem and ABC Logic

Most non-dispersive infrared (NDIR) sensors, the gold standard for low-cost monitoring, suffer from "drift" over time—the zero-point of the sensor shifts due to aging of the light source or accumulation of dust. To counteract this, manufacturers utilize "automatic baseline correction" (ABC) algorithms. These algorithms assume that the lowest CO_2 reading recorded over a specific period (usually 24 h to 7 days) represents unoccupied, outdoor air (approx. 400 ppm). The sensor automatically resets its zero-point to this lowest value [17, 49].

This logic works well for an office that is vacated every night and on weekends. However, in 24/7 environments like hospitals, nursing homes, or residential dormitories, the building may never be fully vacated, and the indoor CO_2 may never drop to 400 ppm. In a continually occupied hospital ward, the lowest reading over a week might be 600 ppm. The ABC algorithm will erroneously "learn" that 600 ppm is the baseline (400 ppm) and subsequently under-report all future readings by 200 ppm. A reading of 800 ppm (indicating good ventilation) would actually be 1000 ppm (indicating potential risk). In such critical settings, sensors must either have ABC disabled and be manually calibrated, or the facility must ensure periods of vacancy/flushing to allow the algorithm to function correctly [17].

5.17.2 The Outdoor Baseline Variable

Calculations of the rebreathed fraction depend on an accurate value for outdoor CO_2 ($C_{outdoor}$). While 400 ppm is the standard global average often used in textbooks, urban environments frequently exhibit elevated local baselines due to traffic and industrial emissions. In city centers or near busy roadways, outdoor levels can range from 450 to 550 ppm [40].

Using a static value of 400 ppm when the actual outdoor level is 500 ppm leads to an overestimation of the indoor-generated contribution. For example, if indoor CO_2 is 1000 ppm, assuming an outdoor level of 400 ppm implies an indoor contribution of 600 ppm. If the true outdoor level is 500 ppm, the indoor contribution is only 500 ppm. This error affects the calculation of the ventilation rate (Q) and the subsequent infection risk estimates. For precision, "differential" monitoring—measuring both indoor and outdoor levels simultaneously—is the gold standard [5, 7].

5.18 Case Study: The "Perfect Storm" in Schools

Schools represent a unique intersection of high occupant density, extended duration of exposure, and often, antiquated ventilation infrastructure. They provide a compelling case study for the application and limitations of CO_2 monitoring.

5.18.1 The Sawtooth Pattern

In a typical classroom, CO_2 levels exhibit a characteristic "sawtooth" profile. Levels rise rapidly when students enter, peak before breaks, drop during recess (if windows are opened or the room is vacated), and rise again during the next lesson. A study by

Batterman [7] in Michigan schools illustrated that relying on a single "spot check" measurement can be deceptively reassuring. A measurement taken at 8:30 AM might show 700 ppm (Green), while by 10:30 AM, the same room could reach 2000 ppm (Red).

5.18.2 Metabolic Rates and "Super-Emitters"

Children have higher metabolic rates per kilogram of body weight compared to adults, but their lower absolute body mass means they produce less total CO_2 per person. Standard ventilation tables (like in some older codes) account for this. However, the infectious output of children, particularly with variants like Omicron, can be significant. Furthermore, classroom activities such as singing or shouting during play can transiently turn a room of low-emitters into high-emitters of both CO_2 and aerosols. A study in Italian schools found that CO_2 concentrations were strongly correlated with the number of pupils and the classroom volume, confirming that CO_2 acts as a robust distinct marker for crowding and potential viral accumulation [18].

5.18.3 The "Open Window" Paradox

In temperate climates, the most common intervention triggered by a high CO_2 alarm is opening windows. The "Fresh Air" study in UK schools found that teachers often compromised on ventilation to maintain thermal comfort, leading to CO_2 accumulation. This behavioral feedback loop limits the efficacy of passive monitoring; without automated systems (e.g., mechanical ventilation with heat recovery), the "human factor" often overrides the biological imperative [52].

In summary, measuring the invisible requires a sophisticated understanding of both the instrument and the environment. CO_2 is not a simple "virus detector," but a dynamic variable that reflects the complex interaction of physiology, physics, and human behavior. When interpreted with an awareness of its limitations—spatial heterogeneity, sensor drift, and the decoupling effect of filtration—it remains the most accessible and powerful tool we have for making the invisible risk of airborne transmission visible.

5.19 The Metabolic Variable: Activity, Vocalization, and the Limits of the Proxy

While carbon dioxide (CO_2) is an excellent tracer for exhaled breath, its utility as a proxy for *infectious* aerosols relies on the assumption that the ratio between exhaled CO_2 and exhaled viral particles remains roughly constant. This assumption holds reasonably well for sedentary activities like office work or quiet classroom study.

However, human physiology introduces a critical non-linearity when activity levels change, creating scenarios where a "safe" CO_2 reading may mask a dangerous viral exposure.

5.19.1 The Physiology of Generation: METs and Emission

The rate of CO_2 generation (G_{CO2}) is a function of the basal metabolic rate and the intensity of physical activity, measured in metabolic equivalents of task (METs). A person sitting quietly (1.0–1.3 METs) generates relatively little CO_2. However, engaging in moderate exercise (3–6 METs) or heavy exertion (>6 METs) drastically increases oxygen consumption and CO_2 production [38].

If a ventilation system is controlled by a CO_2 sensor (demand-controlled ventilation, or DCV), it will ramp up the supply of fresh air as the occupants exercise to maintain the setpoint (e.g., 1000 ppm). In theory, this increased ventilation should also dilute any airborne pathogens. However, this linear compensation fails to account for the disproportionate increase in aerosol emission associated with certain activities.

5.19.2 The "Singing Paradox": When CO_2 Underestimates Risk

Research indicates that while CO_2 production scales linearly with metabolic activity, aerosol emission can scale exponentially with vocalization loudness and respiratory force. Speaking loudly releases approximately 10 times more aerosol particles than breathing; singing or shouting can release 50–100 times more [4, 27].

Consider a choir practice. The singers might increase their metabolic rate (and CO_2 production) by a factor of 2 compared to resting. A ventilation system might double the airflow to keep CO_2 steady at 800 ppm. However, because the singers are vocalizing, their *viral aerosol* emission might have increased by a factor of 50. The ventilation system has compensated for the carbon dioxide, but it may not have been compensated for the virus. In such high-emission scenarios, the "safe" threshold for CO_2 must be lowered drastically, or supplementary air cleaning (which removes virus but not CO_2) must be employed to bridge the gap [26, 36]. This phenomenon explains why super-spreading events frequently occur in choirs, bars, and gyms, even when ventilation appears nominally adequate by standard building codes.

5.20 The Energy-Health Nexus: Tight Buildings and the CO_2 Trap

The history of indoor CO_2 levels is inextricably linked to the history of energy conservation. Following the 1973 oil embargo, the building sector underwent a radical transformation aimed at reducing thermal losses. This era gave birth to the "tight building"—structures sealed to prevent air infiltration, relying entirely on mechanical ventilation which was often throttled down to minimum levels to save fuel [50].

5.20.1 The Legacy of the 1980s Standards

As discussed in previous sections, this drive for efficiency led international agencies in the west to lower minimum ventilation rates in 1981 to 2.5 L/s/person (5 cfm), a level now known to be insufficient for diluting bioeffluents and pathogens. This reduction is widely cited as the primary driver for the emergence of "sick building syndrome" (SBS), a condition characterized by non-specific symptoms (headache, fatigue, mucosal irritation) that correlate strongly with elevated CO_2 and low ventilation rates (Lyles et al. 1991; [20, 47]).

Although standards were subsequently raised, the tension remains. Modern "Green" building certifications often prioritize energy efficiency. While they include IAQ credits, the incentive structure has historically favored energy savings. This creates a "Green Building Paradox" where a building may be carbon-neutral in terms of emissions to the atmosphere, but "carbon-toxic" to its occupants due to accumulated metabolic CO_2 and associated indoor pollutants [2].

5.20.2 Demand-Controlled Ventilation (DCV): Friend or Foe?

To resolve the energy-health conflict, modern HVAC systems increasingly utilize demand-controlled ventilation (DCV). These systems use CO_2 sensors to estimate occupancy and modulate air intake: if the room is empty or sparsely populated (low CO_2), the system reduces outdoor air supply to save energy [17].

While efficient, DCV poses a specific risk during a pandemic. If a single infectious individual enters a large conference room, they will generate insufficient CO_2 to trigger the system to ramp up. The ventilation remains at its minimum setting, allowing the viral concentration in the *local* breathing zone to rise, even if the *average* room CO_2 is low. Furthermore, many DCV sensors are prone to drift or calibration errors. Fisk et al. [17] found that a significant proportion of deployed CO_2 sensors had errors large enough to adversely impact ventilation rates. During outbreaks, guidance often suggests disabling DCV or changing the setpoints to maintain maximum airflow regardless of occupancy, effectively sacrificing energy efficiency for biological safety [11, 12, 41].

5.21 The Diagnostic Power of CO_2: Identifying the "Performance Gap"

Perhaps the greatest value of widespread CO_2 monitoring is its ability to reveal the "performance gap"—the discrepancy between how a building was designed to perform and how it actually operates.

5.21.1 Design vs. Reality

Building blueprints assume specific occupancy densities and ventilation rates. In reality, classrooms designed for 20 students often hold 30; meeting rooms designed for brief occupancy are used for hour-long sessions; and intake dampers break or are manually closed by maintenance staff to fix temperature complaints or save money [7, 24].

CO_2 acts as a "truth serum" for the building. A study in California schools found that despite having mechanical units capable of meeting standards, many were turned off or malfunctioning, leading to CO_2 levels exceeding 1500 ppm in a significant fraction of classrooms [7, 25]. Without sensors, these failures remain invisible. With sensors, the failure becomes quantifiable data.

5.21.2 Continuous Commissioning

The deployment of networked IoT (Internet of Things) CO_2 sensors allows for "continuous commissioning." Instead of balancing the ventilation system once every 5 years, facility managers can identify trends: a spike in CO_2 in the east wing every Tuesday afternoon indicates a scheduling conflict or a damper failure. This data-driven approach shifts ventilation from a static setting to a dynamic response, ensuring that the "lungs" of the building are actually breathing when the occupants need them to [11, 12, 17].

In the final section of this chapter, we will synthesize these findings into a practical framework for implementing CO_2 monitoring strategies in the post-pandemic era, addressing the legal, economic, and behavioral dimensions of making indoor air quality visible.

5.22 A Practical Framework for Implementation: From Theory to Protocol

Moving from the theoretical understanding of carbon dioxide (CO_2) as a risk proxy to its practical deployment requires a standardized protocol. In the absence of rigorous deployment strategies, data can be noisy, misleading, or manipulated. Recent deliberations by expert committees, such as the Joint Committee for Indoor Air Quality Management constituted by the Central Pollution Control Board (CPCB) of India, have begun to crystallize these protocols into actionable guidelines for public spaces [11–13].

5.22.1 The "Goldilocks" Zone for Sensor Placement

The placement of a CO_2 sensor is critical for obtaining a representative sample of the air that occupants are actually breathing. If placed too close to a supply vent, the sensor reads fresh air and underestimates risk. If placed in a stagnant corner or next to a breathing occupant, it overestimates risk. Based on consensus guidelines, the following placement protocols are recommended [11, 12]:

- *Height:* Sensors should be mounted within the "breathing zone," typically 1.1–1.7 m above the floor. Ceiling mounts often read lower concentrations due to stratification and proximity to extraction vents, while floor placement risks damage and dust interference (Mena et al. 2022).
- *Distance from Apertures:* Sensors must be at least 0.5 m away from corners or windows and not within 2 m of doors to avoid drafts that dilute the local concentration.
- *Distance from Occupants:* A critical buffer zone is required. Sensors should be at least 1–2 m away from walls, partitions, and permanent workstations to avoid measuring the direct exhalation plume of a specific individual.
- *Source Avoidance:* Sensors should be kept at least 1 meter away from localized sources of heat or emissions, such as photocopiers or coffee machines, which can disrupt airflow patterns or generate interfering gases [11, 12].

5.22.2 Sampling Duration and Frequency

Spot measurements are insufficient for capturing the dynamic risk profile of a shared space. A classroom might have low CO_2 at 8:00 AM but reach hazardous levels by 11:00 AM. Therefore, guidelines increasingly recommend continuous monitoring, or at minimum, 24-h monitoring cycles that capture both peak occupancy and background levels. The CPCB interim guidelines suggest monitoring covering two seasons (summer and winter) to account for variations in HVAC usage and natural ventilation habits [11, 12]. For routine safety, sampling should occur during peak occupancy hours (e.g., mid-morning and mid-afternoon for schools/offices) to capture the "worst-case" scenario.

5.23 The Policy Landscape: Moving from Recommendations to Regulation

For decades, indoor air quality (IAQ) has been the "Cinderella" of environmental policy—acknowledged but largely unregulated compared to outdoor air. However, the paradigm is shifting. The recognition that "building owners are responsible for building maintenance and services," as codified in documents like the National Building Code (NBC) of India (2016), establishes a liability framework [11, 12].

5.23.1 The Role of Green Building Ratings

Voluntary certifications/green building certifications have historically driven IAQ improvements. The integration of real-time CO_2 monitoring into these certification standards moves IAQ from a design-phase calculation to an operational performance metric. This shifts the focus from *how the building was built* to *how the building is breathing* right now.

5.23.2 Legal Liability and "Safe Workplaces"

In the post-pandemic era, the failure to provide adequate ventilation may increasingly be viewed as a failure to provide a safe working environment. Just as employers must protect workers from chemical hazards or falls, the accumulation of metabolic CO_2 beyond recommended limits (e.g., >1000 ppm) serves as documented evidence of insufficient ventilation. This data could potentially be used in litigation regarding workplace transmission of airborne diseases, pressing facility managers to maintain rigorous documentation of air quality metrics [11, 12, 29].

5.24 The Future: Smart Buildings and the "Digital Twin"

The future of CO_2 monitoring lies in its integration with the Internet of Things (IoT) and Artificial Intelligence (AI). We are moving toward "Intelligent Indoor Environment Monitoring and Management Systems" (IIEMMS) where sensors do not just record data but drive building behavior [53, 54].

5.24.1 Occupancy-Driven Ventilation

CO_2 sensors are increasingly used as proxies for occupancy detection. Mena et al. (2022) reviewed the deployment of environmental sensors and found that CO_2 levels, often combined with temperature and humidity data, can accurately predict the number of occupants in a room. In a "smart" building, this data feeds into the Building Management System (BMS). If the CO_2 rises because five extra people entered a conference room, the BMS algorithms automatically ramp up the ventilation rate or activate supplementary air cleaners in that specific zone. This "demand-control ventilation" (DCV) acts in reverse of its traditional energy-saving mode; instead of reducing air when people leave, it aggressively purges air when people arrive, prioritizing biological safety (Mena et al. 2022).

5.24.2 The "Visible" Building

Perhaps the most transformative change is the democratization of data. New standards advocate for the public display of IAQ metrics. Just as restaurants display hygiene ratings, buildings of the future may display real-time "Air Quality Indices" in lobbies or via apps. This transparency empowers occupants to make informed decisions—choosing to avoid a crowded gym or a stuffy cafe based on the visible CO_2 reading. This behavioral feedback loop creates market pressure for building operators to maintain high-quality indoor environments [29, 53, 54].

5.25 Conclusion: The Proxy Paradox

We conclude this chapter by acknowledging the "Proxy Paradox." Carbon dioxide is simultaneously the best and the most flawed tool we have for infection control.

It is *flawed* because it is not a pathogen. A room can have low CO_2 but high viral load if a super-spreader is singing in a corner [22]. It can have high CO_2 but low viral load if HEPA filters are scrubbing the air clean of particulates [31]. It is a bulk metric that often does not fully capture the dangerous "near-field" transmission between two people talking face-to-face [22].

Yet, it is *the best tool* because it is affordable, ubiquitous, and biologically grounded. It makes the invisible fluid of indoor air visible. It provides a tangible, real-time metric for the nebulous concept of "ventilation." A CO_2 monitor acts as a speedometer for the building's respiratory system, warning us when the air is stagnant and the risk is rising.

Ultimately, CO_2 monitoring is not a "silver bullet", but it is the "essential flashlight" in the dark room of indoor transmission. By understanding its physiology, physics, and limitations, we can use this simple molecule to engineer safer, healthier, and more resilient indoor environments for a world where airborne threats are an enduring reality.

Acknowledgments Many thanks to Dr Rohit Kumar and Manojkumar S. The authors acknowledge the support provided by the institutions including School of Planning and Architecture, New Delhi, Drexel University, and All India Institute of Medical Sciences, New Delhi. Special thanks to Rajshekhar Pullabhatla and Group Captain P Aanand Naidu of ISAC Centre for Built Environment Policy and Tathatara Foundation. Many thanks to all the people who supported this work in many ways. Special thanks to Arthur L Frank.

Declarations The authors Raja Singh, Nirupam Madaan, and Anil Dewan declare no conflict of interests or competing interests in this work. There is no involvement of human participants, animals, human or animal tissue. All authors declare that there was no specific financial support received from any organization for the submitted work. All authors declare that they have no financial relationships at present or within the previous 3 years with any organizations that might have an interest in the submitted work. While all care has been taken in ensuring the accuracy of this work, any inadvertent error may be reported at the earliest. The authors acknowledge the use of supervised language learning models/large language models for enhancement of the work, with responsibility lying with the authors. For more information, the corresponding author may be contacted at email rajaresearch@proton.me.

CRediT Statement The following is the CRediT statement which declares the author credits for this chapter:

Raja Singh: Conceptualization, Methodology, Formal Analysis, Investigation, Data Curation, Writing-Original Draft, Writing-Review & Editing, Visualization, Project Administration.
Nirupam Madaan: Conceptualization, Resources, Validation, Supervision, Project Administration
Anil Dewan: Resources, Validation Supervision.

References

1. ACGIH. Documentation of the threshold limit values and biological exposure indices. American Conference of Governmental Industrial Hygienists; 1991.
2. Allen JG, MacNaughton P, Satish U, Santanam S, Vallarino J, Spengler JD. Associations of cognitive function scores with carbon dioxide, ventilation, and volatile organic compound exposures in office workers: a controlled exposure study of green and conventional office environments. Environ Health Perspect. 2016;124(6):805–12.
3. Apte MG, Fisk WJ, Daisey JM. Associations between indoor CO_2 concentrations and sick building syndrome symptoms in US office buildings: an analysis of the 1994–1996 BASE study data. Indoor Air. 2000;10(4):246–57.
4. Asadi S, Wexler AS, Cappa CD, Barreda S, Bouvier NM, Ristenpart WD. Aerosol emission and superemission during human speech increase with voice loudness. Sci Rep. 2019;9(1):2348.
5. ASTM. Standard guide for using indoor carbon dioxide concentrations to evaluate indoor air quality and ventilation (D6245-18). ASTM International; 2018.
6. Azimi P, Stephens B. HVAC filtration for controlling infectious airborne disease transmission in indoor environments: predicting risk reductions and operational costs. Build Environ. 2013;70:150–60.
7. Batterman S. Review and extension of CO_2-based methods to determine ventilation rates with application to school classrooms. Int J Environ Res Public Health. 2017;14(2):145.
8. Bhattacharya A, Pantelic J, Ghahramani A, Mousavi ES. Assessment of indoor air quality and its biological impacts in the era of COVID-19. Front Built Environ. 2021;7:723460.
9. Buonanno G, Stabile L, Morawska L. Estimation of airborne viral emission: quanta emission rate of SARS-CoV-2 for infection risk assessment. Environ Int. 2020;141:105794.
10. Centres for Disease Control and Prevention (CDC). Guidelines for preventing the transmission of Mycobacterium tuberculosis in health-care settings, 2005. MMWR Recomm Rep. 2005;54(RR-17):1–141.
11. CPCB (Central Pollution Control Board). Report of the Joint committee on indoor air quality management. Ministry of Environment, Forest & Climate Change, Government of India; 2022a.
12. CPCB (Central Pollution Control Board). Minutes of the meetings of the Joint Committee for Indoor Air Quality (IAQ) Management. Government of India; 2022b.
13. CPCB (Central Pollution Control Board). Minutes of the Fifth meeting of the Joint Committee for Indoor Air Quality (IAQ) Management held on March 13, 2023. Government of India; 2023.
14. Du CR, Wang SC, Yu MC, Chiu TF, Wang JY, Chuang PC, et al. Effect of ventilation improvement during a tuberculosis outbreak in underventilated university buildings. Indoor Air. 2019;30(3):422–32.
15. Fisk WJ. The ventilation problem in schools: literature review. Indoor Air. 2017;27(6):1039–51.
16. Fisk WJ, Faulkner D, Palonen J, Seppanen O. Performance and costs of particle air filtration technologies. Indoor Air. 2002;12(4):223–34.
17. Fisk WJ, Mirer AG, Mendell MJ. Do indoor CO_2 sensors for demand-controlled ventilation measure accurate concentrations? ASHRAE Trans. 2010;116(2):162.
18. Gaeta MG, Ropolo M, Pelone F, Gargiulo P, Ricciardi W. Air quality in schools: a systematic review. Ann Ig. 2021;33(3):205–24.
19. Hammond A, Khalid T, Thornton HV, Woodall CA, Hay AD. Should homes and workplaces purchase portable air filters to reduce the transmission of SARS-CoV-2 and other respiratory infections? A systematic review. PLoS ONE. 2021;16(4):e0251049.

20. Hodgson M. Indoor environmental exposures and symptoms. Environ Health Perspect. 2002;110(Suppl 4):663–7.
21. Kurnitski J. Ventilation rate and room size effects on infection risk of COVID-19. REHVA J. 2020;57(3):26–31.
22. Li Y, Cheng P, Jia W. Poor ventilation worsens short-range airborne transmission of respiratory infection. Indoor Air. 2021;32:e12946.
23. Li Y, Leung GM, Tang JW, Yang X, Chao CYH, Lin JZ, et al. Role of ventilation in airborne transmission of infectious agents in the built environment—a multidisciplinary systematic review. Indoor Air. 2007;17(1):2–18.
24. Mendell MJ. Non-specific symptoms in office workers: a review and summary of the literature. Indoor Air. 1993;3(4):227–36.
25. Mendell MJ, Eliseeva EA, Davies MM, Spears M, Lobscheid A, Fisk WJ, Apte MG. Association of classroom ventilation with reduced illness absence: a prospective study in California elementary schools. Indoor Air. 2013;23(6):515–28.
26. Miller SL, Nazaroff WW, Jimenez JL, Boerstra A, Buonanno G, Dancer SJ, et al. Transmission of SARS-CoV-2 by inhalation of respiratory aerosol in the Skagit Valley Chorale superspreading event. Indoor Air. 2021;31(2):314–23.
27. Morawska L, Johnson GR, Ristovski ZD, Hargreaves M, Mengersen K, Corbett S, et al. Size distribution and sites of origin of droplets expelled from the human respiratory tract during expiratory activities. J Aerosol Sci. 2009;40(3):256–69.
28. Morawska L, Tang JW, Bahnfleth W, Bluyssen PM, Boerstra A, Buonanno G, et al. How can airborne transmission of COVID-19 indoors be minimised? Environ Int. 2020;142:105832.
29. Nair AN, Anand P, George A, Mondal N. A review of strategies and their effectiveness in reducing indoor airborne transmission and improving indoor air quality. Environ Res. 2022;213:113579.
30. Nardell EA. Indoor environmental control of tuberculosis and other airborne infections. Indoor Air. 2016;26(1):79–87.
31. Nardell EA. Air disinfection for airborne infection control with a focus on COVID-19: why germicidal UV is essential. Photochem Photobiol. 2021;97(3):493–7.
32. Nardell EA, Keegan J, Cheney SA, Etkind SC. Airborne infection. Theoretical limits of protection achievable by building ventilation. Am Rev Respir Dis. 1991;144(2):302–6.
33. Nathavitharana RR, Rylance J, Nardell E, Lederer P. CO_2 levels may predict TB infection risk. Clin Infect Dis. 2022;75(8):1297–306.
34. Ng DKT, Du H, Singh N. CMOS-compatible mid-infrared ScAlN-based pyroelectric detectors for NDIR CO_2 gas sensing. Sensors. 2020;20(2):376.
35. Ou C, Hu S, Luo K, Yang H, Hang J, Cheng P, et al. Insufficient ventilation led to a probable long-range airborne transmission of SARS-CoV-2 on two buses. Build Environ. 2022;207:108414.
36. Peng Z, Jimenez JL. Exhaled CO_2 as a COVID-19 infection risk proxy for different indoor environments and activities. Environ Sci Technol Lett. 2021;8(5):392–7.
37. Persily A. Challenges in developing ventilation and indoor air quality standards: the story of ASHRAE Standard 62. Build Environ. 2015;91:61–9.
38. Persily A, de Jonge L. Carbon dioxide generation rates for building occupants. Indoor Air. 2017;27(5):868–79.
39. Pettenkofer MV. Über den Luftwechsel in Wohngebäuden. Cotta; 1858.
40. Prill R, Fisk WJ, Turk BH. Evaluation of sensor-based demand controlled ventilation in an office building. Proc ACEEE Summer Study Energy Efficiency Build. 2000;3:289–300.
41. REHVA. REHVA COVID-19 guidance document: how to operate and use building services in order to prevent the spread of the coronavirus disease (COVID-19) in workplaces. Federation of European Heating, Ventilation and Air Conditioning Associations; 2020.
42. Richardson ET, Morrow CD, Kalil DB, Bekker LG, Wood R. Shared air: a renewed focus on ventilation for the prevention of tuberculosis transmission. PLoS ONE. 2014;9(5):e96334.
43. Riley EC, Murphy G, Riley RL. Airborne spread of measles in a suburban elementary school. Am J Epidemiol. 1978;107(5):421–32.

44. Rudnick SN, Milton DK. Risk of indoor airborne infection transmission estimated from carbon dioxide concentration. Indoor Air. 2003;13(3):237–45.
45. Satish U, Mendell MJ, Shekhar K, Hotchi T, Sullivan D, Streufert S, Fisk WJ. Is CO_2 an indoor pollutant? Direct effects of low-to-moderate CO_2 concentrations on human decision-making performance. Environ Health Perspect. 2012;120(12):1671–7.
46. Schuettler T, Waurick I, Hinz B, Gerhards C. Particle decay in public transportation: a field study in trams in Germany. Sci Rep. 2022;12:1–10.
47. Seppänen OA, Fisk WJ, Mendell MJ. Association of ventilation rates and CO_2 concentrations with health and other responses in commercial and institutional buildings. Indoor Air. 1999;9(4):226–52.
48. Shen Y, Li C, Dong H, Wang Z, Martinez L, Sun Z, et al. Community outbreak investigation of SARS-CoV-2 transmission among bus riders in eastern China. JAMA Intern Med. 2020;180(12):1665–71.
49. Shrestha PM, Humphrey JL, Carlton EJ, Adgate JL, Barton KE, Root ED, Miller SL. Impact of outdoor air pollution on indoor air quality in low-income homes during wildfire seasons. Int J Environ Res Public Health. 2019;16(19):3535.
50. Sundell J, Levin H, Nazaroff WW, Cain WS, Fisk WJ, Grimsrud DT, et al. Ventilation rates and health: multidisciplinary review of the scientific literature. Indoor Air. 2011;21(3):191–204.
51. Tran VV, Park D, Lee YC. Indoor air pollution, related human diseases, and recent trends in the control and improvement of indoor air quality. Int J Environ Res Public Health. 2020;17(8):2927.
52. Viner RM, Waddington C, Mytton OT, Booy R, Ho ZJ, Kinra S. Transmission of SARS-CoV-2 by children and young people in households and schools: a meta-analysis of population-based and contact-tracing studies. J Infect. 2022;84(3):361–82.
53. Wiryasaputra R, Yu CT, Lee PY, Kim E. Indoor air monitoring system with CO_2 prediction for COVID-19 risk mitigation. Front Public Health. 2022a;10:1022055.
54. Wiryasaputra R, Huang CY, Kristiani E, Liu PY, Yeh TK, Yang CT. Review of an intelligent indoor environment monitoring and management system for COVID-19 risk mitigation. Front Public Health. 2022b;10:894958.
55. Yang L, Iwami M, Chen Y, Wu M, van Dam KH. Computational decision-support tools for urban design to improve resilience against COVID-19 and other infectious diseases: a systematic review. Prog Plan. 2022:100657.
56. Yaglou CP, Riley EC, Coggins DI. Ventilation requirements. ASHVE Trans. 1936;42:133–62.

Recommendations for Indian Public Buildings

6

Raja Singh, Nirupam Madaan, and Anil Dewan

6.1 Introduction: The Silent Crisis in the Subcontinent

In the bustling metropolises of India—from the humid, coastal sprawl of Chennai to the smog-laden winters of Delhi—a silent physiological battle is being waged every day. It occurs not on the traffic-choked streets, which have long dominated the discourse on air pollution, but inside the glass-and-concrete monoliths that define modern urban India. As millions of citizens seek refuge from the heat and outdoor pollution within malls, corporate offices, schools, and hospitals, they enter an environment that has, until very recently, operated in a regulatory vacuum.

For decades, the Indian narrative on air quality was exclusively outdoors. The National Ambient Air Quality Standards (NAAQS) monitored the pollutants in the streets, yet the air within—where urban Indians spend nearly 90% of their time—remained largely unmonitored and unregulated. This chapter marks a departure from the universal principles discussed in previous chapters to focus specifically on the Indian context. This focus is necessitated not only by India's unique climatic and demographic challenges but by a landmark shift in legal and scientific policy precipitated by the COVID-19 pandemic and citizen activism.

We are witnessing a paradigm shift. The Indian building sector is moving from a seemingly singular obsession with energy efficiency (often achieved by sealing

R. Singh
Founder/Researcher, The Built, New Delhi, Delhi, India

Former Post Doctoral Fellow, Department of Environmental and Occupational Health, Dornsife School of Public Health, Drexel University, Philadelphia, Pennsylvania, USA

N. Madaan
Department of Hospital Administration, All India Institute of Medical Sciences, New Delhi, Delhi, India

A. Dewan
Department of Architecture, School of Planning and Architecture, New Delhi, Delhi, India

R. Singh et al., *Infection Control in the Everyday Built Environment*,
https://doi.org/10.1007/978-981-95-8624-0_6

buildings tightly) to a more holistic requirement for *infection resilience* and *indoor environmental quality (IEQ)*. This chapter narrates the genesis of this shift, analyzing the recent interventions by the National Green Tribunal (NGT), the formation of the Central Pollution Control Board (CPCB) Joint Committee, and the scientific rationale behind the newly proposed interim guidelines for Indian public spaces.

6.2 The Unique Challenge of the Indian Built Environment

To understand why specific recommendations are needed for India, distinct from Western standards like ASHRAE (USA) or REHVA (Europe), one must appreciate the specific conditions of the Indian built environment.

6.2.1 The Density Factor and the Wells-Riley Equation

The first challenge is occupant density. Indian public spaces—particularly transport hubs, hospitals, and educational institutions—operate at occupant densities significantly higher than those assumed in standard Western ventilation models. As established in Chap. 2, the risk of airborne infection is governed by the Wells-Riley equation, where the probability of infection (P) is a function of the number of infectors (I), the quanta generation rate (q), pulmonary ventilation rate (p), exposure time (t), and the volume of clean air (Q):

$$P = 1 - e \wedge \left\{ -\left(\left(I \bullet q \bullet p \bullet t \right) / Q \right) \right\}$$

In the Indian context, the variable S (number of susceptible individuals) per unit volume is exceptionally high. When a metro station in Mumbai or a waiting room in a government hospital in Kolkata is packed to capacity, the "rebreathed air fraction" skyrockets. A ventilation rate of 10 L/s/person, which might be sufficient for a sparsely populated office in Scandinavia, becomes woefully inadequate in a densely packed Indian classroom where the aggregate CO_2 generation outpaces the HVAC system's dilution capacity [25]. The CPCB's Joint Committee explicitly recognized this, noting that CO_2 levels increase synchronously with human presence and serve as a critical surrogate index for ventilation and infection risk [8].

6.2.2 The Outdoor Air Paradox

The second challenge is the quality of the "fresh" air. Standard dilution ventilation assumes that outdoor air is clean. However, in many Indian cities, the outdoor air frequently contains particulate matter ($PM_{2.5}$ and PM_{10}) at concentrations far exceeding WHO guidelines [32]. Ventilating a building by simply opening windows (natural ventilation) in Delhi during November might dilute viral aerosols but simultaneously introduce hazardous levels of combustion byproducts, creating a "double burden" of disease [17]. This necessitates a complex strategy involving hybrid ventilation and heavy filtration, differing from regions with pristine outdoor air. But, most Indian small towns and the rural areas may not have this issue and the practices of the polluted cities may be copied by them without realising that in such situations opening the window may be feasible.

6.2.3 Empirical Validation: What Actually Exists in Indian Buildings

While the preceding sections describe the theoretical and regulatory challenges of the Indian built environment, it is equally important to examine the empirical reality of HVAC and ventilation systems actually deployed in Indian public buildings. To address this gap, the author conducted a series of structured empirical investigations across four categories of Indian public buildings using the Right to Information Act (RTI), 2005 as a formal research instrument.

This methodology enabled the collection of authenticated technical data directly from public authorities responsible for building operations, including details of HVAC typology, presence of fresh air intake, filtration specifications, ultraviolet disinfection, and carbon dioxide monitoring. The studies covered airports, premier educational institutions, mass congregational buildings, and nationally significant administrative buildings.

This approach transforms IAQ research in India from speculative commentary into evidence-based assessment grounded in officially disclosed engineering data.

6.3 The Legal Awakening: The National Green Tribunal Intervention

The genesis of formal indoor air quality (IAQ) guidelines in India is rooted in judicial activism. The narrative begins with two critical legal applications filed before the National Green Tribunal (NGT), the apex judicial body for environmental disputes in India.

6.3.1 OA No. 143/2016 and OA No. 206/2022

The first case, *Dileep Nevatia vs. Union of India* (OA No. 143/2016), sets the stage by arguing that indoor air pollution (IAP) is as serious as outdoor air pollution (OAP). The applicant presented evidence that IAP causes premature deaths due to pneumonia, chronic obstructive pulmonary disease (COPD), and lung cancer, disproportionately affecting women and children [8].

This was followed by *Raja Singh vs. Union of India* (OA No. 206/2022). The applicant in this case argued a profound legal point: that large public buildings are "public places" and thus the air quality within them should be regulated under the Air (Prevention and Control of Pollution) Act, 1981. The applicant contended that sealing buildings and recirculating air through ACs without adequate fresh air intake facilitates the spread of airborne infections like COVID-19 and tuberculosis. They demanded enforceable provisions for window design, CO_2 monitoring, and responsible use of air conditioners [8].

6.3.2 The NGT Verdict: Extending the "Air Act" Indoors

In a historic order dated April 19, 2022, the NGT acknowledged the gravity of the situation. The Tribunal noted that while the Bureau of Indian Standards (BIS) had norms in the National Building Code (NBC), there was a lack of specific, enforceable standards for indoor air pollutants in public spaces. The NGT ruled that "a case is made out for a direction to evolve an appropriate mechanism… to work out appropriate standards and protocols for indoor air quality for safeguarding public health at Public places" [8].

Crucially, the NGT defined "public place" referencing the Noise Pollution (Regulation and Control) Rules, 2000, to include:

- Auditoriums and Cinema Halls
- Hotels and Restaurants
- Public Waiting Rooms and Convention Centres
- Shopping Malls
- Educational Institutions and Libraries
- Public Offices

This judicial order effectively brought the indoor environment of these facilities under the purview of environmental regulation, mandating the formation of a Joint Committee to draft the roadmap for Indian IAQ standards [8].

6.4 The Joint Committee on Indoor Air Quality Management

In compliance with the NGT directive, the Central Pollution Control Board (CPCB) constituted a high-level Joint Committee. The composition of this committee reflects the interdisciplinary nature of the problem, bringing together engineering, medical, and environmental experts.

6.4.1 Composition and Mandate

The committee was chaired by the Member Secretary of the CPCB and included representatives from:

- *Ministry of Environment, Forest and Climate Change (MoEF&CC)*
- *Ministry of Housing and Urban Affairs (MoHUA):* Responsible for building by-laws.
- *Ministry of Health and Family Welfare (MoH&FW)/National Centre for Disease Control (NCDC):* Providing the health and epidemiological perspective.
- *Council of Scientific and Industrial Research (CSIR):* Providing scientific R&D inputs.
- *Bureau of Indian Standards (BIS):* The body responsible for the National Building Code.
- *Academic Experts:* From IIT Delhi, ICMR, and others.

The committee's mandate was to evolve appropriate mechanisms, standards, and protocols. However, during their deliberations (specifically the first meeting on May 19, 2022), the committee recognized a critical data gap. Unlike the robust datasets available for outdoor air, India lacked a comprehensive, long-term database of indoor air pollutants across different climatic zones and building types [8]. Consequently, they decided to adopt a phased approach: first, to release "Interim Guidelines" based on a literature review and international best practices, and second, to commission a long-term monitoring study to establish definitive "Guide Values" or standards [9, 10].

6.5 The Pollutants of Concern for India

One of the first tasks of the Joint Committee was to identify which pollutants required immediate attention in Indian public buildings. This selection process, detailed in the committee's report, offers insight into the specific chemical and biological hazards prioritized by Indian regulators.

The committee categorized pollutants into two primary groups based on their origin [8]:

1. *Indoor Source Pollutants:* Generated by occupant activities, building materials, and furnishings.
2. *Infiltration Pollutants:* Entering from the outdoor environment due to air exchange.

6.5.1 Priority Parameters

After reviewing guidelines from the WHO, US EPA, and other bodies, the committee shortlisted the following parameters for the interim guidelines and the proposed long-term study:

- *Particulate Matter ($PM_{2.5}$ and PM_{10}):* Included because of the high outdoor load in Indian cities and indoor sources like cleaning and dust resuspension.
- *Carbon Dioxide (CO_2):* Accepted as the primary surrogate for ventilation adequacy and human bioeffluent accumulation. High CO_2 indicates overcrowding and poor air change rates, directly correlating with infection risk [8, 30].
- *Carbon Monoxide (CO):* A critical pollutant in spaces with combustion sources, particularly relevant for malls with food courts and hotels [8].
- *Total Volatile Organic Compounds (TVOCs):* Derived from paints, varnishes, cleaning agents, and sanitizers—the use of which increased dramatically during the pandemic [8].
- *Formaldehyde (HCHO):* A known carcinogen emitted by plywood, particleboard, and other composite wood products heavily used in Indian interiors [8].
- *Ozone (O_3):* Included due to its presence in outdoor air and emission from certain office equipment like photocopiers [8].

6.5.2 Excluded

Parameters (For Now) Notably, the committee decided *not* to set standards for radon, biological contaminants, sulfur dioxide (SO_2), and nitrogen dioxide (NO_2) in the initial phase.

- *Radon:* It was argued that radon presence is largely due to construction deficiencies (cracks in piling/foundation) and geological factors, which are difficult to control via standard retrofits. It was relegated to R&D studies [9, 10].
- *Biological Contaminants:* While acknowledging their health impact, the committee noted that these are "complex pollutants." Instead of setting a numerical limit (e.g., CFU per cubic meter), they focused on controlling the *factors* that promote biological growth, specifically dampness and inadequate ventilation [8].
- *SO_2 and NO_2:* The committee concluded that indoor sources for these are not a major concern in most public places in India, unlike residential settings where biomass cooking might occur [9, 10].

6.6 Source Attribution in Indian Public Spaces

To effectively manage IAQ, one must identify the specific sources within different building typologies. The Joint Committee provided a matrix of likely emission sources for different public places, which serves as a diagnostic tool for building managers [8].

- *Malls:* The primary sources identified were cooking activities in food courts (generating CO and PM) and the extensive use of cleaning products and air fresheners (generating TVOCs).

- *Hospitals:* Sources include laboratory consumables, potent disinfectants/cleaning agents (TVOCs), and alcohol-based products like sanitizers. The committee specifically noted the risk of cross-infection in corridors and waiting areas [8].
- *Cinemas/Auditoriums:* The primary pollutants here are TVOCs off-gassing from interior wood products, heavy acoustic furnishings, and carpets.
- *Airports:* Similar to cinemas, formaldehyde from plywood/fiberboard and TVOCs from furnishings are key concerns.
- *Educational Institutions:* Laboratories (chemicals) and canteens (cooking) were identified as specific hotspots, alongside the general bioeffluent load from high student density [8].

This source attribution is critical because it dictates the mitigation strategy. For a cinema hall, increasing ventilation to flush out TVOCs from carpets is the priority. For a hospital, filtration to remove pathogens and chemical neutralization of disinfectants takes precedence.

6.7 The Shift from Energy to Health: A Critique of Green Ratings

A significant aspect of the NGT proceedings was the examination of existing Green Building Rating Systems. The applicant in *Raja Singh vs. MoHUA* (OA No. 466/2022) argued that the current regulatory mechanism for green buildings needs to be expanded. While these ratings incentivize energy efficiency (through FAR/FSI bonuses), these systems need regulation, and further to note is that these may have historically and inadvertently encouraged "tight" buildings with poor air exchange to save cooling costs [8].

The committee noted that while existing codes (NBC 2016) do have ventilation provisions, the *enforcement* and *performance monitoring* of these provisions in terms of actual human health outcomes may have been lacking. The committee suggested that the regulation of the green building rating industry is a policy matter for the Ministry of New and Renewable Energy (MNRE) and MoHUA [9, 10].

6.8 Scientific Foundations of the Interim Guidelines

The "Interim Guidelines for Indoor Air Quality Management in Public Places" released, (to the applicant/first author under RTI) by the committee are built upon a synthesis of global literature (WHO, US EPA) and the specific constraints of the Indian infrastructure. They are designed as a set of "DOs and DON'Ts" to be implemented by building owners immediately, even before final numerical standards are gazetted.

6.8.1 Ventilation and Air Conditioning

The guidelines reinforce the National Building Code (NBC) 2016 (Part 8, Section 3) as the baseline for ventilation rates. However, they introduce crucial modifications for the post-pandemic era:

- *Dilution:* The guidelines explicitly state that recirculated air *must* be diluted with fresh air to avoid the buildup of pollutants. This counters the common practice in Indian commercial buildings of running ACs on virtually 100% recirculation to conserve energy during peak summer, through leakages may incidentally occur [8]. This finding has been empirically confirmed by the author's survey of 58 Indian airports, where 39 reported not to have comprehensive dilution-capable HVAC systems (See Table 6.1).
- *Purging:* A new requirement for "Pre-occupancy Purge" has been introduced. Buildings should run their HVAC systems for a period *before* daily occupancy begins to flush out contaminants that accumulated overnight (e.g., VOCs from cleaning, or biological growth). This aligns with REHVA guidelines for COVID-19 operation [28].
- *Demand Control Ventilation (DCV):* The committee recommended considering DCV systems. These systems use CO_2 sensors to detect occupancy load and automatically modulate fresh air intake. In the Indian context, where occupancy fluctuates wildly (e.g., a mall on a weekend vs. a weekday), DCV offers a mechanism to ensure infection resilience (high ventilation when crowded) while saving energy when empty [8].

6.8.2 Source Control Measures

The guidelines propose specific source control measures that address the Indian market reality:

Table 6.1 HVAC type and ventilation capability across 58 Indian airports

S. No.	Type of air conditioning system	Total number of airports
1.	Centralized H.V.A.C System	18
2.	V.R.V/V.R.F/Packaged/Cassetted type	8
3.	Split/Room Air Conditioner/Tower Type standalone	12
4.	H.V.A.C + Split	8
5.	H.V.A.C + V.R.V	1
6.	Heat Generator System	1
7.	Details not provided	3
8.	H.V.A.C + H.V.L.S Fan	1
9.	No H.V.A.C	4
10.	V.R.F + Split Combination	2

Source: Singh [34]

- *Low-VOC Materials:* There is a strong recommendation to use paints and coatings that conform to *ECOMARK* criteria (issued by MoEF&CC). This is an attempt to steer the market away from high-VOC solvent-based paints which are still prevalent in the Indian construction sector [9, 10].
- *Formaldehyde Limits:* For wood products (MDF, particle board), the guidelines refer to Indian Standards (e.g., IS 12406:2021) for formaldehyde emission. This is critical as cheap composite wood is a massive source of carcinogenic HCHO in Indian offices [8].
- *Photocopiers:* Recognizing ozone and particulate emissions from heavy-duty photocopiers, the guidelines mandate keeping them away from general working areas, preferably in unoccupied, well-ventilated zones [8].

6.9 The Road Ahead: Establishing Indian Standards

The Interim Guidelines are just the first step. The Joint Committee has laid out a roadmap to develop legally binding "Guide Values." This involves a comprehensive monitoring study across different climatic zones of India.

The proposed study will cover six cities representing India's climatic diversity:

1. *Srinagar* (Cold)
2. *Delhi* (Composite/High Pollution)
3. *Chennai* (Warm and Humid/Coastal)
4. *Bengaluru* (Temperate)
5. *Jodhpur* (Hot and Dry)
6. *Shillong* (Cold/Northeast topography)

This geographical spread is scientifically vital. A ventilation strategy that works in the dry heat of Jodhpur (evaporative cooling) will fail in the humidity of Chennai. Similarly, the infiltration of outdoor PM is a massive variable in Delhi but less so in Shillong. By monitoring 10 categories of public places in these cities over two seasons (Summer and Winter), the CPCB aims to generate a representative dataset to define what "clean indoor air" means for India [9, 10].

In the following sections of this chapter, we will delve deeper into the technical implementation of these guidelines, examining the specific engineering interventions required for different building types to meet these emerging standards.

6.9.1 Empirical Assessment of HVAC Systems in Indian Public Buildings

Data were collected using the Right to Information Act, 2005, which legally obliges public authorities to provide authenticated records within 30 days. This was RTI was used as a scientific data collection tool. Unlike questionnaire-based surveys, RTI requests allow only retrieval of existing documentary records, thereby minimizing researcher bias and enhancing data authenticity. This explains the methodology used.

Table 6.2 Filtration adequacy in airports

S. No.	Type of filter integrated in the HVAC system	No. of Airports with filter
1	M.E.R.V < 5–6	5
2	M.E.R.V 5–6	2
3	M.E.R.V < 7–8	8
4	M.E.R.V 7–8	6
5	M.E.R.V 10	1
6	M.E.R.V 8	2
7	M.E.R.V 13	1
8	M.E.R.V 8 + M.E.R.V 14	1
9	M.E.R.V 8 + M.E.R.V 11	1
10	H.E.P.A	2

Source: Singh [34]

The parameters extracted included:

(i) HVAC system typology (centralized vs recirculatory).
(ii) Presence of integrated fresh air intake.
(iii) Filtration grade (MERV/micron rating).
(iv) Presence of ultraviolet germicidal irradiation (UVGI).
(v) CO_2 monitoring capability.

Four independent datasets were generated covering airports, engineering institutes, congregational public buildings, and nationally significant administrative buildings.

Only 19 of 58 airports possessed full central HVAC systems capable of controlled dilution ventilation. The remaining 39 relied partially or entirely on recirculatory systems (split, VRV, packaged), structurally incapable of delivering meaningful fresh air. This demonstrates that even critical national infrastructure such as airports may remain fundamentally underprepared in part for airborne infection resilience (as per when the data was collected).

Of the 43 airports that reported filtration presence, only five deployed filters with MERV ≥ 10 (See Table 6.2). The majority employed MERV 5–8 filters, which are functionally equivalent to dust filters and ineffective against $PM_{2.5}$ and aerosolized pathogens. This exposes a dangerous policy paradox: dilution ventilation is advocated, yet filtration systems are incapable of preventing pollution ingress.

6.10 The Engineering of Safety: Strategies for Healthcare Facilities

The battle against airborne pathogens is most fiercely fought within the walls of healthcare facilities (HCFs). In India, the infrastructure of public health ranges from world-class tertiary care centers to resource-constrained primary health centres. The COVID-19 pandemic mercilessly exposed the vulnerabilities in this heterogeneous landscape, particularly regarding infection control through ventilation. The *Joint Committee on Indoor Air Quality Management*, constituted by the Central Pollution Control Board (CPCB), identified hospitals as a critical category for IAQ monitoring and regulation [9, 10]. However, translating these regulatory intents into engineering reality requires a granular understanding of hospital design, specifically focusing on the "invisible" architecture of airflow.

6.10.1 The "Waiting Area" Vulnerability

While intensive care units (ICUs) and isolation wards often receive the bulk of engineering attention, recent research suggests that the true "Achilles' heel" of Indian hospital infection control may be the waiting area. A study by Singh [33], titled *"The Risk Status of Waiting Areas for Airborne Infection Control in Delhi Hospitals,"* provides a sobering assessment of this overlooked zone. Using the Right to Information (RTI) Act, 2005, researchers queried major government hospitals in Delhi regarding their specific measures for airborne infection control in waiting areas.

The responses were revealing. Major hospitals/institutions either stated that "no requisite information is available on record" or provided generic responses about general cleanliness [33]. This lack of documented engineering controls for waiting areas is critical because these spaces are characterized by:

1. *High Occupant Density:* Indian hospital waiting rooms frequently operate at crush capacity, often exceeding design loads by significant margins.
2. *Mixed Population:* These areas house a volatile mix of undiagnosed infectious patients (index cases) and highly susceptible individuals (immunocompromised patients, relatives).
3. *Transient Occupancy:* Unlike a ward where patients may mostly be static, waiting areas have high turnover, creating complex, turbulent airflow wakes that can disperse pathogens unpredictably.

Singh [33] applied the Wells-Riley equation to a typical waiting area scenario, demonstrating that without specific dilution ventilation (Air Changes per Hour, ACH > 6) or supplementary air cleaning, the probability of infection transmission may remain dangerously high. The study highlighted that while the *National Building Code of India 2016 (NBC 2016)* prescribes ventilation rates, the *operational reality* often involves recirculating air-conditioning (Split ACs) to combat the searing Delhi heat, thereby creating a "closed chamber" for airborne viruses [33].

6.10.2 The Split AC Conundrum in Indian Public Buildings

A pervasive challenge in Indian public infrastructure—including courts, government offices, and smaller clinics—is the reliance on Split Air Conditioning units. Unlike Centralized Air Conditioning plants (HVAC) which *can* be engineered to introduce fresh outdoor air, standard split AC units recirculate 100% of the indoor air, cooling it via a refrigerant coil. They provide *thermal comfort* with negligible effective ventilation (dilution) [36].

During the pandemic, this issue reached the Delhi High Court. In the matter of *Court on its Own Motion vs Union of India*, the court deliberated on the safety of operating air-conditioned courtrooms. Technical committees, including experts from the Council of Scientific and Industrial Research (CSIR) and the Public Works Department (PWD), noted that many rooms in the High Court blocks had no provision for fresh air intake in their AC systems [36].

The Joint Committee report [9, 10] and the proceedings from the High Court highlighted a critical retrofit strategy for such spaces:

- *Modifying Fenestration:* Cutting glass panes to install exhaust fans or fresh air intakes.
- *Hybrid Operation:* Using split ACs for cooling while simultaneously operating exhaust fans to create negative pressure and induce fresh air infiltration, albeit at the cost of energy efficiency (thermal loss).
- *CO_2 Monitoring:* Implementing mandatory carbon dioxide (CO_2) monitoring as a surrogate for ventilation adequacy. If CO_2 levels exceed 800–1000 ppm, it indicates that the split AC is recirculating too much rebreathed breath, triggering a need to open windows or vacate the room [9, 10, 36].

6.10.3 The Role of Anterooms and Buffer Zones

For higher-risk zones within hospitals, such as isolation rooms for tuberculosis or COVID-19, the physical layout plays a decisive role in containment. A systematic review by Andalib et al. [3] emphasized the effectiveness of *anterooms* (vestibules) in controlling hospital infections. An anteroom acts as an airlock or buffer zone between the contaminated patient room and the clean corridor.

The mechanism of protection is twofold:

1. *Pressure Buffer:* It helps maintain the pressure differential (negative pressure in the isolation room) by preventing direct communication between the room and the corridor.
2. *Dilution Zone:* Air escaping from the patient room during door opening is diluted and exhausted in the anteroom before it can reach the corridor.

Andalib et al. [3] noted that the design of the door (hinged vs. sliding) and the speed of door opening significantly affect contaminant leakage. Hinged doors can create a "pumping" effect, pulling contaminated air out of the isolation room. Anterooms mitigate this by providing a secondary barrier. For Indian hospitals, where space is often at a premium, retrofitting temporary anterooms using plastic sheeting or portable partitions during outbreaks is a recommended strategy to enhance "infection resilience" without major structural changes [3].

6.11 Air Filtration and Cleaning: The Second Line of Defense

When ventilation (dilution) is limited by outdoor pollution or thermal constraints—a common scenario in Indian megacities where outdoor PM2.5 levels can be hazardous—*filtration* becomes the primary mechanism for pathogen removal.

6.11.1 HVAC Filtration Standards

The CPCB Joint Committee's interim guidelines recommend that HVAC systems in public places be equipped with appropriate filtration. While HEPA (high-efficiency particulate air) filters are the gold standard, capturing >99.97% of particles at 0.3 microns, they impose a significant pressure drop that many existing Indian HVAC systems may not handle [9, 10, 25]. Further, if not regularly replaced and maintained, these filters may cause more harm than good.

Therefore, a tiered approach is often recommended:

- *MERV 13 (or ISO ePM1):* Upgrading standard pre-filters to MERV 13 is often feasible for commercial systems and provides substantial capture of respiratory aerosols (1–5 microns) [25].
- *In-Room Air Cleaners:* For spaces served by split ACs or with poor ventilation, portable air cleaners with HEPA filters are essential. Research by Mousavi et al. [24] and others indicates that these devices can significantly reduce the "clearance time" of aerosols in a room. However, their placement is critical; they must be positioned to draw air *away* from occupants, not pull contaminated air *past* them [24].

6.11.2 Ultraviolet Germicidal Irradiation (UVGI)

UVGI emerged as a potent technology during the pandemic. In the Delhi High Court deliberations, it was observed that UVGI installed in air handling units (AHUs) only disinfects the inside surface of ducts/ some air *recirculated* through the duct. It may not protect occupants from short-range transmission (face-to-face) within the room [36].

For effective protection in crowded Indian settings (e.g., waiting halls, railway stations), *Upper-Room UVGI* is a superior strategy. This involves creating a zone of high-intensity UV-C light in the upper portion of the room (above occupant heads). Convection currents lift exhaled aerosols into this "kill zone," where they are rapidly inactivated [26]. This technology is particularly robust because it does not rely on air ducts and has a lower energy footprint than increasing mechanical ventilation rates [39]. Yet, there are issues related to high capital costs and need for maintenance which may sometimes be a challenge in low resource settings, where simple dilution ventilation may be easy to follow and cheaper to do.

6.12 The Challenge of Implementation: From Guidelines to Ground Reality

The existence of guidelines (NBC 2016; [9, 10]) does not guarantee compliance. Further, NBC is a recommendatory document, unless specifically notified by state. The gap between policy and practice in India is often bridged—or widened—by economic and behavioral factors.

6.12.1 Behavioral Compliance and "Mask Fatigue"

Even the best-engineered building cannot prevent infection if the occupants do not comply with basic hygiene. A systematic review by Gozdzielewska et al. [13] highlighted that while hand hygiene and surface disinfection are critical, their effectiveness is contingent on consistent adherence. In the Indian context, "mask fatigue" and the discomfort of wearing masks in hot, humid conditions pose significant challenges.

Studies on mask usage in non-patient care areas show that compliance often drops when staff are "off-duty" in breakrooms or offices, which then become hotspots for transmission [27]. Therefore, building design must account for human fallibility. Ventilation and filtration are "passive" controls—they work regardless of occupant behavior—making them more reliable than "active" controls like masking or distancing in the long run. These observations mirror systematic evidence that the built environment itself facilitates—or frustrates—distancing behaviors during outbreaks, strengthening the case for passive, engineering-led protections [1].

6.12.2 Economic Feasibility

Implementing 12 ACH or installing HEPA filtration carries a cost. However, analyses suggest that the cost of *inaction*—measured in lost productivity, healthcare expenses, and mortality—far outweighs the retrofitting costs. For the Indian context, "frugal engineering" solutions are vital. These might include:

- *Exhaust-Only Ventilation:* Using simple exhaust fans to create negative pressure and pull fresh air in through passive vents, rather than expensive balanced ventilation systems.
- *Natural Ventilation Optimization:* Designing windows for cross-ventilation (wind-driven) and stack ventilation (buoyancy-driven) to utilize India's thermal gradients, as discussed in the NBC 2016 [9, 10].

6.13 The Educational Sector: Ventilation in the High-Density Classroom

Schools in India represent a unique and critical category of public infrastructure. Unlike the office towers of Gurugram or the malls of Mumbai, the vast majority of Indian schools—particularly government-run institutions—rely primarily on natural ventilation. However, they also operate at occupant densities that are among the highest in the world, with class sizes often ranging from 40 to 60 students in rooms designed for 30. This creates a seemingly "perfect storm" for airborne transmission, where the metabolic CO_2 generation and potential viral load can rapidly overwhelm the natural air exchange rate. The urgency of reform is no longer hypothetical; it is evidenced by systematic deficiencies documented across airports, universities, public halls, and national governance buildings.

6.13.1 The Limits of Natural Ventilation in Indian Cities

While the National Building Code (NBC) 2016 prescribes window-to-floor area ratios to ensure adequate ventilation, these design standards assume that windows will remain open. In practice, extreme weather (summer heatwaves reaching 45 °C, monsoon rains, and winter smog) and outdoor noise pollution frequently compel teachers to close windows.

In Delhi, during the winter months (November–January), schools often face a "double burden." Opening windows to dilute potential viral aerosols introduces hazardous levels of ambient $PM_{2.5}$ (often >300 micrograms per cubic meter) and cold drafts. Keeping windows closed protects against smog and cold but causes CO_2 levels to skyrocket, often exceeding 3000–4000 ppm, indicating a dangerous accumulation of rebreathed air [5, 29].

6.13.2 Recommendations for Indian Schools

Based on the principles of infection control and the constraints of the Indian context, the following recommendations are proposed:

- *Mechanical Augmentation (Exhaust Fans):* For schools unable to afford full HVAC systems, the most cost-effective retrofit is the installation of high-capacity exhaust fans. Operating exhaust fans creates negative pressure, actively pulling fresh air in through even small openings (cracks, vents) or partially opened windows. This ensures a consistent air change rate (ACH) regardless of wind speed or temperature differences [36].
- *The "Sawtooth" Protocol:* If continuous ventilation is impossible due to extreme heat or cold, schools should adopt a rigorous "purge" protocol. Windows and doors must be fully opened for 10–15 min between every class period. This flushes out the accumulated bio-aerosols, resetting the risk level before the next session. This mimics the "sawtooth" profile of CO_2 decay observed in studies where intermittent airing was effective [12].
- *Outdoor Learning:* Given India's generally high solar UV index (which inactivates viruses outdoors), classes should be moved to open courtyards or playgrounds whenever weather permits. This utilizes the "infinite dilution" of the outdoor environment, virtually eliminating long-range transmission risk [26].

6.13.3 Auditoriums in Premier Institutions: Empirical Results from Model Buildings

A study of 19 auditoriums in premier government-funded engineering institutions revealed systemic ventilation deficiencies. Despite these institutions representing India's highest technical capacity, only:

- 6 of 19 reported achieving NBC-compliant air changes.
- 11 of 19 reported any fresh air integration.
- Only 2 had CO_2 monitoring.
- Only 1 reported UVGI.
- None deployed HEPA filtration.

This demonstrates that even India's most technically advanced campuses may not operationalize airborne infection control in practice. These buildings, which should serve as national exemplars, instead reflect non awareness of ventilation as a public health infrastructure (Table 6.3).

Table 6.3 Ventilation and filtration parameters in premier engineering auditoriums

S. No.	Institute	Whether NCAP non-attainment city	ACH if mentioned 4–8	ACH as per NBC 2016	Whether Fresh Air Provision in HVAC Yes/No	Fresh air quantified	CO_2 monitoring	UVGI	Whether HEPA filter provided	Filter provided	Filter least count/ Efficiency
1	A large congregational library of a premier technology institute in New Delhi	Yes	3–4	Yes	Yes	100 % fresh air, no return	No	No	No	Pre Filter (MERV 8 or less)	Not provided
2	An auditorium of a premier technology institute in New Delhi	Yes	4–6	Yes	Yes	17733 CFM fresh air	No	No	No	Pre Filter (MERV 8 or less)	Not provided
3	The largest auditorium of an premier technology institute in North India	No	12 (in case of fire)	Yes	Yes	17733 CFM fresh air	No	Yes	No	MERV 13 EU 7	3 micron/Not provided
4	A large lecture hall located in the lecture hall complex of a prominent technology institute in Western India	Yes	Not provided	Not provided	No	Not provided	No	No	No	MERV 8	10 micron/90%

(continued)

Table 6.3 (continued)

S. No.	Institute	Whether NCAP non-attainment city	ACH if mentioned 4–8	ACH as per NBC 2016	Whether Fresh Air Provision in HVAC Yes/No	Fresh air quantified	CO_2 monitoring	UVGI	Whether HEPA filter provided	Filter provided	Filter least count/ Efficiency
5	A convention hall of a large premier institute in the metro city of Mumbai	Yes	1	No	Yes	Not provided	No	No	No	MERV 7–8 EU 4	10 micron/Not provided
6	The Main Auditorium in a prominent technology institute in the Indian state of Uttar Pradesh	Yes	>10	Yes	Yes	100 fresh air provision	No	No	No	Not specified (MERV 8 or lesser)	10 micron/80%
7	An auditorium belonging to one of India's largest premier institute located in Eastern India	No		Not provided	No	Not provided	No	No	No	Pre Filter (MERV 8 or less)	Not provided
8	Another auditorium belonging to the Eastern Indian premier institute	No		Not provided	No	Not provided	No	No	No	Pre Filter (MERV 8 or less)	Not provided

S. No.	Institute	Whether NCAP non-attainment city	ACH if mentioned 4–8	ACH as per NBC 2016	Whether Fresh Air Provision in HVAC Yes/No	Fresh air quantified	CO_2 monitoring	UVGI	Whether HEPA filter provided	Filter provided	Filter least count/ Efficiency
9	The main auditorium located in the academic block of a premier institute located in central India	Yes	9 ACPH 2.42 Fresh ACPH	Yes	Yes	2500 CFM fresh air 2.42 fresh ACPH	No	Nɔ	No	MERV 5–6 EU 3	Not provided
10	Main Conference Room located in the Auditorium Building of a prominent North East Indian institute	Yes	1	No	No	Not clear	No	Nɔ	No	Pre Filter (MERV 8 or less)	Not provided/30%
11	Auditorium of a premier institute in Western India	Yes	1	No	Yes	Fresh Air 1 ACPH	Yes	No	No	Pre Filter (MERV 8 or less)	10 micron
12	Auditorium of a premier institute in Northern India	Yes	Naturally Ventilated	N.A.	N.A	Not Applicable	No	No	No	N.A.	Not applicable

(continued)

Table 6.3 (continued)

S. No.	Institute	Whether NCAP non-attainment city	ACH if mentioned 4–8	ACH as per NBC 2016	Whether Fresh Air Provision in HVAC Yes/No	Fresh air quantified	CO_2 monitoring	UVGI	Whether HEPA filter provided	Filter provided	Filter least count/ Efficiency
13	Auditorium in a Student Activity Centre of a premier technology institute of South India	No	1.5	No	Yes	Not provided	Yes	No	No	Not provided (MERV 5–6 or lesser)	Not provided
14	A Seminar Hall, located in a premier institute in Western India	Yes	<1 (because of split a.c.)	No	No	0	No	No	No	OEM filters	2.5 micron OEM/Not provided
15	An Audio Visual Auditorium Located in a premier institute in Central India	No		Not provided	Yes	15% of design condition fresh air	No	No	No	Pre Filter (MERV 8 or less)	5 micron/Not provided
16	An auditorium in a South Indian premier institute	No	12	Yes	No	0	No	No	No	OEM Filters	Not provided
17	An auditorium in a central Indian premier institute	Yes		Not provided	Yes	9800 cfm Fresh air	Not clear	No	No	Pre Filter (MERV 8 or less)	10 micron/90%

S. No.	Institute	Whether NCAP non-attainment city	ACH if mentioned 4–8	ACH as per NBC 2016	Whether Fresh Air Provision in HVAC Yes/No	Fresh air quantified	CO_2 monitoring	UVGI	Whether HEPA filter provided	Filter provided	Filter least count/ Efficiency
18	The main auditorium of a premier institute in Southern India	No	Naturally Ventilated	N.A.	N.A.	Not applicable	Not clear	No	No	N.A.	N.A.
19	The central seminar hall located in a premier institute in Northern India	Yes	Not provided	Not provided	Yes	Return Duct Closed 100% Fresh Air	No	No	No	MERV 7–8 EU 4	Not provided

Note: The name of the institutes in this study has been anonymized
Source: Singh [35]

6.14 The "Split AC" Syndrome: Retrofitting Offices and Small Commercial Spaces

A pervasive challenge in the Indian built environment is the widespread reliance on Split Air Conditioning (or "High-Wall") units. Unlike centralized HVAC systems, which have ducts to bring in outdoor air, standard split ACs recirculate 100% of the indoor air. They provide thermal comfort by cooling the air but provide negligible effective ventilation exhaust. In small offices, courtrooms, and clinics where these units are ubiquitous, the risk of cross-infection is maximal.

6.14.1 The Delhi High Court Case Study

The risks posed by split ACs were judicially recognized during the COVID-19 pandemic. In the matter of *Court on its Own Motion vs Union of India*, the Delhi High Court established a technical committee to assess the safety of its own air-conditioned courtrooms. The committee, including experts from the Council of Scientific and Industrial Research (CSIR) and the Public Works Department (PWD), noted that many chambers relied on split units with no fresh air intake. They concluded that operating these units in a sealed room during a pandemic was unsafe [36].

6.14.2 Engineering Solutions for Split AC Environments

To mitigate this risk without discarding millions of installed units, the following hybrid strategies are recommended by Indian experts and the CPCB Joint Committee:

1. *The "Fan + AC" Hybrid Mode:* If a split AC is used, the room must *not* be sealed. A window should be kept partially open (ajar), and an exhaust fan should be running. While this increases the thermal load (and electricity bill), it induces the necessary fresh air exchange. The Central Public Works Department (CPWD) issued guidelines explicitly recommending this trade-off between energy efficiency and health safety during the pandemic [11, 36].
2. *Structural Retrofit (The "Cut-Glass" Method):* In buildings with fixed glass facades (curtain walls) where windows cannot be opened, the High Court committee recommended "cutting/removing the glass at designated places" to install intake louvers or exhaust fans. This drastic measure highlights the primacy of ventilation over aesthetics in infection control [36].
3. *Filtration Augmentation:* Since split ACs typically have coarse mesh filters that do not capture viral aerosols, standalone portable air cleaners (HEPA) should be deployed in these rooms. The clean air delivery rate (CADR) of the purifier must be sufficient to provide an equivalent of 5–6 ACH for the room volume [9, 10, 26]. But they must not give false sense of safety and must be included with suitable fresh air changes.

6.15 Auditoriums and Cinemas: Managing Super-Spreader Risks

Large volume spaces like cinema halls and auditoriums are economically vital to the Indian entertainment and conference sectors. However, the outbreak of the Delta variant in an auditorium in Hunan, China (investigated by [15]), serves as a cautionary tale relevant to Indian settings. In that event, the virus spread across rows, infecting individuals sitting up to 1.5 m away, despite the large volume of the hall.

6.15.1 The ZADIR Model and Displacement Ventilation

Retrospective modeling of auditorium outbreaks suggests that "mixing ventilation" (where cool air is blown from the ceiling and mixed with room air) can inadvertently spread viral plumes horizontally across the audience. In contrast, *Displacement Ventilation*—where cool air is supplied at the floor level (under seats) and extracted at the ceiling—uses the thermal plumes generated by the warm human bodies to lift exhaled breath upwards, away from other occupants. Huang et al. [15] found that displacement ventilation could significantly reduce infection risks compared to mixing ventilation. For Indian cinemas and auditoriums, which often face high occupancy, retrofitting air distribution to approximate a displacement flow (or at least ensuring upward extraction) is a key recommendation.

6.15.2 The Role of CO_2 Monitoring

In large halls, occupancy fluctuates wildly (e.g., a sold-out movie vs. a morning show). A constant ventilation rate is inefficient. Indian guidelines for these "public places" (as defined by NGT) strongly advocate for *demand control ventilation (DCV)*. CO_2 sensors should monitor the breathing zone; as the audience fills up and CO_2 rises, the fresh air dampers (FAD) should automatically open to increase outdoor air supply. If the system cannot maintain CO_2 below 800–1000 ppm, occupancy limits must be enforced [9, 10, 15].

6.16 Summary of Interim Engineering Recommendations

Table 6.4 synthesizes the engineering recommendations for different Indian building typologies, drawing from the CPCB Joint Committee report, CPWD guidelines, and recent literature.

The implementation of these recommendations requires a shift in mindset from "cooling the space" to "cleaning the air." As emphasized by the NGT and the CPCB, the cost of these interventions is measurable, but the cost of inaction—in terms of public health burden—is incalculable.

Table 6.4 Engineering recommendations for Indian public spaces

Building type	Primary ventilation issue	Recommended intervention
Schools	High density, closed windows (weather/noise)	*Exhaust Fans:* Install to force air exchange. *Purge Protocols:* Open all windows between classes
Govt. Offices/ Cabins	Reliance on Split ACs with 100% recirculation	*Hybrid Mode:* Run Split AC + Exhaust Fan + Window Ajar. *Retrofit:* Cut glass facade to install vents
Hospitals (Waiting Areas)	Undocumented ventilation, high cross-infection risk	*Dilution:* Minimum 6–12 ACH. *Upper-Room UVGI:* Essential for crowded TB/COVID waiting halls
Cinemas/ Auditoriums	Large volume, mixing of breath plumes	*Displacement Ventilation:* Supply air low, extract high. *DCV:* Modulate fresh air based on CO_2 levels
Malls/Shopping Centres	Recirculation to save energy; food court emissions	*Filtration:*MERV 13+ in centralized AHUs. *Source Control:* High exhaust rates in food courts (CO/PM removal)

6.17 Transport Hubs: The High-Velocity Vectors

If hospitals are the front lines of the battle against infection, transport hubs—airports, metro stations, and railway terminals—are the logistical arteries through which pathogens traverse the subcontinent. The sheer scale of passenger movement in India is staggering; the Indian Railways alone transports over 23 million passengers daily (pre-pandemic figures). These spaces represent a unique aerobiological challenge: they are transient spaces characterized by extreme fluctuations in occupant density, often involving high metabolic activity (rushing, carrying luggage) and diverse immunological profiles.

6.17.1 Airports: The Illusion of Safety

Modern Indian airports are often architecturally imposing structures with high ceilings and vast glass facades. While they are generally serviced by centralized HVAC systems, the ventilation effectiveness at the "breathing zone" (the bottom 2 m) can be deceptively low. The *Joint Committee on Indoor Air Quality Management* [9, 10] specifically identified "Boarding pass counters and departure waiting areas" as critical monitoring locations.

These specific zones are bottlenecks. Despite the high volume of the terminal building, passengers congregate in dense queues at check-in and security. If the HVAC system utilizes a "mixing ventilation" strategy (supplying cool air from the ceiling to dilute pollutants), the thermal stratification in a high-ceilinged atrium can prevent fresh air from effectively reaching the occupants at floor level. Furthermore, airports are hotspots for cross-contamination between international travelers carrying novel variants and the local population.

Recommendations

- *Displacement Ventilation:* For high-ceiling terminals, displacement ventilation (supplying cool air at low velocity near the floor) is superior to mixing ventilation. It uses the thermal plumes generated by passengers to lift bioaerosols up to the ceiling extraction points, preventing horizontal spread between people in queues [15].
- *Dedicated Exhaust at Counters:* Check-in counters and immigration desks should ideally have local exhaust ventilation combined with local air cleaners to protect staff who interact with thousands of passengers daily.
- *CO_2 Monitoring:* Continuous CO_2 monitoring at waiting areas is non-negotiable. A rise above 800 ppm in a boarding gate area indicates insufficient fresh air supply for the current passenger load, signaling the need to increase air handling unit (AHU) fan speeds [9, 10].

6.17.2 The Metro and Rail Environment

The Delhi Metro and similar systems in Mumbai, Bengaluru, and Chennai operate closed, air-conditioned environments. While the trains themselves have active ventilation, the underground stations rely on tunnel ventilation systems (TVS) and station air conditioning. The risk here is the "piston effect"—trains pushing large masses of air through tunnels—which can transport aerosols between stations.

For surface rail (Indian Railways), the challenge is often the "General Compartment" or non-AC sleeper class, where ventilation is natural (open windows) but density is extreme. In AC coaches, the windows are sealed. During the pandemic, the Indian Railways experimented with involving roof-mounted exhaust fans to increase air changes.

Recommendations

- *Filtration in AC Coaches:* Retrofitting rail HVAC systems with MERV-13 equivalent filters or UVGI systems in the ducts is essential, as increasing fresh air intake beyond design limits can overwhelm the cooling capacity in India's extreme summer heat [36].
- *Platform Ventilation:* In underground stations, ensuring that platform screen doors (PSDs) are not just safety barriers but also air barriers is crucial to separate the tunnel air pressure from the station air conditioning, allowing for better control of station IAQ.

6.18 The Retail and Recreational Landscape: Malls and Food Courts

The proliferation of shopping malls in Tier-1 and Tier-2 Indian cities has created a new dominant typology for public gathering. These are hermetically sealed, climate-controlled environments where people spend hours. The CPCB Joint

Committee report identifies *Malls* as a priority category, specifically highlighting "Corridors/shops, Food court, underground parking, and Atriums & games parlors" as monitoring sites [9, 10].

6.18.1 The Food Court Paradox

The food court is arguably the most hazardous zone within a mall from an IAQ perspective. It represents a convergence of three risks:

1. *Pollutant Generation:* Cooking activities generate carbon monoxide (CO), nitrogen dioxide (NO_2), and particulate matter ($PM_{2.5}$), particularly from tandoors, grills, and wok frying [9, 10].
2. *Behavioral Vulnerability:* It is the only area where mask removal is socially sanctioned and necessary for eating and drinking.
3. *High Density:* Seating is often packed to maximize revenue per square foot.

If the food court is negatively pressurized to prevent cooking odours from entering the mall atrium (a common design standard), it draws air *from* the mall *into* the food court. If the mall air is laden with viral aerosols from asymptomatic shoppers, the food court becomes a collection point for pathogens. Conversely, if the food court is positively pressurized, it spreads cooking pollutants and potential viral aerosols into the retail areas.

Recommendations

- *Dedicated 100% Fresh Air Systems:* Food courts should ideally operate on dedicated treated fresh air (TFA) units with 100% once-through air, avoiding recirculation.
- *Source Capture:* Aggressive kitchen exhaust hoods are vital not just for odours but to remove combustion products (CO, NO_2) that irritate the respiratory tract and increase susceptibility to viral infections [18].
- *CO Monitoring:* Unlike other zones where CO_2 is the proxy, food courts also require carbon monoxide (CO) monitoring to ensure cooking fumes are not accumulating [9, 10].

6.18.2 Mass Congregational Buildings: Evidence from Public Halls, Museums, Stadiums

Across eight heavily used public buildings—including convention centres, stadiums, museums, transport terminals, and auditoriums—none deployed UVGI systems, only one deployed CO_2 monitoring, and all relied predominantly on pre-filters incapable of capturing fine particulates (See Table 6.5). One municipal banquet hall relied exclusively on multiple split air-conditioners with no fresh air provision

Table 6.5 HVAC and infection-control features in mass congregational public buildings

#	The name and details of the building	HVAC type	Whether fresh air provision integrated	Whether filter provided? If yes, then type of filter provided	Whether UVGI provided, with details	Whether carbon dioxide monitoring is done?
1	The main convention hall of IECC, New Delhi. For public gatherings of up to 7720 people	Centralized HVAC with air handling units	5 CFM/person + 0.6 CFM/sqft. Heat recovery wheel present	Pre Filters only (10 μm/90% efficiency)	UVGI absent	CO_2 monitoring done
2	IGI Indoor Stadium. Used for mass gathering public events as well as a sport facility	Centralized HVAC with multiple air handling units and additional openings with exhaust fans	155452 CMH Fresh air. Total AHU capacity 2025242 CMH. Therefore 7.67 & Fresh Air	MERV 6 Filter (90% arrestance/35–40% efficiency)	UVGI absent	CO_2 monitoring not done
3	Maharana Pratap ISBT in New Delhi. Busy mass rush building which has been retrofitted from a non-air-conditioned space	Central HVAC with AHUs. Split type Air Conditioner in some areas	Fresh air provided. Details not provided	Pre-filter only. EU 4 (MERV 7–8)	UVGI absent	Detail not provided
4	National Museum at Janpath	HVAC with AHUs. VRV also present	8–10% Fresh air provided	Pre-filters only (10 μm)	UVGI absent	CO_2 monitoring not done
5	A marriage banquet hall in Begumpur managed by the municipality of Delhi	Multiple packaged type split air conditioners	No fresh air supply. Internal air in recirculated	No filters present	UVGI absent	Detail not provided
6	The auditorium at Siri Fort Complex for major events, including government events	HVAC with air handling units	Details not provided	Pre filters (5 μm)	UVGI absent	CO_2 monitoring not done
7	The major hall in National School of Drama called Abhimanch Hall	HVAC with air handling units	Details not provided (as the air conditioner is very old, according to managers)	Details not available	UVGI absent	CO_2 monitoring not done
8	A public restaurant at the New Maharashtra Sadan in New Delhi.	HVAC with air handling units	Fresh air supplied. Details not provided	Pre Filters present (5 μm/98%efficiency)	No UVGI	Detail not provided

Source: Singh and Dewan [37]

whatsoever, effectively functioning as a closed recirculation chamber during public events. This represents a systemic public health hazard rather than an engineering oversight.

6.19 Beyond Pathogens: The "Sick Building" and Chemical Toxicity

While the NGT's 2022 order was catalyzed by the pandemic, its mandate covers "indoor air quality" broadly, recognizing that chemical pollutants contribute significantly to morbidity. The phenomenon of *sick building syndrome (SBS)*—characterized by mucosal irritation, fatigue, and headaches that resolve upon leaving the building—is often driven by volatile organic compounds (VOCs) rather than pathogens [14, 16, 18].

6.19.1 The Chemical Soup of Modern Interiors

Modern Indian interiors rely heavily on synthetic materials: PVC flooring, particleboard furniture, synthetic carpets, and solvent-based paints. These materials off-gas a variety of VOCs, including formaldehyde, benzene, and 2-ethyl-1-hexanol (2EH).

Case Study: 2-Ethyl-1-Hexanol (2EH) A comprehensive review by Wakayama et al. [42] highlights 2EH as a prominent cause of SBS. 2EH is a metabolite of DEHP (a common plasticizer in PVC) and is also used in fragrances. Crucially, 2EH emission is exacerbated by *dampness*. When PVC flooring is laid over concrete that has not fully cured or in humid conditions (common in India's monsoon), the alkaline hydrolysis of the plasticizer releases 2EH. Inhalation of 2EH causes mucous membrane irritation and has been linked to asthma-like symptoms [42].

In the Indian context, where construction speeds often compromise curing times and monsoon dampness is pervasive, the risk of chemical SBS is acute. The CPCB guidelines explicitly mention *Formaldehyde (HCHO)* and *Total VOCs (TVOCs)* as parameters to be monitored, identifying "plywood, fiberboard, particle boards" as key sources [9, 10].

6.19.2 Neurogenic Inflammation and Chemical Sensitivity

The mechanism by which these low-level chemicals cause symptoms is increasingly understood to be *neurogenic inflammation*. Meggs [19, 20] proposed that chemical irritants trigger sensory nerves in the airways (cranial nerve V), releasing neuropeptides like Substance P, which induce vasodilation, oedema, and inflammation. This process can sensitize the individual, leading to *multiple chemical sensitivity (MCS)*, where even minute exposures trigger systemic reactions. This highlights why "dilution ventilation" is critical not just for viruses, but for flushing out the "chemical background" that sensitizes occupants [19].

6.20 Interim Guidelines for Chemical Safety in Public Buildings

The Joint Committee's recommendations include specific interventions to mitigate chemical risks, bridging the gap between "Green" ratings and actual health [9, 10]:

1. *Material Selection:* Use of paints and coatings conforming to *ECOMARK* criteria (low VOC). Wood products must meet Indian Standards for formaldehyde emissions (e.g., IS 12406:2021).
2. *The "Bake-Out" Myth vs. Flush-Out:* Historically, "baking out" a building (raising temperature to accelerate off-gassing) was recommended. However, evidence suggests this can damage materials. The current recommendation is a *Pre-occupancy Flush-out*: running the HVAC system at maximum outdoor air capacity for several days *before* the building is occupied to remove the initial burst of VOCs from new furnishings [9, 10].
3. *Moisture Management:* Controlling dampness is the single most effective intervention for both mold (fungal) growth and chemical hydrolysis (like 2EH). Relative Humidity (RH) should be maintained below 65–70% to prevent microbial growth and chemical degradation of building materials [16].

6.21 Mixed-Mode Buildings: The Indian Reality

A significant portion of Indian public buildings—especially government offices, schools, and older universities—are neither fully air-conditioned nor fully naturally ventilated. They are *mixed-mode (MM)* buildings. They may use ceiling fans and open windows in winter, but switch to split ACs with closed windows in summer.

6.21.1 The Regulatory Blind Spot

Most international standards classify buildings as either mechanically or naturally ventilated. Mixed-mode buildings often fall into a regulatory grey area. The CPCB Joint Committee explicitly recognized this, deciding that "Mixed mode buildings... may also be considered under the study" to develop specific standards [9, 10].

6.21.2 Operational Protocols for Mixed-Mode

The challenge in MM buildings is the transition period. When windows are closed to turn on ACs, CO_2 levels rise rapidly if no fresh air intake is provided. The protocol for these buildings must be behavior-based:

- *Visual Indicators:* Installation of CO_2 monitors with "Traffic Light" displays is most effective in MM buildings. When the light turns red (e.g., >1000 ppm), occupants are prompted to open windows or doors for a "pulse" ventilation, even if the AC is running [36].
- *Exhaust Augmentation:* In MM buildings using split ACs, the installation of permanent exhaust fans (running continuously) ensures a baseline air change rate, creating a negative pressure that draws fresh air in through envelope leakage or trickle vents, mitigating the "sealed box" effect [9, 10].

6.22 Religious and Cultural Venues: The Challenge of Faith and Aerosols

India is a land where faith is communal. From the packed *darshan* lines at Tirumala to the congregational prayers at Jama Masjid and the hymn sessions in Gurudwaras, religious spaces represent the highest density mass gatherings in the country. Unlike transient spaces like airports where interaction is limited, religious venues involve prolonged static occupancy, often accompanied by vocalization (chanting, singing, praying), which significantly alters the aerobiological risk profile.

6.22.1 The Aerobiology of Chanting and Singing

The mechanics of viral emission are inextricably linked to respiratory activity. While tidal breathing releases a baseline level of aerosols, vocalization increases aerosol emission by an order of magnitude or more. Studies have shown that singing or loud speaking can release 10–50 times more aerosol particles than quiet breathing [4, 23].

In the Indian context, this has profound implications. A *kirtan* or *bhajan* session in a poorly ventilated hall may effectively turn a "super-emitter" event, even if the index case is asymptomatic. The infamous Skagit Valley Chorale outbreak in the USA, where 87% of choir members were infected by a single index case, serves as a grim template for what can occur in Indian religious settings if ventilation is ignored [22]. The risk is compounded by the fact that many religious buildings in India are designed for acoustic resonance (preserving sound) rather than acoustic damping, which may often correlate with enclosed, hard-surfaced volumes that trap air. These events have social and religious value and must be moved to semi outdoor spaces when possible. The design of religious places must focus on semi open spaces.

6.22.2 Incense and Particulate Matter: A Cultural Paradox

A unique IAQ challenge in Indian places of worship is the intentional generation of particulate matter through the burning of incense (*agarbatti*), camphor, and oil lamps (*diyas*). While spiritually significant, these activities may in some situations be major sources of indoor air pollution (IAP).

Studies have demonstrated that certain incense smoke contains particulate matter $PM_{2.5}$, PM_{10}, volatile organic compounds (VOCs) such as benzene and toluene, and carbonyls like formaldehyde [2, 40]. In enclosed shrines or prayer rooms, the concentration of $PM_{2.5}$ during rituals can exceed 500–1000 micrograms per cubic meter, levels that are hazardous to human health [40]. This creates a respiratory "double burden": the particulate matter irritates the respiratory mucosa, potentially upregulating ACE2 receptors or simply compromising the mucociliary escalator, thereby making occupants more susceptible to airborne viral infections like SARS-CoV-2 [31]. In order to retain important cultural practices, the manufacture of such products most beautiful regulated so that no harmful chemicals are added. Further, when ignited, they should be in well ventilated spaces.

6.22.3 Recommendations for Religious Spaces

The *Joint Committee on Indoor Air Quality Management* [9, 10] and building experts suggest the following mitigation strategies for religious venues:

1. *Source Control (Combustion):* Burning of incense and lamps should ideally be relocated to semi-outdoor areas (verandahs) or zones with dedicated local exhaust ventilation (LEV). If indoor burning is essential, it must be timed with periods of minimum occupancy, followed by a "purge" ventilation cycle before the congregation enters [9, 10].
2. *Ventilation Management During Rituals:* During periods of chanting or singing, mechanical ventilation rates should be maximized. If natural ventilation is used, cross-ventilation must be ensured by keeping doors and windows on opposite walls open. The use of pedestal fans should be managed carefully to ensure they blow air *out* of windows rather than across the faces of people (creating a cross-infection stream) [6, 9, 10].
3. *Occupancy Scheduling:* To maintain the effective ventilation rate (L/s/person), the number of devotees allowed inside the sanctum sanctorum or prayer hall at any one time must be strictly regulated based on the room's volume and air change capacity, not just floor area.
4. *Footwear and Dust:* Since footwear is removed outside, tracking of dust is reduced. However, carpets and rugs used for sitting accumulate dust and bio-aerosols. These should be vacuumed daily with HEPA-filtered vacuum cleaners rather than swept with brooms, which resuspends settled particles [9, 10].

6.23 Residential Common Areas: The Extended Living Room

While the NGT order focused on "public places," the urbanization pattern in India has led to the proliferation of high-rise Group Housing Societies (GHS). These complexes contain "common areas"—lobbies, clubhouses, gyms, and community halls—that function as public spaces for the residents. With the "work from home" (WFH) culture becoming entrenched, these areas have seen increased daytime occupancy.

6.23.1 High-Rise Lobbies and Elevators

Elevators are small, enclosed boxes with poor ventilation, representing a high-risk zone for short-range aerosol transmission. A study on elevator transmission dynamics suggests that viral aerosols can linger for minutes after an infected passenger exits, exposing subsequent users [41].

- *Recommendation:* Lift fans must remain operational at all times. In high-rise buildings, the "piston effect" of the moving car can be utilized to enhance air exchange if vent shafts are kept open. Building managers should program elevator doors to remain open when idle at the ground floor to flush out air [36].

6.23.2 Community Halls and Gymnasiums

Gymnasiums in residential complexes pose a severe risk due to the heavy breathing (high metabolic rate) of users. As established in Chap. 5, exercise can increase aerosol emission and oxygen consumption by a factor of 10–20.

- *CO_2 Monitoring:* Installation of CO_2 monitors in gyms is critical. A threshold of 800 ppm should be strictly enforced. If levels rise, occupancy must be reduced immediately.
- *Air Cleaning:* Given that gyms are often air-conditioned and sealed to control humidity and temperature, the use of portable HEPA air cleaners with a high clean air delivery rate (CADR) is recommended to supplement the HVAC system [25].

6.24 The Indian Monitoring Protocol: Standardizing the Invisible

One of the most significant contributions of the CPCB Joint Committee has been the formulation of a draft *Monitoring Protocol* for Indoor Air Quality. In the absence of a standardized protocol, data collected by different agencies (using varying instruments, sampling heights, and durations) is incomparable and often scientifically invalid. The committee's recommendations provide a unified framework for India [9, 10].

6.24.1 Defining the "Breathing Zone" and Sensor Placement

The committee emphasized that monitoring must reflect human exposure. Therefore, samplers/sensors must be placed in the *breathing zone*, defined as a height of *1.1–1.7 m* above the floor (representing the nose height of seated and standing occupants). Crucially, the protocol specifies exclusion zones to prevent data skewing [9, 10]:

- *Away from Apertures:* Sensors must be at least *1 m* away from doors, windows, and supply air diffusers to avoid measuring fresh air drafts or short-circuiting air.
- *Away from Sources:* Sensors should be at least *1 m* away from localized sources like photocopiers or coffee machines.
- *Wall Distance:* To avoid boundary layer effects and thermal plumes from walls, sensors should be at least *0.5 m* away from corners and walls.

6.24.2 Temporal Sampling Strategy

Recognizing the variability of indoor activities, the committee recommended that sampling should not be a snapshot but a representative profile. In practice, *CO_2 and allied environmental sensors* are a robust proxy for occupancy dynamics when deployed thoughtfully, enabling valid demand-responsive control rather than snapshot "hygiene theatre" [21].

- *Duration:* For comprehensive assessment, *24-h continuous monitoring* is recommended to capture the diurnal variation of pollutants (e.g., CO_2 buildup during the day, off-gassing of VOCs at night).
- *Seasonality:* The study design proposed by the committee mandates monitoring across at least two seasons (Summer and Winter) to account for the drastic differences in ventilation practices (AC use vs. open windows) and ambient air quality in Indian cities [9, 10].
- *Target Parameters:* The primary parameters identified for immediate monitoring are $PM_{2.5}$, PM_{10}, CO_2, CO, total VOCs (TVOCs), formaldehyde (HCHO), ozone (O_3), and nitrogen dioxide (NO_2) [9, 10].

6.25 Chemical Hygiene: The Unintended Consequences of "Deep Cleaning"

The COVID-19 pandemic triggered a massive increase in the use of chemical disinfectants. Fogging with sodium hypochlorite, widespread spraying of quaternary ammonium compounds, and heavy use of alcohol-based sanitizers became routine in Indian public spaces. However, this "hygiene theatre" came at a chemical cost.

6.25.1 The Disinfectant-Toxicity Trade-Off

Research indicates that the cleaning products used to kill surface pathogens are themselves potent sources of indoor air pollutants. Reactions between terpenes (found in scented cleaning products) and ozone (from outdoor air or photocopiers) can generate secondary organic aerosols (SOA) and formaldehyde [40, 43].

- *Recommendation:* The CPCB guidelines implicitly warn against indiscriminate chemical use by emphasizing *Source Control*. Disinfection should be targeted (high-touch surfaces) rather than broadcast (fogging). Application of disinfectants should be scheduled during unoccupied hours, followed by a "Pre-occupancy Purge" of the HVAC system to flush out chemical residues before occupants arrive [9, 10].

6.25.2 Pesticides and Pest Control

In tropical India, pest control (for mosquitoes, cockroaches, termites) is a routine building maintenance activity. The organophosphates and pyrethroids used are semi-volatile organic compounds (SVOCs) that partition into dust and can persist indoors for months [40].

- *Integrated Pest Management (IPM):* Buildings should adopt IPM strategies that prioritize physical barriers (sealing cracks, wire mesh on windows) and sanitation over chemical spraying. When chemical control is necessary, it must be followed by rigorous ventilation [9, 10].

6.25.3 Administrative Power Buildings: Symbolic Failure of National Exemplars

Perhaps the most concerning findings emerged from the assessment of India's most symbolically significant buildings: Parliament, Supreme Court, Rashtrapati Bhavan, Legislative Assembly, and major G20 venues. With the exception of the India International Convention and Expo Centre (IICC), none of the assessed buildings employed filtration capable of removing $PM_{2.5}$, none deployed UVGI, and none used CO_2 monitoring as a feedback control (See Table 6.6).

The paradox is stark: buildings that define national governance, occupied by constitutional authorities, are themselves operated under ventilation regimes that would be considered unsafe by modern infection-resilient standards. This undermines not only occupant safety but also the symbolic legitimacy of public health leadership.

Table 6.6 HVAC and IAQ provisions in nationally significant administrative buildings

Name of building	Type of HVAC system	Whether fresh air provision integrated	Whether filter provided. With details.	Whether UVGI is present.	Whether CO_2 is monitoring	Other observations
The Upper House and the Lower House of the Parliament of India	HVAC system	Fresh air provided; ~10% fresh air by design	Details not provided	Negative	No details provided	There is a scope for increasing fresh air intake; UVGI not available
The chamber of the legislative assembly of New Delhi	HVAC with 2 AHUs 12,000 CFM	Fresh air provided by AHU; quantity not known	Yes; MERV 8 (With least count: ~10 μm)[14]	Negative	No performed	The filter may be ineffective against $PM_{2.5}$ despite fresh air intake due to the least count considerations
Court Number 1 of the Supreme Court of India where the Chief Justice of India presides	VRV system; tower-based packaged split air conditioners in multiple remaining rooms	Fresh air 10–15%; advise given to open windows	Yes; but details not given (With probable presence of in-built OEM filters)	Positive	No provision	In the absence of a treated fresh air unit which allows fresh air intake, VRV systems may only recirculate indoor air
Darbar Hall, President's Estate, New Delhi: Venue of national events	HVAC with 9 AHUs of 3300 CFM each	Fresh air provided; 100% fresh air intake 29,700 CFM (according to facility manager)	Yes; only pre-filter (With least count: 10 μm)	Negative	CO_2 monitoring not performed	Although fresh air intake is good for airborne infection control, the filter may be ineffective against $PM_{2.5}$
Ashoka Hall, The President's House in India	HVAC with AHUs 17,000 CFM × 2	Fresh air provided; 100% fresh air 34,000 CFM	Yes; only pre-filter (With least count: 10 μm)	Negative	CO_2 monitoring not performed	Although fresh air intake is good for air borne infection control, the filter may be ineffective against $PM_{2.5}$

(continued)

Table 6.6 (continued)

Name of building	Type of HVAC system	Whether fresh air provision integrated	Whether filter provided. With details.	Whether UVGI is present.	Whether CO_2 is monitoring	Other observations
Chanakya Hall, Located at Hotel Samrat which is also a venue for government events	HVAC with AHUs 12,000 CFM	Fresh air provided; 79.89 CFM/person	Yes; only pre-filter (With least count: 50 μm)	Negative	CO_2 monitoring not performed	The filter may be ineffective against $PM_{2.5}$ despite fresh air intake
IICC, the planery event hall	District air conditioning system; Centralized	Quantity not given; declared in compliance with ASHRAE 62.1 and NBC 2016[15]	EU 3 and EU 8 provided (Which is equivalent: MERV 6 and MERV 14; ~10 μm and 1 μm respectively)[14]	Used advanced oxidation technique	CO_2 is monitored	This may be appropriate as there is sanitation and filtration, along with fresh air intake

Source: Singh and Dewan [38]

6.26 A Roadmap for Resilient Buildings

The recommendations outlined in this chapter represent a fundamental shift in how Indian public buildings are conceived, operated, and regulated. We are moving away from a paradigm where "comfort" (cooling) was the sole metric, to one where "health" (air quality and infection resilience) is paramount.

The interventions proposed range from the frugal (exhaust fans, window operation) to the sophisticated (HEPA filtration, UVGI, DCV). However, the unifying thread is *Ventilation*. Whether dilution of viral aerosols, flushing of chemical toxins, or removal of metabolic CO_2, the introduction of clean, fresh air remains the single most effective intervention.

The legal mandate from the National Green Tribunal and the technical roadmap from the CPCB Joint Committee provide the necessary scaffold for this transformation. It is now up to architects, engineers, and facility managers to implement these changes. The "Indian Public Building" of the future must be a breathing building—one that protects its occupants not just from the elements outside, but from the invisible threats that accumulate within.

FAQs: Recommendations for Indian Public Buildings

Q1: Why are specific IAQ standards needed for India when global standards like exist? A: India presents unique challenges that global standards often do not address. These include:

1. *High Ambient Pollution:* In many Indian cities, outdoor air is heavily polluted with $PM_{2.5}$, meaning simple ventilation (opening windows) can introduce outdoor toxins. Hybrid strategies of ventilation plus filtration are required.
2. *High Occupant Density:* Public spaces in India often operate at densities far higher than Western design standards, leading to rapid accumulation of bio-aerosols.
3. *Climatic Diversity:* India has varied climatic zones (hot-dry, warm-humid, composite) necessitating region-specific ventilation strategies rather than a "one size fits all" approach.

Q2: What is the significance of the National Green Tribunal (NGT) order regarding indoor air? A: The NGT order dated April 19, 2022, is a watershed moment because it legally recognized indoor air pollution (IAP) as a public health threat comparable to outdoor air pollution. It mandated the government to regulate IAQ in public places under the Air (Prevention and Control of Pollution) Act, 1981, moving IAQ from a voluntary "comfort" issue to a mandatory "health" issue.

Q3: Can Split ACs be used safely in offices and clinics? A: Standard split ACs recirculate indoor air and do not provide fresh air exchange. To use them safely, they must be operated in a "hybrid mode": keeping windows partially open or installing exhaust fans to induce fresh air intake. Relying solely on split ACs in closed rooms creates a high risk of airborne infection transmission.

Q4: What are the primary pollutants of concern in Indian public buildings? A: The CPCB Joint Committee identified the following priority pollutants:

- *Biological:* Respiratory viruses (SARS-CoV-2, Influenza, TB).
- *Particulate:* $PM_{2.5}$, PM_{10} (from outdoor ingress and indoor cleaning/cooking).
- *Chemical:* Carbon dioxide (CO_2—metabolic), carbon monoxide (CO—from pantry/cooking), total volatile organic compounds (TVOCs—from cleaners/paints), and formaldehyde (from furniture).

Q5: How can religious places manage infection risk given the high density? A: Key strategies include:

- *Ventilation:* Maximizing cross-ventilation during rituals involving chanting/singing.
- *Source Control:* Moving incense/lamp burning to outdoor or well-ventilated areas to reduce PM load.
- *Dust Management:* Vacuuming carpets (instead of sweeping) or wet mopping to prevent resuspension of dust and pathogens.

Q6: What is the "Pre-occupancy Purge"? A: This is a ventilation strategy recommended in the new guidelines. It involves running the building's ventilation system at maximum capacity for a period (e.g., 2 h) *before* occupants arrive in the morning. This flushes out contaminants (VOCs, bio-aerosols) that may have accumulated overnight or from cleaning activities.

Q7: Is CO_2 monitoring useful for infection control? A: Yes. While CO_2 is not a pathogen, it is an excellent proxy for ventilation effectiveness and "rebreathed air." High CO_2 levels (above 800–1000 ppm) indicate poor ventilation and overcrowding, correlating with a higher risk of airborne disease transmission. It serves as a "traffic light" warning system for building managers.

Q8: Are "Green Buildings" automatically healthy buildings? A: Not necessarily. "Green" ratings often prioritize energy efficiency, which can lead to sealing buildings tightly to prevent cooling loss. Without adequate active ventilation, this can trap pollutants indoors (the "Green Building Paradox"). The new Indian guidelines emphasize that energy efficiency must not come at the cost of human health; infection resilience is a non-negotiable aspect of sustainability.

6.27 The Indian Monitoring Protocol: Standardizing the Invisible

One of the most significant hurdles in managing indoor air quality (IAQ) in India may have been a lack of a standardized protocol for measurement. Unlike ambient air quality (AAQ), which is governed by strict monitoring mandates under the National Ambient Air Quality Standards (NAAQS) [7], indoor monitoring has largely been ad-hoc, conducted by varied researchers using disparate methodologies, sensor types, and sampling durations. This inconsistency renders data incomparable and legally unenforceable. To address this, the *Joint Committee on Indoor Air Quality Management*, constituted by the Central Pollution Control Board (CPCB) following the National Green Tribunal (NGT) order, has formulated a *"Preliminary Protocol for Monitoring Indoor Air Quality"* [9, 10].

This protocol represents the first step toward a unified national framework for assessing the health of Indian buildings. It moves beyond the vague requirement of "adequate ventilation" found in older building by-laws to quantifiable, verifiable metrics.

6.27.1 Sensor Placement: The "Breathing Zone" Doctrine

The validity of any IAQ assessment hinges on where the sample is taken. A common error in building management is placing sensors near supply air diffusers (where air is cleanest) or near exhaust vents (where air is stagnant), leading to skewed data. The CPCB protocol explicitly defines the sampling location to reflect human exposure [9, 10]:

- *Height:* The inlet of samplers or monitors must be placed at the *breathing zone*, defined as *1.1–1.5 m above the floor*. This corresponds to the nose height of an average adult, whether seated (in offices/schools) or standing (in malls/airports).
- *Proximity to Occupants:* In environments with fixed seating (e.g., offices, schools), the monitor should be placed centrally but not directly in the exhalation plume of a specific individual to avoid measuring concentrated breath rather than mixed room air.
- *Exclusion Zones:* To ensure representative sampling, monitors must be placed:
  - Away from direct sunlight and moisture sources (which can affect sensor accuracy, particularly NDIR CO_2 sensors and laser-scattering PM sensors).
  - At least *1 m away* from localized sources of emissions, such as photocopiers, coffee machines, or restrooms, unless the specific objective is to measure source strength [9, 10].

6.27.2 Sampling Duration and Frequency

Spot measurements (snapshots) are notoriously unreliable in dynamic environments like Indian public buildings where occupancy fluctuates wildly—for instance, a cinema hall is empty at 9 AM but at crush capacity by 11 AM. The CPCB committee acknowledged that "it is difficult to ascertain health effects due to exposure for a few hours in some public place" based on short-term data [9, 10]. Consequently, the roadmap for future standards recommends:

- *24-Hour Monitoring:* To capture the diurnal variation of pollutants, including the buildup of metabolic CO_2 during peak hours and the accumulation of VOCs during non-operational hours (due to reduced ventilation).
- *Seasonal Coverage:* India's diverse climate necessitates monitoring across at least two seasons (Summer and Winter). This accounts for the behavioral shift from "closed-window/AC mode" in summer to potential "open-window/natural

ventilation" or "heating mode" in winter, which drastically alters air exchange rates [9, 10].

6.28 Administrative Controls and Chemical Hygiene

While engineering controls (ventilation, filtration) are paramount, the Joint Committee recognized that source control—limiting what pollutants are introduced into the building—is equally vital. This is particularly relevant in the post-pandemic era, where the fear of surface transmission led to the indiscriminate use of chemical disinfectants, inadvertently creating a secondary respiratory hazard.

6.28.1 The "Hygiene Theatre" Paradox

During the height of the COVID-19 pandemic, many Indian facilities adopted "deep cleaning" protocols involving the fogging of sodium hypochlorite or the extensive use of quaternary ammonium compounds. While effective at killing surface pathogens, these chemicals release significant quantities of volatile organic compounds (VOCs) and can react with indoor ozone to form secondary organic aerosols and formaldehyde [43].

The CPCB Interim Guidelines implicitly address this by emphasizing *Source Control* and *Pre-Occupancy Purge*. The guidelines state:

- *"Application of polishes, varnishes, paints, pesticides or such products, generating VOC emissions, should be scheduled during unoccupied hours or periods of low occupancy."* [9, 10].
- *"Pre-occupancy purge should be carried out to ensure that contaminants, that may build up during construction or during unoccupied periods, are removed prior to occupancy."* [9, 10].

This effectively mandates that if chemical disinfection is performed, the HVAC system must be run in "flush-out" mode (100% fresh air) for a sufficient duration before occupants enter the building, preventing the "chemical soup" syndrome.

6.28.2 Material Selection: The ECOMARK Mandate

In a move to integrate manufacturing standards with health standards, the committee deliberated on adopting international standards for low-emitting materials. However, it was decided to prioritize the *ECOMARK* criteria notified by the Ministry of Environment, Forest and Climate Change (MoEF&CC). The guidelines recommend:

- *Paints and Coatings:* Preference for products conforming to ECOMARK criteria to minimize VOC emissions.
- *Composite Wood:* Use of low-formaldehyde emitting panel products (MDF, particle board) conforming to Indian Standards (e.g., IS 12406:2021) [9, 10]. This is crucial in Indian offices where modular furniture is a major source of formaldehyde, a known carcinogen and respiratory irritant.

6.29 The Way Forward: The 6-City Study and Future Standards

The "Interim Guidelines" released by the CPCB are a stop-gap measure. The ultimate goal, as directed by the NGT, is to establish scientifically robust, legally enforceable "Guide Values" or standards for Indoor Air Quality in India. Complementing field measurements, computational decision-support frameworks can guide scenario testing and retrofit prioritization for infectious-disease resilience across building typologies [44].

To achieve this, the Joint Committee has approved a comprehensive roadmap for a long-term field study [9, 10].

6.29.1 Geographical and Climatic Representation

Recognizing that a "Delhi-centric" standard may not apply to the tropical south or the Himalayan north, the committee selected six cities to represent India's climatic diversity for the baseline data generation:

1. *Srinagar* (Cold climate)
2. *Delhi* (Composite climate, high ambient pollution)
3. *Chennai* (Warm-Humid, coastal)
4. *Bengaluru* (Temperate)
5. *Jodhpur* (Hot-Dry)
6. *Shillong* (Cold/Northeast topography)

6.29.2 Target Public Places

The study will monitor 10 specific categories of public places, identified as high-risk or high-impact zones:

1. *Malls* (Corridors, Food Courts, Atriums)
2. *Hospitals* (Waiting areas, OPDs)
3. *Cinema Halls/Auditoriums*
4. *Museums*

5. *Gymnasiums*
6. *Airports* (Check-in, Departure waiting)
7. *Hotels* (Lobbies, Rooms, Restaurants)
8. *Educational Institutions* (Colleges—Lecture theatres, Labs)
9. *Schools* (Classrooms)
10. *Public Offices* (Workspaces, Conference rooms)

6.29.3 The Parameters of Concern

The study will focus on measuring $PM_{2.5}$, PM_{10}, *CO_2, CO, TVOC, Formaldehyde (HCHO),* and *Ozone (O_3)*. Notably, biological contaminants (bacteria/fungi) and radon were excluded from routine monitoring in this phase due to their complexity, with the recommendation that they be taken up by research institutes for specialized studies [9, 10].

6.30 Conclusion: From "Sick Buildings" to "Resilient Infrastructure"

The journey of indoor air quality in India has evolved from a peripheral concern of thermal comfort to a central pillar of public health policy. The intervention of the National Green Tribunal and the subsequent formation of the CPCB Joint Committee mark a paradigm shift. We are moving away from the era where energy efficiency (the "tight building") was the sole design driver, toward an era of *Infection Resilience* and *Environmental Health*.

The recommendations outlined in this chapter—ranging from the installation of CO_2 monitors and MERV-13 filters to the strategic use of exhaust fans and the "Pre-occupancy Purge"—are not merely theoretical ideals. They are actionable, evidence-based responses to the biological reality that we share the air we breathe. By implementing these measures, Indian public buildings can transition from being potential vectors of disease to being sanctuaries of health.

As India continues its rapid urbanization, the "lungs" of our buildings must be as robust as the lungs of our citizens. The cost of upgrading our ventilation infrastructure is measurable in rupees; the cost of *not* doing so is measured in human lives and societal well-being. The "Invisible Crisis" is no longer invisible; we have the metrics, the methods, and the mandate to solve it.

FAQs: Recommendations for Indian Public Buildings

Q1: Why is there a specific focus on Indian public buildings compared to residential buildings? A: Public buildings (malls, offices, schools, hospitals) have high occupant densities and often rely on centralized HVAC systems that can recirculate pathogens if not properly managed. Furthermore, the National Green Tribunal's order specifically mandated the regulation of IAQ in "public places" as defined under the Noise Pollution Rules, 2000, bringing them under the purview of the Air Act.

Q2: What is the "Pre-Occupancy Purge" and why is it recommended? A: The "Pre-Occupancy Purge" involves running the building's ventilation system (preferably with 100% fresh air) for a specific duration (e.g., 2 hours) before occupants arrive. This practice flushes out pollutants like VOCs that accumulate from cleaning agents, furniture off-gassing, or biological growth during the night or weekend when the system is off.

Q3: Can we use plants to clean indoor air in Indian offices? A: While plants are aesthetically pleasing and have psychological benefits, the CPCB Joint Committee noted that there is currently "inadequate evidence" to suggest that houseplants remove significant quantities of pollutants in real-world building environments compared to the rate of ventilation. They are not a substitute for proper fresh air exchange.

Q4: Why was radon excluded from the immediate monitoring protocol? A: The committee excluded radon from the mandatory monitoring list for public places because the committee stated that its presence is primarily due to geological factors and construction deficiencies (cracks in foundations) rather than daily operational practices. It requires specialized, long-term study rather than routine monitoring by facility managers.

Q5: What is the recommended height for installing IAQ sensors? A: Sensors should be installed at the *breathing zone*, which is approximately *1.1–1.5 m* above the floor. This ensures the data reflects the air actually being inhaled by occupants. Sensors placed on ceilings or near supply vents often provide misleadingly "clean" readings.

Q6: Are there specific guidelines for split ACs in offices? A: Yes. Since standard split ACs recirculate indoor air without adding fresh air, they can allow CO_2 and pathogens to build up. Recommendations include using them in "hybrid mode" (keeping a window partially open and using an exhaust fan) to induce fresh air exchange, even though this slightly reduces energy efficiency.

Q7: What is the role of the "ECOMARK" in IAQ? A: The ECOMARK is a certification by the Bureau of Indian Standards (BIS) for environmentally friendly products. The guidelines recommend using paints, coatings, and wood products that meet ECOMARK criteria because they have lower emissions of volatile organic compounds (VOCs) and formaldehyde, which are major indoor pollutants.

Q8: Who is legally responsible for maintaining IAQ in a building? A: According to the National Building Code (NBC) 2016, and reiterated by the CPCB Joint Committee, the *building owner* is responsible for the maintenance and services of the building, including the ventilation systems and indoor air quality.

Q9: What are the priority pollutants to monitor in Indian public spaces? A: The CPCB has identified $PM_{2.5}$, PM_{10} (particulate matter), CO_2 (carbon dioxide), CO (carbon monoxide), TVOC (total volatile organic compounds), HCHO (formaldehyde), and ozone (O_3) as the priority parameters for monitoring.

Q10: How does outdoor air pollution affect indoor ventilation strategies in India?
A: In cities with high outdoor pollution (like Delhi), simply opening windows can introduce dangerous levels of $PM_{2.5}$. Therefore, a *hybrid strategy* is recommended: using mechanical ventilation with high-grade filtration (MERV 13/HEPA) to clean the outdoor air before bringing it inside, rather than relying solely on natural ventilation during high-pollution days.

Acknowledgments Many thanks for Dr Prakash Swaminathan, Gaurav Shorey and Oluyemi Toyinbo. The authors acknowledge the support provided by the institutions including School of Planning and Architecture, New Delhi, All India Institute of Medical Sciences, New Delhi, and Drexel University. Special thanks to Rajshekhar Pullabhatla and Group Captain P Aanand Naidu of ISAC Centre for Built Environment Policy and Tathatara Foundation. Many thanks to Dr Arthur L Frank, MD. Many thanks to all the people who supported this work in many ways.

Declarations The authors Raja Singh, Nirupam Madaan, and Anil Dewan declare no conflict of interests or competing interests in this work. There is no involvement of human participants, animals, human or animal tissue. All authors declare that there was no specific financial support received from any organization for the submitted work. All authors declare that they have no financial relationships at present or within the previous 3 years with any organizations that might have an interest in the submitted work. While all care has been taken in ensuring the accuracy of this work, any inadvertent error may be reported at the earliest. The authors acknowledge the use of supervised language learning models/large language models for enhancement of the work, with responsibility lying with the authors. For more information, the corresponding author may be contacted at email rajaresearch@proton.me.

CRediT Statement The following is the CRediT statement which declares the author credits for this chapter:

Raja Singh: Conceptualization, Methodology, Formal Analysis, Investigation, Data Curation, Writing-Original Draft, Writing-Review & Editing, Visualization, Project Administration.
Nirupam Madaan: Conceptualization, Resources, Validation, Supervision, Project Administration.
Anil Dewan: Resources, Validation Supervision.

References

1. Akinci Z, Epton T, Tsimpida D. Impact of the built environment on social distancing during the COVID-19 pandemic: a systematic review. BMC Public Health. 2022;22(1):1–22.
2. Amoatey P, Omidvarborna H, Baawain MS, Al-Mamun A. Indoor air pollution and exposure assessment of the gulf cooperation council countries: a critical review. Environ Int. 2018;121:491–506.
3. Andalib S, Faghani M, Zia Ziabari SM, Shenagari M, Salehiniya H, Keivanlou M, Rafat Z. The effectiveness of the anteroom on hospital infection control. Front Public Health. 2022;10:828845. https://doi.org/10.3389/fpubh.2022.828845.
4. Asadi S, Wexler AS, Cappa CD, Barreda S, Bouvier NM, Ristenpart WD. Aerosol emission and superemission during human speech increase with voice loudness. Sci Rep. 2019;9(1):2348.
5. Batterman S. Review and extension of CO_2-based methods to determine ventilation rates with application to school classrooms. Int J Environ Res Public Health. 2017;14(2):145.

6. Centres for Disease Control and Prevention (CDC). Ventilation in buildings. 2020. Retrieved from https://www.cdc.gov/coronavirus/2019-ncov/community/ventilation.html.
7. CPCB (Central Pollution Control Board). National Ambient Air Quality Standards. New Delhi; 2009.
8. CPCB (Central Pollution Control Board). Report of the Joint Committee on Indoor Air Quality Management (In Original Application 143/2016 (WZ) with Original Application 206/2022). Ministry of Environment, Forest & Climate Change, Government of India; 2022.
9. CPCB (Central Pollution Control Board). Minutes of the Fifth meeting of the Joint Committee for Indoor Air Quality (IAQ) Management held on March 13, 2023. Government of India; 2023a. Annexure V: Preliminary Protocol for monitoring indoor air quality
10. CPCB (Central Pollution Control Board). Minutes of the Fourth and Fifth meetings of the Joint Committee for Indoor Air Quality (IAQ) Management. Government of India; 2023b.
11. CPWD (Central Public Works Department). Guidelines for running of air circulation, air cooling and air conditioning equipment during COVID-19. Government of India; 2020.
12. Ferrari S, Blázquez T, Cardelli R, Puglisi G, Suárez R, Mazzarella L. Ventilation strategies to reduce airborne transmission of viruses in classrooms: a systematic review of scientific literature. Build Environ. 2022;222:109366.
13. Gozdzielewska L, et al. Interventions to prevent the transmission of respiratory viral infections in home and community settings: a systematic review. BMC Public Health. 2022;22:1283.
14. Horvath EP. Building-related illness and sick building syndrome: from the specific to the vague. Cleve Clin J Med. 1997;64(6):303–9.
15. Huang J, Hao T, Liu X, Jones P, Ou C, Liang W, Liu F. Airborne transmission of the Delta variant of SARS-CoV-2 in an auditorium. Build Environ. 2022;219:109212.
16. Joshi SM. The sick building syndrome. Indian J Occup Environ Med. 2008;12(2):61–4.
17. Liu Y, Ma H, Zhang N, Li Q. A systematic literature review on indoor PM2.5 concentrations and personal exposure in urban residential buildings. Heliyon. 2022;8(1):e10174.
18. Lyles WB, Greve KW, Bauer RM, Ware MR, Schramke CJ, Crouch J, Hicks A. Sick building syndrome. South Med J. 1991;84(1):65–75.
19. Meggs WJ. Neurogenic inflammation and sensitivity to environmental chemicals. Environ Health Perspect. 1993;101(3):234–8.
20. Meggs WJ. Hypothesis for induction and propagation of chemical sensitivity based on biopsy studies. Environ Health Perspect. 1997;105(Suppl 2):473–8.
21. Mena AR, Ceballos HG, Alvarado-Uribe J. Measuring indoor occupancy through environmental sensors: a systematic review on sensor deployment. Sensors. 2022;22:3770.
22. Miller SL, Nazaroff WW, Jimenez JL, Boerstra A, Buonanno G, Dancer SJ, et al. Transmission of SARS-CoV-2 by inhalation of respiratory aerosol in the Skagit Valley Chorale superspreading event. Indoor Air. 2021;31(2):314–23.
23. Morawska L, Johnson GR, Ristovski ZD, Hargreaves M, Mengersen K, Corbett S, et al. Size distribution and sites of origin of droplets expelled from the human respiratory tract during expiratory activities. J Aerosol Sci. 2009;40(3):256–69.
24. Mousavi ES, Kananizadeh N, Martinello RA, Sherman JD. COVID-19 outbreak and hospital air quality: a systematic review of evidence on air filtration and recirculation. Environ Sci Technol. 2021;55(7):4134–47. https://doi.org/10.1021/acs.est.0c03247.
25. Nair AN, Anand P, George A, Mondal N. A review of strategies and their effectiveness in reducing indoor airborne transmission and improving indoor air quality. Environ Res. 2022;213:113579. https://doi.org/10.1016/j.envres.2022.113579.
26. Nardell EA. Air disinfection for airborne infection control with a focus on COVID-19: why germicidal UV is essential. Photochem Photobiol. 2021;97(3):493–7.
27. Patterson PD, Mcilvaine QS, Nong L, et al. Masking by health care and public safety workers in non-patient care areas to mitigate SARS-CoV-2 infection: a systematic review. JACEP Open. 2022;3:e12699. https://doi.org/10.1002/emp2.12699.
28. REHVA. REHVA COVID-19 guidance: document on how to operate and use building services in order to prevent the spread of the coronavirus disease (COVID-19) in workplaces. Federation of European Heating, Ventilation and Air Conditioning Associations; 2021.

29. Richardson ET, Morrow CD, Kalil DB, Bekker LG, Wood R. Shared air: a renewed focus on ventilation for the prevention of tuberculosis transmission. PLoS ONE. 2014;9(5):e96334.
30. Rudnick SN, Milton DK. Risk of indoor airborne infection transmission estimated from carbon dioxide concentration. Indoor Air. 2003;13(3):237–45.
31. Setti L, Passarini F, De Gennaro G, Barbieri P, Pallavicini A, Ruscio M, et al. Airborne transmission route of COVID-19: why 2 meters/6 feet of inter-personal distance could not be enough. Int J Environ Res Public Health. 2020;17(8):2932.
32. Silva ACT, Branco PTBS, Sousa SIV. Impact of COVID-19 pandemic on air quality: a systematic review. Int J Environ Res Public Health. 2022;19(4):1950.
33. Singh R. The risk status of waiting areas for airborne infection control in Delhi hospitals. Cureus. 2022a;14(3):e23211.
34. Singh R. Studying the double paradox in air conditioning at Indian airports for airborne infection prevention and filtration of harmful suspended particulate matter. Cureus. 2022b;14(4):e23748. https://doi.org/10.7759/cureus.23748. PMID: 35509738; PMCID: PMC9058289
35. Singh R. Public health issue of indoor dilution ventilation for disease prevention versus PM2.5 in intake air in auditoriums of premier engineering institutes in India. Cureus. 2022c;14(5):e25258. https://doi.org/10.7759/cureus.25258. PMID: 35755566; PMCID: PMC9217168
36. Singh R, Dewan A. Case study of the indoor air quality of the Delhi High Court: a critical review of the building envelope and HVAC systems. J Commun Dis. 2022a;54(1):30–5.
37. Singh R, Dewan A. Implementation of the Right to Healthy Environment: regulations for running air conditioners in public buildings and recognition of biological pollutants. Res Square. 2022b; https://doi.org/10.21203/rs.3.rs-1270717/v1.
38. Singh R, Dewan A. Air conditioners, airborne infection prevention and air pollution in buildings in New Delhi. Int J Tuberc Lung Dis. 2022c;26(3):288–90. https://doi.org/10.5588/ijtld.21.0704. PMID: 35209974
39. Thornton GM, Fleck BA, Fleck N, Kroeker E, Dandnayak D, Hartling L. The impact of heating, ventilation, and air conditioning (HVAC) design features on the transmission of viruses, including the 2019 novel coronavirus (COVID-19): a systematic review of humidity. PLoS ONE. 2022;17(10):e0275654.
40. Tran VV, Park D, Lee YC. Indoor air pollution, related human diseases, and recent trends in the control and improvement of indoor air quality. Int J Environ Res Public Health. 2020;17(8):2927.
41. van Rijn C, Somsen GA, Hoffer S, Boon S. Reducing aerosol transmission of SARS-CoV-2 in hospital elevators. Int J Indoor Environ Health. 2020;30(6):1361.
42. Wakayama T, Ito Y, Sakai K, Miyake M, Shibata E, Ohno H, Kamijima M. Comprehensive review of 2-ethyl-1-hexanol as an indoor air pollutant. J Occup Health. 2019;61(1):19–35.
43. Wolkoff P, Wilkins K, Clausen PA, Nielsen GD. Organic compounds in office environments—sensory irritation, odour, measurements and the role of reactive chemistry. Indoor Air. 2006;16(1):7–19.
44. Yang L, Iwami M, Chen Y, Wu M, van Dam KH. Computational decision-support tools for urban design to improve resilience against COVID-19 and other infectious diseases: a systematic review. Prog Plan. 2022:100657.

Control of Mosquito-Based, Vector-Borne Infections in the Built Environment

7

Raja Singh, Nirupam Madaan, and Anil Dewan

When you are in your house, each exhaled breath of yours carries carbon dioxide and lactic acid. This is the sign for a mosquito to be attracted and depend on your warm body to feed on your blood and sustain life for itself as a species. But, as a separate species, we humans have also suffered from the side effect of this mosquito feeding process. This side effect in mosquito-borne diseases has not only plagued mankind since the last 500,000 years, but is getting lethal with every passing day [54]. There is a long list of vector-borne diseases where the vector is a mosquito of different species. Some of the most common diseases that are mosquito-borne are Malaria, Dengue, Zika, Chikungunya, Japanese encephalitis virus disease, West Nile virus disease, Rift Valley fever, lymphatic filariasis, and yellow fever [70].

There is a multitude of vector-borne disease control methods and prevention techniques that have been prevalent, but for the sake of this chapter, we have concentrated our focus on the interventions for prevention of mosquito-borne diseases that are possible through the built environment and its changes. This means that any intervention that can be done in the building, after it is constructed, which can be integrated into the design, is the main focus. There are also inclusions of certain interventions that can be done during occupation of the building, but our focus remains on the design-based interventions that can be done in buildings at the drafting board stage. The most obvious among these measures are given as follows, as

R. Singh
Founder/Researcher, The Built, New Delhi, Delhi, India

Former Post Doctoral Fellow, Department of Environmental and Occupational Health, Dornsife School of Public Health, Drexel University, Philadelphia, Pennsylvania, USA

N. Madaan
Department of Hospital Administration, All India Institute of Medical Sciences, New Delhi, Delhi, India

A. Dewan
Department of Architecture, School of Planning and Architecture, New Delhi, Delhi, India

R. Singh et al., *Infection Control in the Everyday Built Environment*,
https://doi.org/10.1007/978-981-95-8624-0_7

suggested in the Manual on Integrated Vector Management in India prepared by the National Centre for Vector Borne Diseases Control [36]:

1. Mosquito-proofing of houses by fixing wire mesh on windows and doors.
2. Improved design to avoid undue waterlogging and access to overhead tanks, roof tops, etc.
3. Safe rainwater harvesting, by using covered tanks.

In a previous version of the Guidelines for Integrated Vector Management for Control of Aedes Mosquito [24], the National Vector Borne Disease Control Programme also suggested Environmental Management measures as follows:

1. Environmental modification which includes long-lasting transformation of vector habitats which includes water supply changes, mosquito-proofing of water tanks, cisterns of underground reservoirs.
2. Environmental manipulations like temporary changes to vector habitats that involve management of required and non-required containers and also the removal of natural breeding sites in and around human habitation.
3. Changes in human habitations which aim to reduce man-virus contact by mosquito proofing of houses with screens on doors and windows.

There is also a guideline for legislative measures, about which we will talk in detail, but the gist is that legislative measures include suitable laws and byelaws that should be enacted and implemented for regulation of storage/utilization of water by communities, various agencies, and avoiding mosquito- genic conditions at all sites, before, during, and after the construction. There is a specific mention to have building byelaws which include the above changes so that these become enforceable by law.

An example of this is the Delhi Municipal Corporation (Malaria and other Mosquito Borne Diseases) Bye-laws, 1975 which states duty of persons in occupation of premises to:

1. Prevent any collection of standing or flowing water in which mosquito may breed or are likely to breed, unless the water has been treated effectively to prevent such breeding.
2. Prevention of presence of any container or receptacle which allows to collect and retain water which may breed mosquitoes.

But the mere existence of the above byelaws was not considered enough, as there was an outbreak of mosquitoes in Delhi in the recent years. Let us look at the dengue cases recorded in New Delhi over the past few years in Table 7.1, which showed a blast of cases of dengue in the year 2021. This led the Hon'ble Delhi High Court to take this rise into cognizance and initiated a *suo moto* Public Interest Litigation case in Delhi [59]. The cases were even rising in the winter months, when usually the mosquitoes would not earlier be available due to the dip in temperature, but there was

Table 7.1 Tabulation of Dengue and Chikungunya cases in Delhi from 2010 to 2021

Year	Dengue cases in Delhi	Chikungunya cases in Delhi
2010	6259	120
2011	1131	110
2012	2093	6
2013	5574	18
2014	995	8
2015	**15,867**	64
2016	4431	**12,279**
2017	9271	940
2018	7136	407
2019	5077	520
2020	1269	126
2021	**13,089**	112
Total	**72,192**	**14,710**

a connection to the adaptation of the mosquitoes to the temperatures. If we try to investigate the reason for this rise, some experts state that the reason is related to climate crisis [11], i.e., an extended rain cycle and high humidity levels. Though this was considered only as a strong driving factor, with the main reason being urban intensification and potential inclusion of new virus [21]. A reaction to this in response by the Delhi Government was the notification of the Delhi Prevention and Control of Malaria, Dengue, Chikungunya or any Vector Borne Disease Regulation, 2021 [15] which in its preamble stated that the government was in the opinion that ordinary provisions of the law for the time being in force were in sufficient to prevent the outbreak and spread of vector borne diseases namely Malaria, Dengue, Chikungunya, etc. In this, the notification very specifically stated that "No person shall occupy a new building unless an occupation certificate is obtained from the respective local body requiring the provision of anti-mosquito system in such premises."

But if we look beyond Delhi, which is a metropolitan city in one of the somewhat tropical country in the world with a burgeoning population, we can look at the example of an Indian state which is majorly rural. The data spans over 2 years and is of four diseases caused by the mosquito. This data is given in Table 7.2.

In this, notably, the Visakhapatnam district has the maximum number of cases. This district has 52.5% rural population according to the 2011 census [17]. It is important to note that the majority of cases on malaria are from the tribal and rural areas, which forms 52% of the population and the rising diseases caused by the Aedes mosquito are due to the urban population as Aedes is mostly an urban vector and the district has seen rapid urbanization [4]. There is also forest area in the district as well as proximity to the forested area, which still stands as an area with malaria presence [47].

But as part of this book, this chapter focuses on the relation of vector control measures specifically in the built environment. The most common ones have already been listed above, but it is important to look at two important issues. One is the scientific basis of the vector control measures that have been stated to be related to

Table 7.2 Cases of mosquito-borne diseases in Andhra Pradesh 2020–2021 [18]

		Malaria		Dengue		Chikungunya		Japanese Encephalitis	
S. No.	District	2020	2021	2020	2021	2020	2021	2020	2021
1	Srikakulam	34	38	23	191	1	0	0	0
2	Vizianagram	120	103	16	268	0	1	0	0
3	Visakhapatnam	1259	841	211	1213	25	31	0	0
4	East Godavari	283	102	91	792	1	0	0	0
5	West Godavari	133	78	82	354	1	9	1	0
6	Krishna	21	11	44	225	0	0	0	0
7	Gunturu	26	15	182	653	0	2	0	0
8	Prakasam	34	3	81	155	0	3	0	0
9	Nellore	11	11	28	139	0	0	0	0
10	Chittor	3	29	25	213	0	0	0	0
11	Kadapa	30	21	21	90	0	0	0	0
12	Ananthapuram	41	15	105	178	0	0	0	0
13	Kurnool	32	47	16	289	0	2	0	0
Total		2027	1314	925	4760	28	48	1	0

the built environment, as to make sure that the evidence that exists is certain and scientifically sound.

The second issue was to look at the mosquito control and its relation to airborne infection control which we have covered in earlier chapters. The relation exists because we need fresh air changes for airborne infection control, and in order to take in this fresh air in non-centralized air-conditioned setting, the windows need to be opened. This is all the more relevant in geographies where people depend entirely on natural ventilation. Here there needs to be a gap creation between mosquitoes and humans which can be done by blocking access to mosquitoes while letting in fresh air. This can be done by using wire screening in doors and windows as well as other techniques which we shall discuss.

In order to first have an evidence-based approach, a review was performed, which followed the following methodology:

1. Once the need to investigate the evidence across studies was established, the keywords needed for literature study were identified.
2. The PubMed database was chosen as a reliable database of health-based studies and was fed in with the following keywords or search terms:
   "building interventions for prevention of vector borne disease" OR, OR "built environment and vector borne diseases" OR, OR "malaria" OR, OR "dengue" OR, OR "chikungunya" OR, OR "zika" OR, OR "wire mesh" OR, OR "mosquito screening"
3. Out of the multiple results, the top 199 most relevant as stated automatically were chosen from the PubMed database. This may be a limitation as papers beyond these were not screened. But for the sake if informing the reader, it sets the correct tone of the direction of the idea.

4. Out of the 199, the title and abstract of these papers were screened on the following criteria:
   (a) Relation to the built environment.
   (b) Mention of the changes or interventions that are required to be made to buildings or components of buildings.
   (c) Mention of mosquito screening, mosquito nets, and wire mesh as a direct component that can be identified as a measure of the built environment.
5. Out of the 199, 36 were finalized, but 3 were rejected as they were not available in the English language as a full record. 33 records were derived and checked in detail for evidence.
6. The 33 studies have been listed in a tabulated form along with the major derived information in Table 7.3.

The flow diagram of the studies included in the narrative review has been given in Fig. 7.1. There is a limitation as all the studies were not screened and 199 first relevant studies were screened which make this as a narrative review and not a scoping or a systematic review.

First, let us look at the analysis of the 33 papers that were studied and classify these based on the most common conclusions derived from these. These are given in Table 7.4.

Let us look at the papers that focused entirely on built environment interventions with respect to control of vector-borne diseases, or rather mosquito-borne diseases which form the focus of our study. The main setting -the-tone was done by the fact that due to high insecticide prevalence, there has been an overlooking of the preventive measures that could be done through improved housing, especially when malaria and other mosquito-related diseases are concerned. This concern has been shared by many studies. One paper quoted a randomized controlled trial which showed an anemia reduction by 47% by the use of full house screening, which is one of the most important interventions apart from the other housing-related interventions [65]. The landmark study out of the 6 studies focused on the built environment gave a mnemonic called DELIVER which stands for Doors, Eaves, Lifted, Insecticide-treated Bed-nets, Ventilation (and Screening), Environmental Management and Roofs, as all the parts of the building which need intervention for effective building-related intervention for control of vector-borne diseases [35]. This study resonated the concern about dependence on insecticides which may not only affect human beings but are also subject to insecticide resistance. This study quoted the concept of modern housing vs. traditional housing as shown in 15,000 studies that were reviewed and the results quoted. There were 45–65% fewer malaria cases reported when compared to traditional homes. The DELIVER approach suggested in the study in some brief detail is as follows:

1. Doors: Provision of screened doors and closed eaves should be done as this would mean a reduction of 59% of malaria mosquitoes and reduce human and mosquito contact. The door needs to be tight-fitting and preferably have self-closing hinges.

Table 7.3 The included studies in the review listed according to title and description of information

S. No.	Author	Title	Description
1	Canana [7]	A cost analysis to address issues of budget constraints on the implementation of the indoor residual spray program in two districts of Maputo Province, Mozambique	This paper specifically focuses on indoor residual spraying in two districts in Mozambique. It talks about the national plan which includes indoor residual spraying as an effective way of malarial control. The paper acknowledged insecticidal resistance, and there is a monitoring mechanism and there was a change in insecticide, and will keep using older insecticides where resistance is not reported. This is possible due to the monitoring mechanism
2	Okumu et al. [41]	Key characteristics of residual malaria transmission in two districts in South-Eastern Tanzania—implications for improved control	The study stated that most malaria transmission still occurs indoors even though there is a sizable proportion Anopheles mosquitos biting outdoors. The study says that even though the outdoor proportion of biting should no doubt be talked effectively even though it may be marginal. But even the mosquitoes that bite outdoors regularly enter houses at some time at least in their lives. Therefore, effective indoor intervention is required not only for indoor proportion but also for outdoor proportion of malaria vectors
3	Ven Den Berg et al. [68]	Recent trends in global insecticide use for disease vector control and potential implications for resistance management	The study stated that increased consideration should be given to alternative vector control tools that prevent the development of insecticide resistance. The central problem has been reliance on few insecticides and the following insecticide resistance. This calls for immediate switch to alternative path to vector control. This is in line with WHO's global vector control response 2017–2030
4	Canavati et al. [8]	Targeting high-risk forest goers for malaria elimination: a novel approach for investigating forest malaria to inform program intervention in Vietnam	In this forest dwellers not using mosquito nets even though there was availability and higher chance of malaria. Their willingness despite availability was low and hence a cause of concern. There was also a category that was sleeping in huts without walls Having vector measures that require least effort, unlike insecticide nets may be most useful in these cases

5	Lindsay et al. [35]	Recommendations for building out mosquito-transmitted diseases in sub-Saharan Africa: the DELIVER mnemonic	There is a concern that dependence on insecticides was insufficient and improved housing is required. Modern housing had 47% lower odds of malaria infection and 45–65% few malaria cases than in traditional homes. Another important point is that a less ventilated house produces more carbon dioxide and attracts more mosquitoes indoors. The study suggests the DELIVER approach. This mnemonic is as follow: 1. Doors: providing screen doors and closed eaves meant a reduction of 59% of malaria mosquitoes. The doors need to be tight fitting with screens and self-closing hinges 2. Eaves: in a study closing the eaves of thatched houses resulted in 94% fewer malaria mosquitoes. Closing of eaves will make the house hotter and hence screen eaves are a better idea 3. Lifted: Some studies performed show that the mosquitoes often don't predominantly reach heights and the conclusion is that there is compelling evidence that raising a house off the ground will reduce mosquito house entry. This can be on platforms or stilts 4. Insecticide-treated bed nets: Or, ITNs were linked to 42% reduction in malaria compared with untreated bed nets 5. Ventilation (and screening): In tropical climates, ventilation is important for cooling the house. Screening is important in these windows, which must be larger. A study showed screening doors and windows reduced malaria episodes by 61% 6. Environmental Management: This involves prevention of any stagnant water by means of preventing any water utensils, tires or containers. This means appropriate management in and around houses including in the water management systems 7. Roofs: Some roofs like metal roofs instead of thatch may prevent the growth of mosquitoes, but this cannot be generalized warrants further research Multisectorial integrations are required. The training on the medical side to engineers and architects and vice versa is required. The UN SDGs promote multisectorial collaboration. Global levels policies are required like housing guidelines or urban guidelines which integrate vector control in the building design The gaps highlighted are how mosquitoes enter buildings, micro financing homes case studies, scaling up of the same and more evidence on health benefit of tweaking habitats

(continued)

Table 7.3 (continued)

S. No.	Author	Title	Description
6	Kigozi et al. [34]	Rapid shifts in the age-specific burden of malaria following successful control interventions in four regions of Uganda	With respect to the built environment, this study suggests two interventions like long lasting insecticidal nets and indoor residual spray, but also mentions the issue of insecticide resistance by showings results where such resistance occurs. Because of this the study suggests needs for alternative measures
7	Hildon et al. [27]	"We have this, with my husband, we live in harmony": exploring the gendered decision-making matrix for malaria prevention and treatment in Nampula Province, Mozambique	This study focuses on the gender based approach to vector control
8	Russell et al. [49]	Capacity of National Malaria Control Programmes to implement vector surveillance: a global analysis	The study looks at the limitations and challenges faced by the national malaria control programs of about 36 countries in Africa, Asia and Americas. The study states that major interventions include vector surveillance, long lasting insecticidal nets, indoor residual spraying and larval source management, The study states that there is also an issue of insecticide resistance acknowledged in the study
9	Keys et al. [33]	Prevalence of malaria and lymphatic filariasis in bateyes of the Dominican Republic	No direct relation of built environment-related factors. There is some reference to bed nets, but it is part of an unrelated study protocol
10	Murta et al. [38]	Misperceptions of patients and health workers regarding malaria elimination in the Brazilian Amazon: a qualitative study	With respect to vector control in the built environment, the paper talks about long lasting insecticide nets and its usage. People have misconceptions on its usage. Health education, including cultural notions about vector control and community mobilization of various social actors will be required for the penetration of scientific knowledge to the public
11	Seger et al. [53]	Community assessments for mosquito prevention and control experiences, attitudes, and practices - U.S. Virgin Islands, 2017 and 2018	This study shows the concerns of Zika outbreak associated with hurricanes in the US Virgin islands. 40% households were concerned about contracting Zika during the outbreak and hurricanes in the islands. More than 70% households were concerned about getting Zika or other mosquito borne diseases during this time. There was a decrease in built environment factors integrity during hurricane response. Percentage of houses with undamaged window screens decreased from 64.4% to 30% during this time. The percentage of houses with undamaged door screen decreased from 39.9% to 22.7% and households with air conditioning decreased from 41% to 19.8%. Vector control decreases during natural disasters. This study used community assessment to find out these shifts and these must be repeated and reported

12	Derua et al. [16]	Bacterial larvicides used for malaria vector control in sub-Saharan Africa: review of their effectiveness and operational feasibility	This study talks about a novel way of larva management using bacterial larvicides in sub-Saharan Africa. This complements techniques like insecticide treated bed nets and indoor spraying. Larval source management is an important strategy in malaria control. This is most relevant in habitats that originate due to agriculture, mining and constructions. Out of many, manmade habitats are created due to construction activities
13	Adhikari et al. [1]	Perceptions of asymptomatic malaria infection and their implications for malaria control and elimination in Laos	This paper talks about the perception of asymptomatic malaria infections in Laos, especially mass drug administration for built environment related issues, the closest this article talks about is mosquito nets which 97.5% participants recalled using at home. 91.1% participants recalled sleeping under one the previous night of the survey
14	Van Eer et.al [69]	Decreased endemic malaria in Suriname: moving towards elimination	This study shows a decrease in malaria in Suriname after interventions measures for malaria prevention and control were introduced. These included impregnated bed nets for children and pregnant women, which is one of the factors that led to the eradication of malaria between 2002 and 2007
15	Doda et al [19]	A qualitative study of use of long-lasting insecticidal nets (LLINs) for intended and unintended purposes in Adami Tullu, East Shewa Zone, Ethiopia	The study looks at long-lasting insecticidal nets and found that though 64% of households owned at least one, there were cases of misuse and repurpose, were some people liked it for fences, roping, wall plastering etc. Proper training, improving perceptions, education and creating ownership were some solutions suggested
16	Pacheco et al. [43]	The 2016 Earthquake in Ecuador: Zika Outbreak After a Natural Disaster	This paper deals with the spread of vector disease Zika after the built environment getting destroyed due to a natural disaster, earthquake in this case. There are concerns regarding open pots and water collection in debris leading to breeding of mosquitoes. Therefore, there must be an interdisciplinary response to vector disease increase after natural disasters when health services are also hit
17	Muriuki et al. [37]	A comparison of malaria prevalence, control and management strategies in irrigated and non-irrigated areas in eastern Kenya	The study was about non-irrigated areas in Kenya to check for malaria prevalence, control and management. This study acknowledges the relation to building material and construction type. It does not include the same in the study. This study shows that environmental management is an effective way for malaria. Mosquito nets and bed nets have been discussed, along with clearing of bushed for malaria prevention along with management of breeding sites around house, indoor residual spraying and lighting fires along with mosquito coils

(continued)

Table 7.3 (continued)

S. No.	Author	Title	Description
18	Tusting et al [65]	Building malaria out: improving health in the home	The paper highlights the fact that overlooking of housing related interventions was there due to insecticide prevalence. The paper reports a randomized control trial, where there was anemia reduction by 47% when full house is screened, and hence this is an important intervention among others for malaria prevention through the built environment. The study raises four concerns related to window screening: Firstly, basic questions on housing related interventions and their validation. Secondly, questions of safety and other unintended consequences. Thirdly was the concern of acceptability of housing interventions. Fourthly, there are implementation and policy related concerns
19	Donnelly et al. [20]	A systematic, realist review of zooprophylaxis for malaria control	This study looks at zooprophylaxis which talks about having animals in proximity so that they divert mosquito bites away from humans. In this review, 20 articles were included in the final review out of 75 documents initially screened. Out of 9 studies, 6 studies reported a positive relationship between animal ownership and malaria risk. The optimal placement of animals in not specified as such, and there are concerns that there may be zoopotentiation in certain cases of species of mosquitoes. Further research is needed in this area. The study also acknowledges other built environment interventions like screening of windows, bed nets and closed roofing, though this has not been quantified or was the main focus
20	Tusting et al. [64]	The evidence for improving housing to reduce malaria: a systematic review and meta-analysis	The study is about whether improved housing can reduce malaria by decreasing house entry by malaria mosquitoes. This paper is a systematic review and meta analyses that has included 90 studies out of 15,526 screened. 53 reported epidemiological outcomes and 39 showed somewhat lower risk. This study states there is paucity of evidence. The primary comparison was between modern home and traditional home for relation to reduction of malaria by reducing house entry of mosquitoes. With respect to home screening, one randomized control test, there was a 48% reduction in anemia, with no effect on malaria. Three cohort studies were associated with lower incidence of clinical malaria. There were no lower odds of malaria or anemia in screened case-control studies, cohort studies or cross-sectional studies. The evidence on roof, wall and floors is inconsistent. Closed eaves were associated with quarter reduction. Presence of ceiling showed third reduction and house elevation shows no association. The GRADE (Grading of recommendations, assessment, development and evaluation) shows that evidence is low. The direction and consistency of effects indicate that housing is an important risk factor for malaria

21	Chanda et al. [10]	Addressing malaria vector control challenges in South Sudan: proposed recommendations	This paper mainly focuses on vector control measures like LLIN, epidemiological monitoring, and establishing intersectoral integrated vector management. It also talks about larval control measures like predator fish. The paper in general is not directly linked to built environment interventions except mainly bed nets mainly
22	Pulford et al. [45]	Feasibility and acceptability of insecticide-treated plastic sheeting (ITPS) for vector control in Papua New Guinea	This study looks at the feasibility and acceptability of a vector control product, which is a sheet that is integrated into the interior of the house. It is an insecticide treated plastics sheets, which is claimed to last for 3–5 year period. The participants reported a perceived reduction in the number of mosquitoes in and around the house and also a reduction in bites after installation. There was a perceived change of increase in temperature and a unusual smell. The authors state that this must be integrated along with a range of vector control measures. There was feasibility shown, and the study was funded indirectly by the company manufacturing the ITPS. It was declared suitable in the study for the Papua New Guinea context
23	Joshi et al. [32]	Can visceral leishmaniasis be eliminated from Asia?	This paper focuses on sand flies as a vector. The relation of vector control for sand flies and its relation to mosquito control needs further research but there may be commonalities. Indoor residual spraying and insecticide treatment of bed nets is a suggested measure against sandflies. There was also a mention of use of lime plastering which reduced sand-fly density in the Indian site but the same effect was not seen when mud plastering was used
24	Siegert et al. [56]	The effect of socioeconomic factors and indoor residual spraying on malaria in Mangaluru, India: a case-control study	This study found that housing is one of the factors influencing malaria. Living in a building with tiled roof and indoor residual spraying helped reduce malaria. Roof type was chosen as the overall proxy parameter for quality of housing. While living in tiled roof, decreased the odds of malaria, the cement roof doubled the odds compared to poor quality roofs like hut, mud, straw and thatch. This is counter intuitive and challenges existing studies. This may be due to cement roof with no preventive measures like eaves blockings and window screenings. Window screenings play a contributory role. The roof type proxy had three options: Cement, tile or poor quality roofs like thatch, hut mud, straw and metal sheet

(continued)

Table 7.3 (continued)

S. No.	Author	Title	Description
25	Brady et al. [5]	Vectorial capacity and vector control: reconsidering sensitivity to parameters for malaria elimination	The paper suggests that an integrated approach to vectoral control for malaria elimination is required. It states that where there is insecticide resistance, a single mode of vector control may be need to be replaced by other methods like larval source control which achieves comparable reductions in transmission comparable in costs to insecticide treated bed nets and indoor residual spraying. This paper also suggest use of genetically modified mosquitoes
26	Santos et al. [52]	A perspective on inhabited urban space: land use and occupation, heat islands, and precarious urbanization as determinants of territorial receptivity to dengue in the City of Rio De Janeiro	This study looks at the urban scale level of dengue receptivity by including built environmental parameters. The study divides the urban area into four territorial dimensions: heat islands, unconsolidated urban sprawl area, urban connections and slum area The heat islands provide good niches for proliferation of Aedes vectors. The unconsolidated urban sprawls may help in dengue settlement process. The urban connections help in spreading of dengue spread due to high circulation of people from different areas. The slums with their high density, also seem to have greater risk for dengue
27	Curtis et al. [14]	Insecticide treated nets: impact on vector populations and relevance of initial intensity of transmission and pyrethroid resistance	The paper states the advantages of using insecticide treated nets in reducing malaria transmission. It also states that there is a scope of insecticide resistance by use of the insecticide treated nets. The study state that though treated nets are valuable, continued monitoring and research are still necessary
28	Nguela et al. [40]	The effect of improved housing on indoor mosquito density and exposure to malaria in the rural community of Minkoameyos, Centre Region of Cameroon	This study is an entomological study that lasted for 12 months where the main intervention was housing modification through systematic random sampling of houses. The modifications were windows, door and eaves, walls and roofs to limit mosquito access into houses. In Cameroon where the study was performed, the only interventions was long lasting bed nets, and due to insecticide resistance, there is a need to focus on other vector interventions. The main intervention was screened doors with metallic netting and a wooden frame. In difference species, the improved houses and reduction in mosquito density by 1.7 or 1.8 fold. There was also a reduction of bites. There is also a clear reduction of human vector contact in houses due to screening and blocking, Policy may include aspects of housing design as vector control

29	Saha et al. [50]	Knowledge, attitudes, and practices regarding malaria control among the slash and burn cultivators in Rangamati Hill tracts of Bangladesh	As far as built environment factors are concerned, the study only looked at the need of insecticide treated nets and cleanliness ion surroundings of the house., that too from the point of view of the attitudes of the slash and burn cultivators in a particular hilly area of Bangladesh
30	Sanou et al. [51]	Insecticide resistance and behavioural adaptation as a response to long-lasting insecticidal net deployment in malaria vectors in the Cascades region of Burkina Faso	This paper mainly focuses on long-lasting insecticidal net deployment in Burkina Faso w.r.t malarial vectors. The study states that insecticidal resistance increases after the distribution of long lasting insecticidal nets. This means there is need for effective alternative indoor interventions, which may be non-insecticidal
31	Waite et al. [71]	Eave tubes for malaria control in Africa: a modelling assessment of potential impact on transmission	This paper talks about a modelling assessment of using eaves tubes in Africa. Eaves tubes use house odors to attract mosquitoes which die due to contact with the insecticide coated netting. 'Eaves tubes' is the combined package of screening of doors and windows, closing of eaves and putting the insecticide based tubes. The study was a population model to find out epidemiological outcomes at large scale outside of the laboratories. Eaves tubes show a community level effect. An example is that when there is 70% mortality, and if only 20% of the houses have eaves tubes, the properties without eaves tubes also see reduction of 50% in relative transmission potential. The eaves tubes not only kill, but also deflect the mosquitoes. There is scope for further research on eaves tubes
Excluded as out of scope			
32	Urner et al. [67]	Hunters' view on the control of African swine fever in wild boar. A participatory study in Latvia	This paper was not related to vector control but suggested physical control measures rather than other control measures
33	Monique et al. [39]	A 12-year follow-up of intestinal schistosomiasis in pre-school-aged children in Assoni Village, Eastern Senegal	This is not related to vector borne diseases, but is related to a disease where the worms create disease through water. This also means built environment interventions like pit latrines that need to be constructed

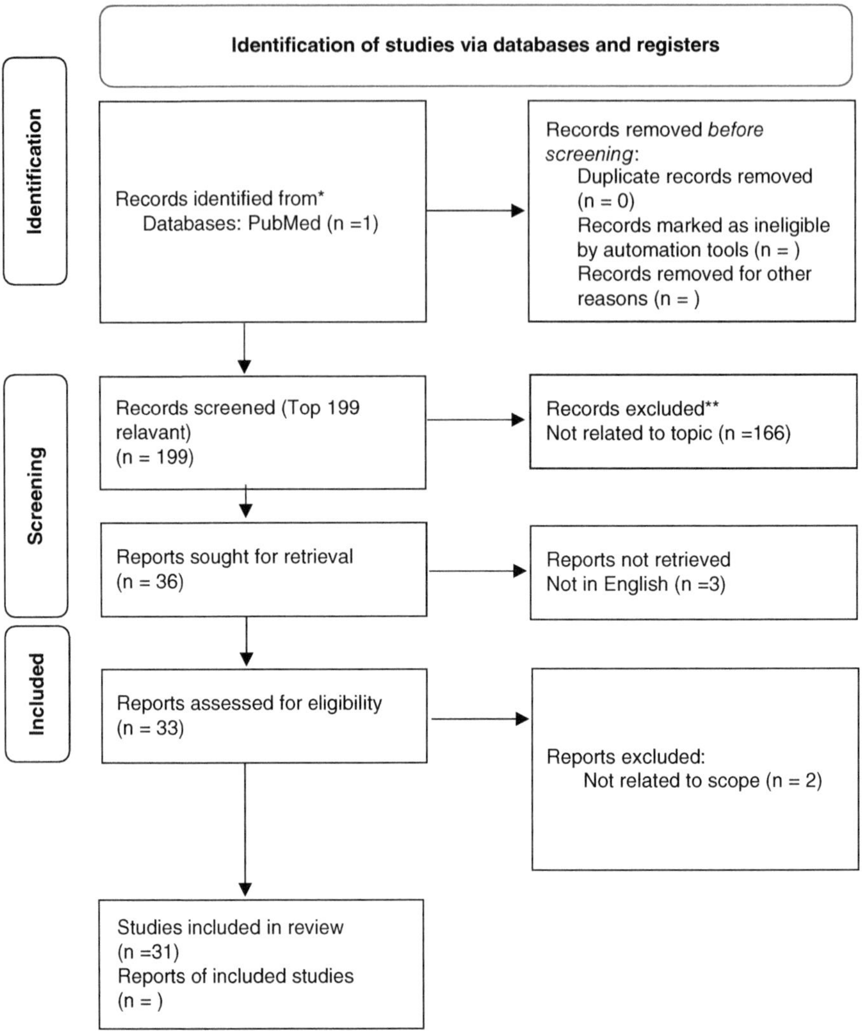

Fig. 7.1 PRISMA 2020 flow diagram for new systematic reviews has been used in this narrative review

2. Eaves: This is the area between the wall and the roof, which was studied and a study was reported to have 94% reduction in malaria mosquitoes when the eaves were closed. But, opening the eaves would mean the house would get hotter as these eaves were an outlet for the hot rising air generated indoors leading to convection current and being replaced by outside cooler air. Therefore, the suggestion of screened eaves was made. This has been further enhanced and will be discussed later, as this feature may be restricted to certain geographies and may not be a universal feature across geographies.

Table 7.4 The analysis of the papers studied under different topical subheadings

S. No.		Issue	No. of studies	Studies in question
1		The papers that fully concentrated on built environment-related interventions as the main focus	6	Lindsay et al., Tusting et al. (2 papers), Siegert et al., Santos et al., Nguela et al. [12, 25, 27, 31, 33, 35]
2		Papers that dealt with other related issues which are mentioned as follows:		
	a	The intervention, mosquito nets, is mentioned, dealt with, or studied	16	Canavati et al., Kigozi et al., Russell et al,, Murta et al., Keys et al., Derua et al., Adhikari et al., Van Eer et al., Doda et al., Muriuki et al., Donnelly et al., Joshi et al., Brady et al., Curtis et al., Saha et al., Sanou et al. [1, 5, 8, 14, 16, 19, 20, 32–34, 37, 38, 49–51, 69]
	b	Papers that mentioned, dealt, or studied the effect of disaster in built environment and vector control.	2	Seger et al., Pacheco Barzallo et al. [43, 53]
	c	Papers that dealt with, studied, or mentioned indoor residual spraying.	8	Canana et al., Kigozi et al., Russell et al., Derua et al., Muriuki et al., Joshi et al., Brady et al., Curtis et al. [5, 7, 14, 16, 32, 34, 37, 49]
	d	Papers that raised the issue of insecticide resistance (which has been taken as a reason for alternative vector control measures)	6	Canana et al., Van Den Berg et al., Kigozi et al., Russell et al., Brady et al., Curtis et al., Sanou et al. [5, 7, 14, 34, 49, 51, 68]
	e	Papers that showcase a new or a different or an innovative concept	3	Eaves Tubes: Waite et al. [71] Use of Insecticide-Treated Plastic Sheeting: Pulford et al. [45] Zooprophylaxis: Donnelly et al. [20]
	f	Larval Source Management	4	Russell et al., Derua et al., Chanda et al., Brady et al. [5, 10, 16, 49]

3. Lifted: This means that there is evidence that mosquitoes often don't predominantly reach heights. This may be platform-raised or stilt-raised houses.
4. Insecticide-Treated Ned Nets: These are various references to this like bed nets, mosquito nets, insecticide-treated nets (ITNs), or long-lasting insecticidal nets (LLINs). But the focus is on insecticide-treated ones which shows 42% reduction in malaria compared with untreated bed nets.
5. Ventilation (and screening): In tropical climates, ventilation is important for cooling the indoors, for which screening is important in these windows which must be large in size. Study shows that screening doors and windows reduced malarial episodes by 61%

Study also recommended multisectorial interdisciplinary integrations that may be required. The training is required to be given to engineers and architects, and vice versa. The study also quotes the United Nations Sustainable Development Goals [63] which also promote multisectorial collaboration as well. The study states that global policies are required like housing guidelines or urban guidelines which integrate vector controls in the building design. The gaps that the study has highlighted are further study on how mosquitoes enter buildings, about micro-financing of homes and related case studies, about scaling up of the house level interventions and implementations, and on the health benefit of tweaking habitats.

The next study which focused on the Indian context and took place in Mangalore in Karnataka, India [56]. This study found that housing is one of the key factors that influenced malaria and this study went on to create proxy for housing type. The study stated that living in a building with tiled roof and indoor residual spraying helped reduce malaria. Roof type was the selection made in the study as the overall proxy for quality of housing. The study observed that while living in tiled roof decreased the odds of malaria, the cement roof doubled the odds compared to poor quality roofs like hut, mud, straw, and thatch. The roof type used as proxy has classified the roofs into three types: First, poor quality roofs like thatch, hut, or straw; second, cement roof; third, tile roof; and fourth, metal roof. This is counterintuitive as compared to the study stated just before this one and challenges the conclusions drawn by existing studies. This is attributed to the fact that the cement roof may be used with no other preventive measures like eaves blocking and window screenings. The study clearly shows that window screenings play a strong contributory role.

There was another important entomological study that lasted for 12 months where the main intervention in the study was housing modification through systematic random sampling of houses [40]. The modifications made in the houses were windows, doors, eaves, walls, and roofs to limit mosquito access into the houses. This study was performed in the rural community of the Minkoameyos region in Cameroon. Before the interventions mentioned in the study, the main intervention in Cameroon were only long-lasting insecticidal bed nets. But due to insecticide resistance there was a need for focus on other vector control interventions through an integrated approach. The main intervention mentioned was screened doors with metallic netting and a wooden frame. With respect to the different species of mosquito, the improved houses, the reduction in mosquito density was in the range of

1.7–1.8 fold. There was also a reduction in bites. There was also a reduction of human vector contact in these houses due to screening and blocking. The study concluded that housing design and related interventions were important part of policy formulation for vector control in human habitations.

It is also very important to mention another study which looked at housing and built environment interventions at the larger planning scale instead of localized house-based interventions only [52]. The study looked at the urban scale level of dengue receptivity by including built environment parameters. The study divided the urban area in the city of Rio de Janeiro in Brazil into four territorial dimensions, i.e., heat islands, unconsolidated urban sprawl area, urban connections, and slum area. The study stated that heat islands provided good niches for the proliferation of Aedes mosquito which was responsible for Dengue. The unconsolidated urban sprawls help in the dengue settlement process. The urban connection areas, usually of transit utility, help in spreading of dengue due to high circulation of people from different areas. The slums, with their high density, were also believed in the study to have a greater risk for dengue.

But the most important paper included in the the chapter is a systematic review which found out the evidence for improving housing to reduce malaria [64]. The question asked was whether improved housing can reduce malaria by decreasing the house entry by malaria mosquitoes. This systematic review and meta-analyses included 90 studies out of the 1526 screened. 53 studies reported epidemiological outcomes and 39 showed somewhat lower risk. The primary comparison was between modern and traditional home for reduction of malaria by reducing house entry of mosquitoes. With respect to home screening, the study quoted one randomized control trial which stated that there was a 48% reduction in anemia with no effect on malaria. Three cohort studies were associated with a lower incidence of clinical malaria. There were no lower odds of malaria or anemia in screened case-control studies, cohort studies, or cross-sectional studies. The evidence on roof, wall, and floors is inconsistent. Closed eaves were associated with quarter reduction. Presence of ceiling showed third reduction and house elevation shows no association. The study declares that there is a paucity of evidence in general and also by the GRADE (Grading of recommendations, assessment, development and evaluation) framework, the evidence was low, yet the study declares in the conclusion that the direction and consistency of effects indicate that housing is an important risk factor for malaria. There is another study [65], already quoted which also listed the potential concerns related to one of the housing interventions for vector control, namely, window screening. These are, firstly, basic questions on housing-related interventions and their validation. Secondly, questions of safety and other unintended consequences. Thirdly was the concern regarding acceptability of housing interventions and lastly, the larger concerns regarding implementation and policy changes required.

Apart from the above papers with major focus on building-related or housing-related intervention, there were papers that focused on integrated approach or other approaches with mention of, inclusion of, or discussion about one specific intervention. This singular most important intervention was a bed net, most specifically the one that was treated with insecticide. This was either simply the insecticide-treated nets or the long-lasting insecticidal-treated nets. The most common intervention that was shared across the studies, even though these may not be directly related to the built environment, was the nets against mosquitoes like bed nets, which have been known by different names in the studies but aim at the same typology, though having changes in types and features. This is a bed net composed of the fabric which has the insecticide integrated into the weave and this bed net lasts for a long time as there is no insecticide which has to be constantly supplied. The use of such nets as compared to the normal nets is based on the fact that when a mosquito comes and lands on a bed net which has insecticidal treatment, the mosquito will die, and there will be community reduction of adult mosquitoes. The problem with untreated bed nets as stated in Indian guidelines is that ordinary mosquito nets may provide limited physical barrier between mosquito and man and the mosquitoes may still bite through the net or get inside the net following improper use. The advantages of these nets are that these may also keep other insects that cause nuisance like cockroaches, bedbugs, houseflies, fleas, etc. also at a distance. The long-lasting ones last for up to 20 washes and last for 3–5 years [25].

But it must also be noted that the use of bed nets requires the potential victims of mosquitoes to be proactive, which may not be the case in geographies around the world where malaria does not evoke the same response as the rest of the world would have [54]. This was visible in the study related to forest dwellers in Vietnam which stated that these dwellers were not using mosquito nets; even though there was a higher chance and availability of malaria. They were less willing even though there was availability. There was also a category which was sleeping in huts without any walls. This raised the issue of the use of vector measures which would require minimal effort by victims, and insecticide use was not the best option in this case [8] and other methods like larval source management may also be used, like stated in a sub-Saharan study [16]. But even in this case of using insecticide-treated nets, there are concerns of insecticidal resistance and alternative measures are still sought after as stated in a study from Uganda [34] and this was studied in detail in another study talking about pyrethroid resistance [14]. When the national malaria control programs of about 36 countries across Africa, Asia, and America were studied, the major interventions included vector surveillance, indoor residual spraying, larval source management, and most of all long-lasting insecticidal nets, though with the rider of possibility of resistance of mosquitoes developed for the insecticides [49]. In another study from the Dominican republic there was some reference to bed nets [33]. But one of the major issues with bed nets has been studied in a Brazilian Amazon study which states that people have misconceptions on the usage of the bed nets. The study went on to suggest that health education, including cultural notions about vector control and community mobilization of various social actors will be required for the penetration of scientific knowledge to the public [38]. A study in Suriname shows that there was a decrease in malaria between 2022 and 2007 after interventions for malaria control and prevention were introduced. The major intervention was impregnated bed nets specially for children and pregnant women [69]. In another related study in Laos, 97.5% participants recalled using it at home with

91.1% participants recalling using sleeping under one on the previous night of the survey [1]. But there are also concerns of misuse as in a study in Adami Tullu, East Shewa Zone in Ethiopia, though 64% houses owned one, these were repurposed to be used for wall plastering, fences, roping, etc. There was a need stated for proper training, improving perceptions, education, and creating ownership as some of the solutions [19]. There are other studies which also include bed nets of the insecticidal type [5, 20, 37], but there are certain more specific studies. This includes the one in hilly areas of Rangamati Hills in Bangladesh [50], and another one in Burkina Faso [51]. The Burkina Faso study shows the issue of insecticidal resistance. But, it is not only mosquitoes that can be dealt with by the insecticidal nets as stated before. Even sand flies can be dealt as a vector by insecticidal nets along with lime plastering instead of mud plastering in building as stated in a study from Asia [32].

There are two notable studies that deal with the new and innovative methods of vector control with respect to mosquitoes, along with a third one talking about zooprophylaxis. The first one uses Eaves tubes, which has been an important innovation dealing with malaria. The study mentioned talks about a modeling assessment of using eaves tubes in Africa. These tubes use house odors to attract mosquitoes which are subsequently killed due to contact with the insecticide-coated netting which is placed in the middle of these tubes, allowing air to pass through without letting the mosquitoes pass through. These "eaves tubes" are a combined package of screening of doors and windows, closing of eaves, and putting the insecticide-based tubes on the "eaves." In the study, a population model was used to find out the epidemiological outcomes at large scale outside of the laboratories. These eaves tubes show a community-level effect. This can be demonstrated by the fact that when there is 70% mortality and if only 20% of the houses have eaves tubes, the properties without these eaves tubes also see a reduction of 50% in relative transmission potential. The eaves tubes not only kill, but also deflect the mosquitoes. There is future scope of research in this method of using eaves tubes [71].

The second innovative method in the papers included was insecticide-treated plastic sheeting. An intervention study was done to look at the feasibility and acceptability of the vector control product, which is a sheet that is integrated into the interior of the house. This is an insecticide-treated plastic sheet, which is claimed to last for 3–5-year period. The participants reported a perceived reduction in the number of mosquitoes in and around the house and also a reduction in bites after installation. There was a perceived change of increase in temperature and an unusual smell. Their use was advised along with other vector control measures. Though funded by the manufacturer, the study shows that this innovation was suitable in the Papua New Guinea context [45].

There was also the strategy of using zooprophylaxis for malaria control. Zooprophylaxis means the use of animals (such as cattle) to divert disease-carrying insects such as mosquitoes from humans. In this case the disease is malaria. In this systematic review, 20 articles were included in the final review out of the 75 documents initially screened. Out of the 9 studies, later selected, 6 studies reported a positive relationship between animal ownership and malaria risk. The optimal placement of animals is not specified as such, and there are concerns that there may be zoo potentiation in certain cases of species of mosquitoes. Further research is needed in this area. The study also acknowledges other built environment interventions like screening of windows, bed nets, and closed roofing, though this has not been quantified or was not the main focus [20].

There were two studies which also looked the vector control after disaster, mostly natural disasters, and how prevention and control mechanisms can be framed and implemented. The first study based in the United States Virgin islands, performed in 2017 and 2018, shows the concerns regarding Zika outbreak associated with hurricanes in the islands [53]. 40% of the households were concerned about getting Zika or other mosquito-borne diseases during this time. There was a decrease in the built environment factors integrity during the hurricane response. The percentage of houses with undamaged window screens decreased from 64.4% to 305 during this time. The percentage of houses with undamaged door screens decreased from 41% to 19.8%. The study is a clear indication to the fact that vector control decreases during natural disasters. The use of community assessment was done in this study to find out the shifts as stated before. These community assessments must be repeated across geographies and reported for policy directions. The second study is based on the Zika outbreak following the 2016 earthquake in Ecuador. This paper deals with the effect of vector control post disaster. There are concerns regarding open pots and water collection in debris leading to the breeding of mosquitoes. Therefore, there must be an interdisciplinary response to vector disease increase after natural disasters when the health services are also hit [43].

There are other studies which stated the use of indoor residual spraying, which is when inside of dwellings is sprayed with an insecticide to kill mosquitoes that spread malaria [30]. Some of the studies include the one set in two districts of Mozambique. This paper talks about the national plan which includes residual spraying as an effective way of malarial control. The paper had acknowledged the insecticidal resistance, and there is a monitoring mechanism and there was a change in insecticide, and will keep using older insecticides where resistance is not reported. This is only possible due to monitoring mechanism that must be put in place elsewhere too [7]. There was another study from two districts in Tanzania which acknowledges that even though there are indoor malarial vectors, the outdoor proportion of mosquitoes is also sizeable. This states that effective indoor intervention is required not only for indoor but also for the outdoor proportion of the malarial vectors as there is a constant in and out of mosquitoes from the houses to the outside [41].

There are also studies which deal with the intervention of larval source management [5, 10, 16, 49]. This means that the mosquitoes will be controlled at the growth stage itself, before they become adults and be enabled to feed on humans and carry vector-borne diseases. This has been taken up in multiple national malaria control programs and is also taken up in individual papers which also talk about predators fish, like this paper from South Sudan [10]. Larval source management is suggested to be most required for habitats that originate due to agriculture, mining, and construction. Out of many other ways, manmade mosquito habitats are created due to construction activities [16]. There are also suggestions for genetically modified mosquitoes [5] which are beyond the scope of our discussion.

But even with the use of insecticide-treated nets, there is a concern as highlighted before of insecticide resistance [5, 14]. This has led to increased consideration that should be given to alternative vector control tools that prevent the development of this insecticidal resistance. The central issue is the reliance on few insecticides and the following insecticide resistance. This is also in line with the World Health Organisation's Global Vector Response 2017–2030 [42, 68]. This acknowledgement of the insecticide resistance issue is there in major national malaria control programs [49]. The insecticide-treated nets have been in general recognized my multiple studies and the need for alternative vector methods is clear [1, 5, 8, 14, 16, 19, 20, 32–34, 37, 38, 49–51, 69]. Housing interventions are a promising solution for the same [12, 25, 27, 31, 33, 35].

There is one study which was not included in the study and was later added. This is most particularly focused to the screening of doors and windows for excluding mosquitos from houses. This study was performed in Rural Gambia and remains one of the few intervention studies. This study has shown that the screened prototype doors reduced the number of house-entering mosquitoes by 59–77% [31]. This has been validated by the Vector Control Research Centre of the Indian Council of Medical research, which further states that Screened doors and windows may be a useful intervention for minimizing exposure to vector mosquitoes [28]. The screening of doors and windows has been advised as one of the vector control options. This has been reinstated by the National Centre for Vector Borne Diseases Control and reinstated that wire screening of doors and windows is a protection method for minimizing vector contact to prevent mosquito borne diseases [55].

Now, we need to talk about the nexus between airborne infections and vector-borne infections. This may sound a little bit of an overstatement, but the fact will be illustrated in detail. Dilution ventilation was suggested as a means of prevention of airborne spread of diseases by major Heating, Ventilation and Air Conditioning organizations of the world like the Federation of European Heating, Ventilation and Air Conditioning Associations or REHVA, the Society of Heating, Air Conditioning and Sanitary Engineering in Japan or SHASE, the American Society of Heating, Ventilation and Air Conditioning Engineers or ASHRAE and related societies from China. This has also been suggested by the Indian Society of Heating, Refrigeration and Air Conditioning Engineers. These guidelines were studied together in a study comparing the guidelines suggested during the COVID 19 pandemic [13, 22, 26, 29]. Dilution Ventilation as stated before means supply of fresh air which dilutes the aerosolized disease pathogens like tuberculosis, COVID-19, measles, influenza, and others. The traditional centralized air conditioners may have mechanism for dilution ventilation built into the air-conditioning systems, but in smaller units, there may be use of smaller recirculation-based air conditioning systems which used split air conditioning where there is an indoor unit and an outdoor unit with no air exchange possible in these units [57]. These split air conditioners are also used in larger community spaces where the windows are sealed and there is recirculation of the indoor air [46, 60]. In these cases the only way for dilution ventilation may be by opening of windows. But there is a possibility that people may not open the windows more frequently. The cause of not opening the windows was to be investigated.

This led to the development of an online-based window openability pilot survey with the major objectives being to get an indication as to whether people open their windows or not, and if they don't, the reason why they don't.

To perform this study, we followed the following steps:

1. Calculating Sample Size.
   The number of households in India is 25,00,00,000. For this number, the sample size calculated at confidence level of 95% with margin of error of 8.3% was 140.
2. An Online Survey was formulated on Google Forms and circulated among users of buildings.
3. The results were gathered and reported.

The results show that 77 of the 140 respondents had "Mosquitoes/Bees/Insects can come in through the window" as their major concern. The most obvious solution to such a problem was to have a window which lets in fresh air and also prevents mosquitoes/bees and animals from entering.

But then we wanted to find out the urban context of openability of windows, and the reasons as to why people would not open their windows, but for that a reality check was needed whether this was also the on-ground reality. For this a pilot study was performed in a posh South Delhi locality, where 210 randomly selected houses were observed unobtrusively [58, 61].

Each house was visually checked for the presence of the windows, their opening, and the presence of wire mesh. Out of 210 houses visually surveyed, only 88 had a window/door with a wire mesh. This indicated that no wire mesh in windows means less opening of windows, esp. when recirculation-based air conditioner is used. This means an increased chance of airborne transmission risk, but also means that when windows were to be opened, there would be direct access of mosquitoes as there was an absence of the wire mesh. This would discourage people to open the windows due to the mosquito scare and therefore the objective of fresh air supply may suffer. This pilot study encouraged the undertaking of a full-fledged study with more parameters in small plots. 265 house plots in a focus neighborhood in New Delhi were selected randomly. The following main objectives were:

1. To appraise the type of door and window with respect to the material of the construction.
2. To relate the type of window choice to the type of construction.
3. To check for the presence of wire mesh in the door/window as a factor for allowing for openability related to dilution ventilation.

The methodology followed was that a visual field study was conducted. Another south Delhi, somewhat densely populated locality, was chosen randomly. The reason for choosing the locality was that it is a dense locality which falls under the Delhi Bye laws as all the plots require approval and fall within the house tax jurisdiction of the South Delhi Municipal Corporation, one of the biggest municipal bodies which enforces the implementation of the Unified Building Byelaws, 2016.

Table 7.5 The number of house plots with type of construction

Type of house construction	Number
New stilt type	40
New (Pre stilt era)	138
Old houses	36
Renovated/Face-lifted	24
Very old (No change since 1960–1970)	24

There have also been new houses constructed here. Another reason for choosing this locality was that it has houses from different eras, including the ones which followed the pre 1962 norms with increased setbacks and height limits [66].

The study results are in Table 7.5.

The study concluded that 40 out of the 265 were newly constructed ones. Out of these 16 has no openable window. Only 9 out of 40 had a wire mesh in the openings. There was no wire mesh in plots having PVC-based windows. The choices made of the window opening frames lead to less openability and lesser chance of having a wire mesh. These windows decrease dilution ventilation and increase the probability of infection spread.

The limitations to openability also need to be discussed in detail as there are critical factors associated with openability of windows: till now issue was the use of recirculation-based air conditioners and how spaces that use the same behave with respect to transmission of airborne infection. Use of outside air in the inside is a critical factor which depends on multiple determinants. In smaller units which use room air conditioner that determinant is the presence of openings which allow outside air to enter. These openings may or may not be opened by inhabitants due to various factors as follows:

Firstly, the entry of noise when windows are open: Occurrence of high levels of noise [23] is a factor in urban settings, mostly due to the traffic that exists.

Secondly, thermal Comfort in the extreme climate of New Delhi. New Delhi which has extreme climate [6]. Many studies have been done linking thermal comfort and natural ventilation [2, 3, 44] and this is an important factor why architects and building professionals must consider in planning of spaces.

Thirdly, a further challenge confronting urban centers in developing countries such as New Delhi is the persistently high level of ambient air pollution. Among the various pollutants, fine particulate matter, particularly PM2.5, constitutes a significant public health risk in New Delhi as well as in many global cities [48]. Research suggests that shutting windows offers only limited protection from indoor $PM_{2.5}$ exposure, as these fine particles infiltrate indoor environments irrespective of window position. Such infiltration occurs through mechanisms such as Brownian motion [72] and air leakage through unavoidable building gaps and cracks. Consequently, strategies that rely solely on preventing outdoor air from entering indoor spaces are unlikely to produce substantial improvements.

Similarly, downstream technological interventions, such as the use of portable air purifiers, may lead to increased energy consumption at the community level.

Therefore, long-term improvements in ambient air quality remain the most effective solution [62]. Even though air purifiers can reduce particulate concentrations, gaseous pollutants including sulfur dioxide, nitrogen oxides (NOx), and carbon monoxide may persist indoors and require mitigation at their emission sources. Evidence from developed nations and cities such as Beijing demonstrates that governmental policy interventions targeting ambient pollution can result in measurable improvements and represent a viable path forward.

Interestingly, certain studies have observed that opening windows can, under specific conditions, reduce indoor particulate levels by enabling their dispersion outdoors [59]. Window opening also facilitates the reduction of indoor-generated volatile organic compounds (VOCs), which are commonly emitted from cleaning agents, paints, varnishes, and furniture finishes. Such reductions occur through dilution ventilation processes. However, in larger public facilities in New Delhi that rely on centralized air-conditioning systems, inadequate filtration systems remain a concern [60]. The installed filters in many public assembly buildings may not be sufficiently effective in removing PM2.5 particles. Access to clean and healthy air is increasingly recognized as a fundamental human right [46], underscoring the urgent need for comprehensive measures aimed at reducing ambient pollution as a long-term strategy to improve indoor air quality.

Fourth, another concern may be the sense of security when the windows are open. Though there is a presence of steel grill on the inside. This is below the glass pane shutter which is an anti-theft measure.

Fifth, the reason that people may not open windows is the lack of openability. This means that the designer or the building owner has installed windows with fixed glass panes or partially openable glass windows. Another factor in window openability can be lack of wire mash/wire screening which may prevent people from opening operable windows. Wire screening is the key vector-borne disease prevention measure in major tropical cities. People may not install wire mesh due to a variety of concerns like lack of aesthetic appeal, extra expense, non-prescription by architect or building designer. While taking decisions about construction, the occupants or the designers may neglect this factor. The newer materials available for facades like PVC may also not have wire mesh as a default attachment. It may be an additional fitment costing more money, taking more space, or looking less aesthetic. People may tend to have an aesthetic connect with large uninterrupted glass panes.

Based on the above studies and literature-based evidence, the following recommendations can be derived:

1. The building professionals, designers, architects, engineers, and hospital administrators must first and foremost at the drafting board stage pay full attention to all details in the working drawings of all projects that there are following considerations with respect to the water and public health engineering:
   (a) All the terraces, balconies, parapets, porches, verandas, open courtyards, and metaled ground areas must have a definitive slope so that there is always a flow of water present in these structures. In case the sloping is missed during the laying of flooring, it will be observed, as is often seen, that there may

be patches of water that may not flow and remain stagnant. This must be remedied at the stage of design by giving appropriate slope in the specifications and not relying upon the contractor or the building executioner to do on their own. For this, reference must be made to Part IX of the National Building Code which deals with Drainage and Sanitation [6].

(b) All the points that have the end of the slope must have appropriate outlet pipe which is covered and ends in a covered receptacle which is sealed. The piping should be as per the standards laid out in the National Building Code of 2016.

(c) If there are overhead tanks, or septic tanks, or water tanks at the ground level, or inspection chambers for water and or sewage, it must be either sealed or in case when air flow in required, must be covered with a wire mesh which is openable. This may also be part of the local building byelaws for certain localities [66].

The above measures will serve as a source management intervention as the adult mosquitoes will not be provided with the water that is essential to lay eggs which will again create the next generation of mosquitoes.

2. At the stage of the design, there must also be inclusion of adult mosquito-related interventions, especially the ones where the contact between the mosquito and human is minimized. For this the following provisions need to be made:

(a) All the windows must be openable and operable with control provided to the user. The windows must be affixed with appropriate wire screening or netting which will prevent the entry of the mosquitoes from the outside to the inside. This will also be relevant where there is a source of mosquito breeding where the building user may not be able to intervene. This may be a large water body, an abandoned house, or any other such building premises. This wire mesh on windows is also included in the Central Public Works Department Guidelines for residential houses, but on an optional basis [9]. There is also an application in this matter filed by the first author before the Hon'ble Delhi High Court for the inclusion in the Unified Building Bye Laws of Delhi as a mandatory provision [12, 59].

(b) The inside of the buildings, especially rooms where beds are placed, must have appropriate provisions for the design for easy installation of bed nets as needed by any user at any time. The provision of appropriate provisions like hooks will be an encouraging factor for a user to install bed nets in the indoors.

(c) The screened doors should be tight-fitting and must have screened panel whenever possible in order to have provisions for natural ventilation without the entry of mosquitoes and flies. The door should also be equipped with self-closing hinge so that the door remains close for most part.

(d) The eaves, or "*jaalis*" or lighting shafts at the higher level on the wall for ventilation should be screened with a wire mesh instead of simply sealing it as it has an important purpose in the passive cooling of the house.

It seems many times that these interventions are placed after the building has been constructed, as these were not included in the design of the building pre construction. This is because these details are not usually considered as the standard part of the building construction module and are seen as something that is to be retrofitted later (like adding an additional jaali door).

3. In order to make sure buildings are made mosquito-proof from the day one, i.e., at the drafting board stage itself, there is a need for integrating the mosquito control measures in the building byelaws, building codes as well as all the statutory inspections and check checklists for buildings. This has also been suggested by the Vector Control authority of various governments including the one in India. The byelaws must not have an indirect specification which is clubbed with the specifications of the water management and furniture or envelope design, but must be integrated as a separate stand-alone enforceable part of provisions that are recognized as mosquito prevention and control interventions which will need to be followed. This will not only put a pressure on architects, builders, and house owners to put the mosquito control provisions, but will also make clear penal offences that are listed and need no special explanation, or are not a subset of some other provision. The presence in the enforceable building byelaws will give mosquito control measures the importance that these may need and may not have always been provided.
4. Finally, as a bottom up approach, the mosquito control measures must become part of the popular discourse through various outreach measures. This also includes the interventions in the curricula of students at the various levels for mosquito control self-help measures. At a more technical level, these must be included in the curriculum of design schools and architectural and engineering courses so that the new generation of building creators are sensitized at the early states and vector control will be the option by default in the built environment.

Acknowledgments Many thanks to Dr Sweta Bhan of ICMR-NIMR. The authors acknowledge the support provided by the institutions including School of Planning and Architecture, New Delhi, All India Institute of Medical Sciences, New Delhi, and Drexel University. Special thanks to Rajshekhar Pullabhatla and Group Captain P Aanand Naidu of ISAC Centre for Built Environment Policy and Tathatara Foundation. Many thanks to Dr Arthur L Frank, MD. Many thanks to all the people who supported this work in many ways.

Declarations The authors Raja Singh, Nirupam Madaan, and Anil Dewan declare no conflict of interests or competing interests in this work. There is no involvement of human participants, animals, human or animal tissue. All authors declare that there was no specific financial support received from any organization for the submitted work. All authors declare that they have no financial relationships at present or within the previous 3 years with any organizations that might have an interest in the submitted work. While all care has been taken in ensuring the accuracy of this work, any inadvertent error may be reported at the earliest. The authors acknowledge the use of supervised language learning models/large language models for enhancement of the work, with responsibility lying with the authors. For more information, the corresponding author may be contacted at email rajaresearch@proton.me.

CRediT Statement The following is the CRediT statement which declares the author credits for this chapter:

Raja Singh: Conceptualization, Methodology, Formal Analysis, Investigation, Data Curation, Writing-Original Draft, Writing-Review & Editing, Visualization, Project Administration.
Nirupam Madaan: Conceptualization, Resources, Validation, Supervision, Project Administration.
Anil Dewan: Resources, Validation Supervision.

References

1. Adhikari B, Phommasone K, Pongvongsa T, Soundala X, Koummarasy P, Henriques G, Peto TJ, Seidlein LV, White NJ, Day NPJ, Dondorp AM, Newton PN, Cheah PY, Mayxay M, Pell C. Perceptions of asymptomatic malaria infection and their implications for malaria control and elimination in Laos. PLoS One. 2018;13(12):e0208912. https://doi.org/10.1371/journal.pone.0208912.
2. Ahmed T, Kumar P, Mottet L. Natural ventilation in warm climates: the challenges of thermal comfort, heatwave resilience and indoor air quality. Renew Sust Energ Rev. 2021;138:110669. https://doi.org/10.1016/j.rser.2020.110669.
3. Ali SF, Lakshya S, Dibakar R, Bishwajit B. Influence of passive design parameters on thermal comfort of an office space in a building in Delhi. J Archit Eng. 2020;26(3):04020017. https://doi.org/10.1061/(ASCE)AE.1943-5568.0000406.
4. Andhra Pradesh: Dengue and malaria sting Vizag more than other districts. The Times of India. 2022. https://timesofindia.indiatimes.com/city/visakhapatnam/dengue-and-malaria-sting-vizag-more-than-other-dists/articleshow/88783513.cms.
5. Brady OJ, Godfray HCJ, Tatem AJ, Gething PW, Cohen JM, McKenzie FE, Perkins TA, Reiner RC, Tusting LS, Sinka ME, Moyes CL, Eckhoff PA, Scott TW, Lindsay SW, Hay SI, Smith DL. Vectorial capacity and vector control: reconsidering sensitivity to parameters for malaria elimination. Trans R Soc Trop Med Hyg. 2016;110(2):107–17. https://doi.org/10.1093/trstmh/trv113.
6. Bureau of Indian Standards. National Building Code 2016. 2016.
7. Canana N. A cost analysis to address issues of budget constraints on the implementation of the indoor residual spray programme in two districts of Maputo Province, Mozambique. Malar J. 2021;20(1):8. https://doi.org/10.1186/s12936-020-03556-3.
8. Canavati SE, Kelly GC, Quintero CE, Vo TH, Tran LK, Ngo TD, Tran DT, Edgel KA, Martin NJ. Targeting high risk forest goers for malaria elimination: a novel approach for investigating forest malaria to inform program intervention in Vietnam. BMC Infect Dis. 2020;20(1):757. https://doi.org/10.1186/s12879-020-05476-8.
9. Central Public Works Department. Manual on Door and Window Details for Residential Buildings Volume 1. Central Public Works Department; n.d. Retrieved November 14, 2021, from https://www.cpwd.gov.in/Publication/manualdw.pdf.
10. Chanda E, Doggale C, Pasquale H, Azairwe R, Baba S, Mnzava A. Addressing malaria vector control challenges in South Sudan: proposed recommendations. Malar J. 2013;12(1):59. https://doi.org/10.1186/1475-2875-12-59.
11. Climate crisis, year-long dengue cases in Delhi linked: South MCD. Hindustan Times. 2022. https://www.hindustantimes.com/cities/delhi-news/climate-crisis-year-long-dengue-cases-in-delhi-linked-south-mcd-101648492705055.html.
12. Court on its own Motion (Mosquito Infestation in Delhi) vs. North Delhi Municipal Corporation and Ors. 2022. http://delhihighcourt.nic.in/dhcqrydisp_o.asp?pn=148630&yr=2022.
13. CPWD. General specifications for heating, ventilation & air-conditioning (HVAC) works. 2017.
14. Curtis CF, Jana-Kara B, Maxwell CA. Insecticide treated nets: Impact on vector populations and relevance of initial intensity of transmission and pyrethroid resistance. J Vector Borne Dis. 2003;40(1–2):1–8.

15. Delhi Prevention and Control of Malaria, Dengue, Chikungunya or Any Vector Borne Disease Regulation, 2021, No. 6/DGHS/2019/PHW-IV/NVBDCP/Notification of VBDs/4714. 2021. https://egazette.nic.in/WriteReadData/2021/230488.pdf
16. Derua YA, Kweka EJ, Kisinza WN, Githeko AK, Mosha FW. Bacterial larvicides used for malaria vector control in sub-Saharan Africa: review of their effectiveness and operational feasibility. Parasit Vectors. 2019;12(1):426. https://doi.org/10.1186/s13071-019-3683-5.
17. District Census Handbook Visakhapatnam (Part XII-A; 29). Directorate of Census Operations, Andhra Pradesh. 2011.
18. District Wise and Year Wise VBDs Andhra Pradesh (Rc. No. 8101/HEO.3/NVBDCP/2022). Director of Public Health and Family Welfare. 2022.
19. Doda Z, Solomon T, Loha E, Gari T, Lindtjørn B. A qualitative study of use of long-lasting insecticidal nets (LLINs) for intended and unintended purposes in Adami Tullu, East Shewa Zone, Ethiopia. Malaria J. 2018;17(1):69. https://doi.org/10.1186/s12936-018-2209-5.
20. Donnelly B, Berrang-Ford L, Ross NA, Michel P. A systematic, realist review of zooprophylaxis for malaria control. Malar J. 2015;14(1):313. https://doi.org/10.1186/s12936-015-0822-0.
21. Experts examine climate crisis, dengue link in Delhi. Hindustan Times. 2022. https://www.hindustantimes.com/cities/delhi-news/experts-examine-climate-crisis-dengue-link-in-delhi-101645380260581.html.
22. Francisco PW, Emmerich SJ, Schoen LJ, Hodgson MJ, Mccoy WF, Miller SL, Li Y, Kong H, Olmsted RN, Sekhar C, Parsons SA, Wargocki P. ASHRAE position document on airborne infectious diseases by ASHRAE Board of Directors. Ashrae Standard. 2020;26. www.ashrae.org.
23. Ghiaus, Christian, Allard, editors. Natural ventilation in the urban environmental assessment and design. Earthscan; 2005.
24. Guidelines for Integrated Vector Management for Control of Aedes Mosquito. National Vector Borne Disease Control Programme, Government of India. n.d. Retrieved May 15, 2023, from https://main.mohfw.gov.in/sites/default/files/79767166351454408152_0.pdf.
25. Guidelines for ITNs and LLINs. National Vector Borne Disease Control Programme, Government of India. n.d. Retrieved May 15, 2023, from https://nvbdcp.gov.in/WriteReadData/l892s/Guidelines-for-ITNS-LLINS.pdf.
26. Guo M, Xu P, Xiao T, He R, Dai M, Miller SL. Review and comparison of HVAC operation guidelines in different countries during the COVID-19 pandemic. Build Environ. 2021;187:107368. https://doi.org/10.1016/j.buildenv.2020.107368.
27. Hildon ZJ-L, Escorcio-Ymayo M, Zulliger R, Arias De Aramburú R, Lewicky N, Harig H, Chidassicua JB, Underwood C, Pinto L, Figueroa ME. "We have this, with my husband, we live in harmony": exploring the gendered decision-making matrix for malaria prevention and treatment in Nampula Province, Mozambique. Malaria J. 2020;19(1):133. https://doi.org/10.1186/s12936-020-03198-5.
28. ICMR-VCRC/RTI-4/SCI/2022/D-190 RTI No. VCRCP/R/E/22/00004. Vector Control Research Centre. Indian Council of Medical Research; n.d.
29. Indian Society of Heating, refrigertaion and Air Conditioning Engineers. ISHRAE COVID-19 guidance document for air conditioning and ventilation. Indian Society of Heating, refrigeration and Air Conditioning Engineers. 2020. https://ishrae.in/mailer/ISHRAE_COVID-19_Guidelines.pdf.
30. Indoor residual spraying. Wikipedia. 2022. https://en.wikipedia.org/w/index.php?title=Indoor_residual_spraying&oldid=1129746538.
31. Jawara M, Jatta E, Bell D, Burkot TR, Bradley J, Hunt V, Kandeh B, Jones C, Manjang AM, Pinder M, Stone S, D'Alessandro U, Knudsen J, Lindsay SW. New prototype screened doors and windows for excluding mosquitoes from houses: a pilot study in rural Gambia. Am J Trop Med Hygiene. 2018;99(6):1475–84. https://doi.org/10.4269/ajtmh.18-0660.
32. Joshi A, Narain JP, Prasittisuk C, Bhatia R, Hashim G, Jorge A, Banjara M, Kroeger A. Can visceral leishmaniasis be eliminated from Asia? J Vector Borne Dis. 2008;45(2):105–11.

33. Keys HM, Noland GS, De Rochars MB, Blount S, Gonzales M. Prevalence of malaria and lymphatic filariasis in bateyes of the Dominican Republic. Infect Dis Poverty. 2019;8(1):39. https://doi.org/10.1186/s40249-019-0547-3.
34. Kigozi SP, Kigozi RN, Epstein A, Mpimbaza A, Sserwanga A, Yeka A, Nankabirwa JI, Halliday K, Pullan RL, Rutazaana D, Sebuguzi CM, Opigo J, Kamya MR, Staedke SG, Dorsey G, Greenhouse B, Rodriguez-Barraquer I. Rapid shifts in the age-specific burden of malaria following successful control interventions in four regions of Uganda. Malar J. 2020;19(1):128. https://doi.org/10.1186/s12936-020-03196-7.
35. Lindsay SW, Davies M, Alabaster G, Altamirano H, Jatta E, Jawara M, Carrasco-Tenezaca M, Von Seidlein L, Shenton FC, Tusting LS, Wilson AL, Knudsen J. Recommendations for building out mosquito-transmitted diseases in sub-Saharan Africa: the DELIVER mnemonic. Philos Trans R Soc B Biol Sci. 2021;376(1818):20190814. https://doi.org/10.1098/rstb.2019.0814.
36. Manual on Integrated Vector Management in India. National Vector Borne Disease Control Programme, Government of India. n.d. Retrieved May 15, 2023, from https://ncvbdc.mohfw.gov.in/Doc/Guidelines/Manual-Integrated-Vector-Management-2022.pdf.
37. Muriuki JM, Kitala P, Muchemi G, Njeru I, Karanja J, Bett B. A comparison of malaria prevalence, control and management strategies in irrigated and non-irrigated areas in eastern Kenya. Malar J. 2016;15(1):402. https://doi.org/10.1186/s12936-016-1458-4.
38. Murta FLG, Mendes MO, Sampaio VS, Junior ASB, Díaz-Bermúdez XP, Monteiro WM, Lacerda MVG. Misperceptions of patients and health workers regarding malaria elimination in the Brazilian Amazon: a qualitative study. Malar J. 2019;18(1):223. https://doi.org/10.1186/s12936-019-2854-3.
39. N'Diaye M, Keita BF, Danfakha F, Keita F, Keita G, Senghor CS, Diop B, Diawara L, Bessin F, Vernet C, Barbier D, Dewavrin P, Klotz F. A 12-year follow-up of intestinal schistosomiasis in pre-school-aged children in Assoni Village, Eastern Senegal. Infect Dis Poverty. 2021;10(1):89. https://doi.org/10.1186/s40249-021-00867-8.
40. Nguela RL, Bigoga JD, Armel TN, Esther T, Line D, Boris NA, Frederic T, Kazi R, Williams P, Mbacham WF, Leke RGF. The effect of improved housing on indoor mosquito density and exposure to malaria in the rural community of Minkoameyos, Centre Region of Cameroon. Malar J. 2020;19(1):172. https://doi.org/10.1186/s12936-020-03232-6.
41. Okumu F, Finda M. Key characteristics of residual malaria transmission in two districts in south-eastern Tanzania-implications for improved control. J Infect Dis. 2021;223(12 Suppl 2):S143–54. https://doi.org/10.1093/infdis/jiaa653.
42. Organization WH, Research UBSP, for, Diseases T in T. Global vector control response 2017–2030. World Health Organization; 2017.
43. Pacheco Barzallo D, Pacheco Barzallo A, Narvaez E. The 2016 earthquake in Ecuador: Zika outbreak after a natural disaster. Health Secur. 2018;16(2):127–34. https://doi.org/10.1089/hs.2017.0099.
44. Patil KN, Kaushik SC, Aggarwal A. Evaluation of natural ventilation potential for indoor thermal comfort in a low-rise building in arid and semi-arid climates of India. In: Zhang G, Kaushika ND, Kaushik SC, Tomar RK, editors. Advances in energy and built environment. Singapore: Springer; 2020. p. 203–21.
45. Pulford J, Tandrapah A, Atkinson J-A, Kaupa B, Russell T, Hetzel MW. Feasibility and acceptability of insecticide-treated plastic sheeting (ITPS) for vector control in Papua New Guinea. Malar J. 2012;11(1):342. https://doi.org/10.1186/1475-2875-11-342.
46. Raja S, Dewan A. Implementation of the Right to Healthy Environment: Regulations for running air conditioners in public buildings and recognition of biological pollutants. Res Square. 2022; https://doi.org/10.21203/rs.3.rs-1270717/v1.
47. Ranjha R, Sharma A. Forest malaria: the prevailing obstacle for malaria control and elimination in India. BMJ Glob Health. 2021;6(5):e005391. https://doi.org/10.1136/bmjgh-2021-005391.
48. Rizwan S, Nongkynrih B, Gupta SK. Air pollution in Delhi: its magnitude and effects on health. Indian J Community Med. 2013;38(1):Article 1. https://doi.org/10.4103/0970-0218.106617.

49. Russell TL, Farlow R, Min M, Espino E, Mnzava A, Burkot TR. Capacity of National Malaria Control Programmes to implement vector surveillance: a global analysis. Malar J. 2020;19(1):422. https://doi.org/10.1186/s12936-020-03493-1.
50. Saha A, Sarker M, Kabir M, Lu G, Müller O. Knowledge, attitudes, and practices regarding malaria control among the slash and burn cultivators in Rangamati Hill tracts of Bangladesh. Malar J. 2019;18(1):216. https://doi.org/10.1186/s12936-019-2849-0.
51. Sanou A, Nelli L, Guelbéogo WM, Cissé F, Tapsoba M, Ouédraogo P, Sagnon N, Ranson H, Matthiopoulos J, Ferguson HM. Insecticide resistance and behavioural adaptation as a response to long-lasting insecticidal net deployment in malaria vectors in the Cascades region of Burkina Faso. Sci Rep. 2021;11(1):17569. https://doi.org/10.1038/s41598-021-96759-w.
52. Santos JPC, Honório NA, Barcellos C, Nobre AA. A perspective on inhabited urban space: land use and occupation, heat islands, and precarious urbanization as determinants of territorial receptivity to dengue in the city of Rio De Janeiro. Int J Environ Res Public Health. 2020;17(18):6537. https://doi.org/10.3390/ijerph17186537.
53. Seger KR, Roth J, Schnall AH, Ellis BR, Ellis EM. Community assessments for mosquito prevention and control experiences, attitudes, and practices—U.S. Virgin Islands, 2017 and 2018. MMWR Morb Mortal Wkly Rep. 2019;68(22):500–4. https://doi.org/10.15585/mmwr.mm6822a3.
54. Shah S. The fever: how Malaria has ruled Humankind for 500000 years. 2018.
55. Sharma R. RTI Request No.: NVBDC/R/E/22/00019. National Centre for Vector Borne Diseases Control; 2022.
56. Siegert K, van Loon W, Gai PP, Rohmann JL, Piccininni M, Näher A-F, Boloor A, Shenoy D, Mahabala C, Kulkarni SS, Kumar A, Wedam J, Gai P, Devi R, Jain A, Kurth T, Mockenhaupt FP. The effect of socioeconomic factors and indoor residual spraying on malaria in Mangaluru, India: a case-control study. Int J Environ Res Public Health. 2021;18(22):11853. https://doi.org/10.3390/ijerph182211853.
57. Singh R, Dewan A. Rethinking use of individual room air-conditioners in view of COVID 19. Creat Space. 2020;8(1):15–20. https://doi.org/10.15415/cs.2020.81002.
58. Singh R, Dewan A. Openability of windows and presence of wire mesh in residences in a New Delhi neighbourhood as a factor of dilution ventilation required for prevention of airborne diseases and vector borne diseases. Cities Health. 2022a:1–8. https://doi.org/10.1080/23748834.2022.2036003.
59. Singh R, Madaan N, Kumar A, Kishore J, Kaipilyawar S, Singh G, Mathur M, Grant M, Dewan A. Mosquito control interventions in the built environment: how the Delhi High Court supported the first step towards the wire mesh policy. Cities Health. 2022a:1–4. https://doi.org/10.1080/23748834.2022.2102179.
60. Singh R, Mondal T, Dewan A. Investigating the effect of an open window vs. A closed window on the concentrations of suspended particulate matter in the indoors with respect to the outdoors. Authorea Preprints; 2022b.
61. Singh R, Dewan A. Air conditioners, airborne infection prevention and air pollution in buildings in New Delhi. Int J Tuberculosis Lung Dis. 2022b;26(3):288–90. https://doi.org/10.5588/ijtld.21.0704.
62. Spears D. AIR: pollution, climate change and India's choice between policy and pretence. HarperCollins India; 2019.
63. THE 17 GOALS | Sustainable Development. n.d.. Retrieved May 15, 2023, from https://sdgs.un.org/goals.
64. Tusting LS, Ippolito MM, Willey BA, Kleinschmidt I, Dorsey G, Gosling RD, Lindsay SW. The evidence for improving housing to reduce malaria: a systematic review and meta-analysis. Malar J. 2015;14(1):209. https://doi.org/10.1186/s12936-015-0724-1.
65. Tusting LS, Willey B, Lines J. Building malaria out: improving health in the home. Malar J. 2016;15(1):320. https://doi.org/10.1186/s12936-016-1349-8.
66. Unified Building Bye Laws for Delhi. 2016. http://119.226.139.196/tendernotices_docs/july2018/COMPENDIUM%20OF%20UBBL%20201605082020.pdf.

67. Urner N, Seržants M, Užule M, Sauter-Louis C, Staubach C, Lamberga K, Oļševskis E, Conraths FJ, Schulz K. Hunters' view on the control of African swine fever in wild boar. a participatory study in Latvia. Prevent Vet Med. 2021;186:105229. https://doi.org/10.1016/j.prevetmed.2020.105229.
68. Van Den Berg H, Da Silva Bezerra HS, Al-Eryani S, Chanda E, Nagpal BN, Knox TB, Velayudhan R, Yadav RS. Recent trends in global insecticide use for disease vector control and potential implications for resistance management. Sci Rep. 2021;11(1):23867. https://doi.org/10.1038/s41598-021-03367-9.
69. Van Eer ED, Bretas G, Hiwat H. Decreased endemic malaria in Suriname: moving towards elimination. Malar J. 2018;17(1):56. https://doi.org/10.1186/s12936-018-2204-x.
70. Vector-borne diseases. n.d. Retrieved May 14, 2023, from https://www.who.int/news-room/fact-sheets/detail/vector-borne-diseases.
71. Waite JL, Lynch PA, Thomas MB. Eave tubes for malaria control in Africa: a modelling assessment of potential impact on transmission. Malar J. 2016;15(1):449. https://doi.org/10.1186/s12936-016-1505-1.
72. Wang F, Meng D, Li X, Tan J. Indoor-outdoor relationships of PM2.5 in four residential dwellings in winter in the Yangtze River Delta, China. Environ Pollut. 2016;215:280–9. https://doi.org/10.1016/j.envpol.2016.05.023.

8 Epilogue: Living with the Invisible—A Manual for the Post-pandemic Built Environment

Raja Singh, Nirupam Madaan, and Anil Dewan

8.1 Introduction: The Awakening to the Air We Share

If the history of public health has taught us anything, it is that the invisible eventually becomes visible, usually through the lens of catastrophe. In the nineteenth century, John Snow made the invisible cholera bacterium visible by mapping the Broad Street pump, fundamentally shifting our understanding of waterborne disease [32]. The twentieth century saw the realization that "miasma" was not the enemy, but that invisible vectors like mosquitoes and microscopic particulates and pathogens in the air were killing us. The COVID-19 pandemic of the early twenty-first century has served as a similarly brutal awakening regarding the air we share in our indoor environments. We have abruptly transitioned from an era where, with liberty taken to state that, buildings were designed primarily for thermal comfort and energy efficiency to an era where the "immune system" of a building—its dilution ventilation and filtration capacity among other things—is a matter of life and death [53].

This epilogue serves not merely as a conclusion to the scientific principles detailed in the preceding chapters, but as a practical manifesto for the future. It bridges the gap between high-level fluid dynamics and the daily decisions made by homeowners, facility managers, teachers, and office workers. We move from the theoretical *R-nought* (R_0) to the practical *reality*. How do we live, work, and play in

R. Singh
Founder/Researcher, The Built, New Delhi, Delhi, India

Former Post Doctoral Fellow, Department of Environmental and Occupational Health, Dornsife School of Public Health, Drexel University, Philadelphia, Pennsylvania, USA

N. Madaan
Department of Hospital Administration, All India Institute of Medical Sciences, New Delhi, Delhi, India

A. Dewan
Department of Architecture, School of Planning and Architecture, New Delhi, Delhi, India

R. Singh et al., *Infection Control in the Everyday Built Environment*, https://doi.org/10.1007/978-981-95-8624-0_8

a world where we acknowledge that every breath we exhale contributes to a shared biological commons?

The following sections translate the rigorous science of bioaerosols, filtration, and ventilation into actionable, "everyday" scenarios. We will dismantle the complex physics of airflow into simple heuristics for safety, focusing first on the domestic sphere—our homes—before moving to workplaces, schools, and public transport.

8.2 The Domestic Fortress: Infection Control at Home

For decades, the home was viewed as a safe sanctuary, immune to the industrial hygiene standards applied to factories or hospitals. However, the pandemic blurred the lines between home, office, and school. Our residences became high-density, multi-functional spaces where the risk of household transmission may exceed that of the community [42]. "Notably, vaccination reduces—but does not eliminate—secondary household transmission risk [29]."As we move forward, the "healthy home" must be redefined not just by the absence of mold or asbestos, but by its ability to flush out metabolic and pathogenic aerosols.

8.2.1 The "Toilet Plume" and Bathroom Hygiene

One of the more overlooked potential sources of indoor contamination can be the bathroom environment. While respiratory transmission is the primary driver of SARS-CoV-2, the potential for fecal-oral and fecal-aerosol transmission could be deemed a possible concern, particularly for pathogens such as Norovirus and potentially SARS-CoV-2 [85].

- *The Science:* When a toilet is flushed without the cover/lid, the turbulence creates a "toilet plume"—a cloud of thousands of aerosol droplets containing fecal matter and possible pathogens. These droplets can rise up to a meter and remain suspended in the air for minutes to hours, or settle on surfaces like toothbrushes and towels [2, 85]. Research has indicated that SARS-CoV-2 RNA can be found in the faeces of infected individuals, even those who are asymptomatic or lack gastrointestinal symptoms [28, 90]. "Beyond bowl aerosols, sanitary plumbing stacks can also aerosolize pathogen-laden air under fault conditions [27]."
- *Real-World Scenario:* Consider a shared apartment or a multi-generational home where one family member is isolating with a mild infection. They share a bathroom. The infected individual uses the toilet, flushes with the lid up, and leaves. Five minutes later, a healthy family member enters to brush their teeth. They inhale the lingering bioaerosol plume and touch surfaces contaminated by settled droplets.
- *Actionable Recommendation:* The "Lid-Down" Protocol.
  - *Behavioral:* The single most effective, zero-cost intervention is to *close the toilet lid before flushing*. This simple mechanical barrier reduces the dispersion of droplet nuclei into the room's air and onto surfaces [85].

- *Engineering:* Ensure the bathroom exhaust fan is functional and, crucially, *leave it running for at least 20 min after use*. Most residential exhaust fans are undersized; extended run times are necessary to achieve the air changes required to clear the plume. If no fan exists, the window must be opened during and after use. The toilet should be passively designed to face the outdoors with louvers for air exchanges while retaining privacy.
- *Hygiene:* Remove personal hygiene items (toothbrushes, towels) from open countertops near the toilet or store them in closed cabinets to prevent fomite deposition [69].

8.2.2 The "Sealed Box" Dilemma: Split Air Conditioners and Bedroom Safety

In many climatic regions, particularly in Asia and the Middle East, the split-unit air conditioner (AC) is the commonly perceived standard for thermal comfort. Unlike centralized HVAC systems that can introduce fresh outdoor air, split ACs typically recirculate 100% of the indoor air to cool it. This creates a "sealed box" effect where metabolic carbon dioxide (CO_2) and viral aerosols accumulate rapidly [78].

- *The Science:* An infected person resting in a bedroom breathes out infectious quanta. In a sealed room with a split AC, there is minimal effective dilution. The viral concentration rises linearly with time. CO_2 levels in such rooms often exceed 2500 ppm overnight, which may indicate that occupants are inhaling a significant percentage of rebreathed air [68]. What is important to note is that it is a common sight to have libraries, public offices, waiting halls where strangers interact to have these recirculation based air conditioners.
- *Real-World Scenario:* In many scenarios, family may often sleep in a single air-conditioned room to save electricity during a heatwave. One parent is pre-symptomatic. By morning, the probability of cumulative exposure can become substantial for the spouse and children due to 8 h of breathing recycled, virus-laden air. This is especially in issue in slums. But, the bigger issue is public spaces where split air conditioners are used due to easy procurement by repeat order. In these spaces one large space has multiple stand alone split air conditioners attached and all the windows are sealed.
- *Actionable Recommendation:* Hybrid ventilation (The "Crack-Open" Method).
  - *Operational:* We must abandon the notion that AC rooms must be hermetically sealed. The recommendation is to run the split AC for thermal comfort but keep a window or door partially open, especially in circumstances when the room is used by more than one person, and if there are strangers, who may be unknowingly infected by an airborne spreading disease [76, 77].
  - *Mechanism:* This introduces a "leak" in the system. While it slightly increases energy consumption (cooling load), it induces necessary air exchange. If a ceiling fan is also running, it aids in mixing the air, preventing stagnant viral pockets and encouraging dilution through the open aperture [37]. Though, it

may be true that many ACs sold may be oversized in terms of capacity and the energy consumption increase may actually be less, if properly studied.

- *Monitoring:* Install a low-cost NDIR (non-dispersive infrared) CO_2 monitor in the bedroom. Aim to keep levels below 800–1000 ppm (Ideally below 500 ppm). If the alarm triggers, open the window further. The CO_2 monitor acts as the "fuel gauge" or a surrogate for your home's air freshness [62].

8.2.3 The Kitchen as a Negative Pressure Zone

Kitchens are often sources of particulate matter ($PM_{2.5}$) from cooking, but they can also be engineered to protect the home from cross-infection. This depends upon the location of the kitchen and other parameters which work case to case, but in general can be stated as follows:

- *The Science:* Exhaust fans or range hoods in kitchens expel air outdoors. This depressurizes the kitchen relative to the rest of the house.
- *Real-World Scenario:* A family member is isolating in a bedroom but needs to enter common areas. Or, guests are visiting, and the host is cooking.
- *Actionable Recommendation:* Use the kitchen exhaust to create directional airflow. When guests are present, or when a sick family member opens their door, run the kitchen exhaust on high. Open a window in a *clean* zone (e.g., the living room). Air will flow from the clean zone, through the house, and out of the kitchen exhaust, sweeping contaminants away rather than letting them stagnate [57]. Alternatively, simply have compartmentalisation in spaces such that each room may have independent windows and cross-ventilation, as this will be most suitable for most Indian situations.

8.3 The Threshold of Safety: Understanding "Clean" Air

A recurring theme in this book has been the definition of "clean" air. Historically, this may have meant air free of offensive odors or industrial dust. The new definition must include "infection resilience"—the capability of an environment to mitigate the transmission of airborne pathogens.

8.3.1 The "6 ACH" Target

For healthcare settings, the CDC recommends 6–12 air changes per hour (ACH) [11, 58]. In a typical home, natural ventilation might provide only 0.5–1.5 ACH when windows are closed [83]. To make a home infection-resilient, we may not need hospital-grade infrastructure, but we need to aim higher than the status quo.

- *Tip:* Achieving 6 ACH in a home solely through mechanical means is expensive and noisy. The most practical approach for the layperson is *cross-ventilation*. Opening windows on *opposite* sides of a room/home creates a pressure differential that can under favorable wind and temperature conditions achieve very high exchange rates (may even reach 10–20 ACH), rapidly flushing out viral aerosols [17]. From a fluid-mechanics perspective, the benefit comes from enhanced mixing and dilution, which lowers far-field concentrations and the rebreathed fraction [8].
- *Protocol:* Implement a "Flush Out" cycle. If visitors leave your home, or before a vulnerable person enters a room, open all windows and doors for 10–15 min. This creates a rapid decay of airborne contaminants, resetting the risk level [10, 13].

8.3.2 Filtration: The HEPA Standard

When outdoor air is polluted (e.g., wildfires, urban smog) or weather prevents window opening, we must rely on cleaning the indoor air.

- *The Science:* SARS-CoV-2 and other viruses travel in respiratory aerosols ranging from <1 micron to >100 microns. While the naked virus is tiny (~0.1 micron), it is almost always carried in larger respiratory fluid droplets. HEPA (high-efficiency particulate air) filters are rated to capture 99.97% of particles at 0.3 micron, which is the most penetrating particle size; they may actually be *more* efficient at capturing smaller (diffusion) and larger (impaction) particles [60].
- *Actionable Recommendation:* Portable air cleaners (PACs).
  - *Selection:* Buy a HEPA-based cleaner. Avoid only "ionizers," "plasma," or "ozone-generating" cleaners, which are believed to produce byproducts believed to be harmful like ozone or formaldehyde, etc. [94].
  - *Placement:* Place the unit in the center of the room or in proximity to the occupants, not ideally hidden in a corner. Ensure the clean air delivery rate (CADR) is appropriate for the room size (aiming for at least the "two-thirds" rule: the CADR (in CFM, etc) should be at least two-thirds of the room's floor area in square feet) [3]. The actual calculation should be done based on the specifications provided.

8.4 The Sociology of Indoor Hygiene: Navigating Social Scenarios

The hardest part of infection control is often not the engineering, but the social dynamics. How do we implement these measures without destroying the social fabric of our lives?

8.4.1 The "Dinner Party" Risk

Eating requires mask removal. Talking, laughing, and potentially singing (e.g., Birthday Songs) may increase aerosol emission rates by 10–50 times compared to breathing [5, 54].

- *The Solution:* The "Swiss Cheese" defense indoors.
  1. *Ventilation:* Before guests arrive, purge the air. During the event, keep windows ajar/open.
  2. *Filtration:* Run a HEPA filter in the dining room. It reduces the background concentration of aerosols.
  3. *Humidity:* If it's winter, use a humidifier to keep relative humidity (RH) between 40% and 60%. Low humidity (<40%) may cause aerosols to shrink (evaporate) and stay airborne longer, while also drying out our nasal mucosa, making us more susceptible to infection [45, 84]. At the same time, over humidification is also risky as condensation can happen in surfaces. A balance is necessary.
  4. *Duration:* Limit the duration of the riskiest activity (like eating). Move, if possible, to a better-ventilated area (or outdoors) for conversation after the meal.

8.4.2 The "Sick Building" Awareness

We must develop a cultural "sixth sense" for sick building syndrome (SBS) and infection risk. If a room feels stuffy, with smells (of body odour, undried carpets or wall dampness) or has condensation on windows, it may be considered a high-risk environment. These are sensory proxies for poor ventilation and high CO_2 [72].

- *Empowerment:* Carry a portable CO_2 monitor. Just as we check the weather before going out, checking the "weather" of the indoor air should become normalized. If a restaurant reads 1500 ppm, it may indicate that 1 in every ~40 breaths you take has been recently exhaled by someone else [62]. This simple data point allows individuals to make informed risk assessments: stay, leave, or put on a high-quality mask (N95/FFP2).

8.5 The Return to Work: Re-engineering the Office Ecosystem

As we transition from the domestic sphere to the professional environment, the complexity of infection control increases exponentially. The modern office building is a hermetically sealed machine, designed primarily for thermal consistency and energy conservation rather than biological safety. For decades, the guiding principle of office design was the minimization of air exchange to reduce heating and cooling loads, a legacy of the 1970s energy crisis [83]. This architectural paradigm inadvertently increased the accumulations of indoor pollutants and biological agents, giving rise to the phenomenon known as sick building syndrome (SBS) [30, 48].

In the post-pandemic era, the "healthy office" is no longer a luxury branding exercise but an occupational health and safety imperative. The following sections dissect the risks inherent in shared workspaces and offer evidence-based strategies for mitigation, drawing on the parallels between SBS and airborne viral transmission.

8.5.1 The "Tight Building" Legacy and the Ventilation Deficit

To understand the risk of viral transmission in offices, one must understand the history of the air we breathe at work. Following the oil embargo of 1973, building codes were revised to seal envelopes and reduce outdoor air intake. Consequently, concentrations of indoor pollutants—ranging from volatile organic compounds (VOCs) emitted by photocopiers and carpets to bioaerosols exhaled by occupants—increased dramatically [41]. A large body of multidisciplinary evidence links higher ventilation rates with lower airborne transmission risk [38].

Research by Sundell et al. [83] and Seppänen et al. [73] established a robust association between low ventilation rates and adverse health outcomes. Specifically, ventilation rates below 10 litres per second per person (L/s/person) are consistently associated with a significantly higher prevalence of SBS symptoms and increased sick leave [73, 83].

- *The Science of "Rebreathed Air":* In a poorly ventilated office, the air you inhale contains a calculated fraction of air that was recently inside the lungs of your colleagues. Rudnick and Milton [68] utilized the Wells-Riley equation to demonstrate that the risk of airborne infection transmission is directly proportional to this "rebreathed fraction," which can be accurately proxied by indoor carbon dioxide (CO_2) concentrations [68].
- *Real-World Scenario:* Consider a "green" certified office building that utilizes demand-controlled ventilation (DCV) to save energy. On a day with moderate occupancy, the DCV system may reduce fresh air intake to maintain CO_2 at 1000 ppm. However, an asymptomatic individual with a high viral load (a super-emitter) enters a conference room. Because the overall building CO_2 is within limits, the ventilation does not ramp up. The viral concentration in the conference room spikes, but the energy-saving algorithm is blind to this biological situation.
- *Actionable Recommendation: Decoupling Ventilation from Occupancy.*
  - *Operational Shift:* Facility managers must override energy-saving protocols during for example critical periods. Ventilation systems should run at nominal speed (design capacity) regardless of partial occupancy. The goal is to maximize the dilution of aerosols, aiming for CO_2 levels closer to outdoor ambient levels (approx. 400 ppm) + 400 ppm, i.e., <800 ppm indoors [57, 62].

- *The "Purge" Cycle:* HVAC systems should be operated for at least 2 h before and after building occupancy. This flushes out airborne droplets (containing possible pathogens) and VOCs that may have accumulated or settled [57].

8.5.2 The Open-Plan Fallacy: Aerosol Dynamics in Shared Spaces

The open-plan office was championed for fostering collaboration, but from an aerobiological perspective, it facilitates the unimpeded transport of aerosols. While large droplets fall within 1–2 m, finer aerosols (<5 microns) behave like a gas, riding thermal plumes generated by body heat and computers, dispersing throughout the zone [44].

- *The Barrier Myth:* A common response to COVID-19 was the installation of glass/acrylic barriers between desks. However, fluid dynamics simulations suggest that while these block ballistic droplets (from a sneeze), they may disrupt airflow patterns, creating stagnant pockets where aerosols accumulate rather than being swept away by the ventilation system [57].
- *Real-World Scenario:* An employee sits in a cubicle surrounded by high plastic shields. The office air supply diffusers are located in the ceiling. The shields prevent the conditioned air from effectively mixing with the air in the cubicle and prevent the exhaust of exhaled breath. The employee is effectively sitting in a bucket of their own (and potentially neighbors') aerosols.
- *Actionable Recommendation: Zonal Filtration.*
  - *Strategy:* Instead of physical barriers that impede airflow, deploy localized air cleaning. Portable air cleaners with HEPA filters placed in high-density zones (e.g., call centers, break rooms) can act as "kidneys" for the room, scrubbing viral particles from the air without relying on the central HVAC system [16, 57].
  - *Calculation:* Ensure the clean air delivery rate (CADR) of the units is sufficient to add 3–6 equivalent air changes per hour (eACH) to the specific zone.

8.6 The Sick Building Syndrome (SBS) Convergence

It is crucial to recognize that the measures required to mitigate SARS-CoV-2 transmission are largely identical to those required to prevent sick building syndrome. SBS is characterized by mucosal irritation (eyes, nose, throat), neurotoxic effects (fatigue, headache), and asthma-like symptoms, often linked to the accumulation of indoor pollutants like formaldehyde, VOCs, and bioeffluents [30, 63].

8.6.1 Neurogenic Inflammation and Chemical Sensitivity

Research by Meggs [47, 48] suggests that chemical irritants in indoor air may trigger "neurogenic inflammation" in some people. This is a process where sensory nerves release neuropeptides (like substance P) in response to irritants, causing inflammation not just in the airway but potentially systemically via "neurogenic switching" [48]. This mechanism explains why poor indoor air quality (IAQ) can be linked to systemic malaise and productivity loss, not just respiratory issues (pending more studies establishing that link) [24].

- *The Convergence:* By increasing ventilation to remove viral aerosols, we simultaneously dilute the chemical irritants that cause SBS. Therefore, the "airborne pandemic-resilient" office is also the "high-productivity" office. The economic argument for enhanced ventilation should thus account for reduced absenteeism from both infectious disease and SBS-related illness [22, 73].

8.6.2 The Role of Humidity

Both viral transmission and SBS symptoms are exacerbated by low relative humidity (RH).

- *The Science:* At low RH (<40%), respiratory aerosols evaporate rapidly, shrinking into smaller "droplet nuclei" that remain suspended in the air for hours [44, 54]. Furthermore, dry air desiccates the mucous membranes of the nose and throat, reducing the efficacy of the mucociliary escalator—our primary innate defense against inhaled pathogens. Conversely, extremely high humidity may favour mold growth, one of key triggers for SBS and asthma [43].
- *Actionable Recommendation: The 40–60% Goldilocks Zone.*
  - Maintain indoor RH between 40% and 60%. This range may contribute to minimizing viral stability, optimizing immune defense, and reducing eye/throat irritation associated with SBS [44, 84]. Though this may also depend on the climate of the region in general.

8.7 The Commute: Transport Hygiene in a Mobile World

Public transport represents a unique challenge: high occupant density, small enclosed volumes, and transient populations. The risk of transmission in buses and trains is well-documented, influenced heavily by ventilation rates and duration of travel [1].

8.7.1 The Bus and Train Microenvironment

Studies analyzing air quality in public transport have shown that CO_2 levels can rise rapidly during peak hours, indicating poor ventilation.

- *The Science:* A study of a COVID-19 outbreak on a bus in China demonstrated that the virus could transmit over distances greater than 2 m, driven by the recirculation of air by the bus's AC system [1, 74]. Environmental sampling has detected SARS-CoV-2 RNA in public buses and subways, consistent with shared-air exposure pathways [55].
- Conversely, trains with high-efficiency filtration and frequent door openings (piston effect) may present lower risks if masks are worn.
- *Real-World Scenario:* A commuter takes a 45-min bus ride. The windows are sealed for AC efficiency. The bus is at 80% capacity. An asymptomatic passenger sits in the rear. The AC system takes air from the rear, cools it, and blows it to the front. The viral load may be effectively distributed to all passengers.
- *Actionable Recommendation: The "Open Window" Policy.*
  - *Behavioral:* Whenever possible, open windows on buses, taxis, and trains. Even a small aperture creates significant air exchange due to the pressure differential caused by the vehicle's movement.
  - *Administrative:* Transport operators should disable recirculation modes on AC systems, forcing 100% fresh air intake, and upgrade cabin filters to MERV-13 or higher where system pressure allows [57]. The same was done by Delhi Metro, which created a layered system based on the time of the day with maximum air changes during early hours when the thermal comfort was not challenged much by the fresh air intake.
  - *Personal:* Commuters should wear high-quality respirators (N95/FFP2) rather than cloth masks on public transport. The high viral load potential in these dense settings overwhelms the limited filtration efficiency of cloth masks [34, 35, 61]. While respirators add physiologic load during exertion, the protection benefit outweighs these costs in high-risk settings [91].

8.7.2 The False Security of Private Vehicles

Carpooling and taxis pose a concentrated risk due to the extremely small air volume of a car cabin (~3 m^3).

- *The Science:* In a closed car with two occupants, CO_2 (and viral aerosols) can rise rapidly, indicating accumulation of rebreathed air and increased potential exposure.
- *Actionable Recommendation:* Cross-ventilation.
  - Open windows on *opposite* sides of the car (e.g., front-left and rear-right) to create a cross-draft that flushes the cabin without blowing air directly from one passenger to another. This must be not be done in a busy traffic intersec-

tion or on days when the outdoor air is heavily polluted (but even then there may be time where infection control will outweigh the issue of pollution entry).

8.8 Practical Protocols for Shared Spaces

To navigate the post-pandemic built environment safely, we must adopt a hierarchy of controls that prioritizes engineering and administrative measures over reliance on individual behavior.

8.8.1 The "Traffic Light" System for Rooms

Just as we use traffic lights for road safety, buildings should employ visual indicators of air safety.

- *Implementation:* Install NDIR CO_2 monitors in all shared meeting rooms and classrooms.
  - *Green (<800 ppm):* Ventilation is likely adequate under typical assumptions. Safer to occupy. This is ideally below 500 ppm.
  - *Yellow (800–1200 ppm):* Ventilation is struggling. Open windows, reduce occupancy, or turn on portable air cleaners.
  - *Red (>1200 ppm):* Ventilation has failed. Vacate the room immediately. This acts as a biological "fire alarm" [62, 68].

8.8.2 Evaluating Air Cleaners: Beware of "Hygiene Theatre"

The market has been flooded with air-cleaning devices, many of which offer dubious protection or generate harmful byproducts.

- *The Trap:* Technologies labeled as "bipolar ionization," "plasma," "hydroxyl radical," or "ozone generating" may often lack rigorous peer-reviewed efficacy data in real-world settings and may produce byproducts, including but not limited to ozone and formaldehyde, which may be lung irritants [57, 94].
- *The Solution:* Stick to *Mechanical Filtration (HEPA)*. HEPA filtration is among the most reliable and well-validated technologies, if maintained properly and if the filter is changed at regular intervals. If viral inactivation is required, *UV-C (ultraviolet germicidal irradiation)* within the ductwork or upper-room fixtures is scientifically validated for ductwork surface, provided it is installed to avoid direct eye/skin exposure [58, 84]. The HEPA filters, if not changed and maintained as per the manufacturer's guidelines, as often is the case in many developing world scenarios, may end up being breeding grounds for more indoor air quality issues, than solving those issues. UVGI inside ducts helps sanitize the

surfaces of the inside of HVAC systems, but may not be able to fully sanitize the flowing air, in the absence of the correct airflow rate and efficacy of the UVGI optimized to such airflow.

8.9 The Educational Imperative: Schools as Resilient Sanctuaries

If the home is the domestic fortress and the office the engine of economy, the school is the cradle of society's future. However, from an aerobiological perspective, schools represent a unique and formidable challenge. They are characterized by high occupant density, prolonged exposure times, vocalization (teaching and peer interaction), and a population that may be less compliant with strict hygiene protocols than adults. The COVID-19 pandemic forced a global re-evaluation of the school environment, shifting the focus from "energy-efficient classrooms" to "infection-resilient learning spaces" [19].

This section applies the physics of airflow and the biology of transmission to the educational sector, offering practical strategies for teachers, administrators, and parents to navigate the "new normal" of school attendance.

8.9.1 The "Winter Classroom" Dilemma and the Wells-Riley Reality

A pervasive scenario in temperate climates involves the conflict between thermal comfort and ventilation. In winter or in cold countries, windows are shut to conserve heat; in summer, they are often shut to retain air-conditioned cooling. This creates a "sealed box" effect.

- *The Science:* The risk of airborne infection in a classroom is governed by the Wells-Riley equation. The probability of infection increases with the number of infectors, the quanta generation rate (q), and the time of exposure (t), and decreases with the volume of clean air supplied (Q) [68]. Children, while often having smaller lung capacities than adults, have higher respiratory rates and, in school settings, engage in high-emission activities like singing, shouting, or loud talking, which can increase aerosol emission rates by orders of magnitude compared to quiet breathing [5].
- *Real-World Scenario:* It is November. A classroom of 30 students is heated to 22 °C with windows closed. The ventilation relies on infiltration (cracks in the building envelope), resulting in an air change rate of only 0.5 air changes per hour (ACH). Carbon dioxide (CO_2) levels rise to 2500 ppm by midday. An asymptomatic student is present. By the end of the 6-h school day, the "rebreathed air fraction" is high enough that the probability of secondary infection is significant. The same may be applicable for a small conference room or a mini auditorium.

- *Actionable Recommendation: The "Sweater Protocol" and Intermittent Purging.*
  - *Behavioral:* We must culturally reframe thermal comfort. During airborne-based epidemic peaks, it is safer to be slightly cold and ventilated than warm and infected. Schools should encourage students to wear extra layers ("The Sweater Protocol") to allow for window opening even in cooler months. The same is true with summer months and climate-appropriate dressing for summers. This includes rebooking the school dress for summers, where traditional vernacular concepts from dresses may be incorporated so that it provides thermal comfort.
  - *Operational:* If continuous window opening is not feasible due to extreme weather or noise, implement *intermittent purging*. Evidence suggests that opening windows and doors fully for 10–15 minutes between classes (during breaks) can rapidly dilute accumulated bioaerosols and reset the risk level, creating a "sawtooth" pattern of contaminant decay [19].
  - *Monitoring:* Use CO_2 monitors as a proxy for ventilation. A study in Indian classrooms demonstrated that without active ventilation, CO_2 dissipation is slow (0.5 ACH), whereas active measures are needed to meet the National Building Code standard of 5–7 ACH [78]. Keep CO_2 below 800–1000 ppm, ideally below 500 ppm.

8.9.2 The "Silent Spread" in Canteens and Lunchrooms

While classrooms can be managed with masks, lunchrooms present an unavoidable risk: masks must be removed to eat. Furthermore, lunchrooms are social spaces where students talk loudly, projecting aerosols.

- *The Science:* Unmasking removes source control. Loud vocalization increases the release of both large droplets and fine aerosols [5]. In a crowded cafeteria, the "near-field" transmission risk (direct ballistic droplets) and "far-field" risk (aerosol accumulation) both spike.
- *Real-World Scenario:* Students sit face-to-face at long tables. They talk and laugh while eating. A pre-symptomatic student laughs, expelling a cloud of aerosols. The ventilation system, designed for odour control rather than infection control, mixes this air across the room.
- *Actionable Recommendation: De-densification and Directionality.*
  - *Engineering:* Shift from "mixing ventilation" to displacement or natural cross-ventilation where possible. If using HVAC, maximize outdoor air intake.
  - *Administrative:* Implement *staggered lunch times* to reduce occupant density by 50%.
  - *Layout:* Eliminate face-to-face seating. Arrange seats in a checkerboard pattern or all facing the same direction to prevent direct projection of respiratory plumes onto another person's face [93]. This will require some innovation from the teacher's end as it should not compromise with the newer concepts of face to face seating for collaborative learning.

- *Silence:* Encourage "quiet eating" periods, or play music at a volume that discourages shouting but allows listening, reducing the quanta generation rate [5].

8.9.3 Upper-Room Ultraviolet Germicidal Irradiation (UVGI): A Historic Solution

When ventilation upgrades are too expensive or structurally impossible (e.g., older buildings, extreme climates), history offers a solution. In 1942, Wells and Wilder demonstrated that upper-room UVGI could help in preventing measles spread in schools [64, 88].

- *The Science:* UV-C light (254 nm) damages the DNA/RNA of microorganisms, preventing replication. In upper-room UVGI, fixtures shield the occupants below but irradiate the air in the upper zone of the room. Natural convection currents or ceiling fans lift aerosols from the breathing zone into the "kill zone" [21, 59].
- *Actionable Recommendation:* For schools with poor ventilation (<3 ACH), installing upper-room UVGI fans/lights is a cost-effective retrofit. It can provide an *equivalent* of 10–20 ACH in terms of pathogen removal without the energy cost of conditioning outside air [49, 64]. But, this must be borne in mind that airflow may be required so that air is mixed in these rooms for it to reach the UVGI. The risks of UVGI should also be studied and its cost-effectiveness, maintenance in developing world should be studied. It should be used only when ventilation is not an option at all, which is seldom the case.

8.10 The University Context: Dormitories and Shared Living

Universities function like small cities, with high-density living in dormitories (halls of residence) posing distinct risks. The communal nature of bathrooms, kitchens, and social spaces facilitates rapid transmission.

8.10.1 Wastewater Surveillance: The Early Warning System

Unlike individual clinical testing, which is reactive and resource-intensive, wastewater surveillance may offer a proactive, aggregate view of infection on campus.

- *The Science:* SARS-CoV-2 and other pathogens are shed in faeces, often days before symptoms appear or in asymptomatic individuals [90]. Detection of viral RNA in sewage can serve as a leading indicator of outbreaks.
- *Real-World Scenario:* A university dormitory houses 500 students. Clinical testing is voluntary. An outbreak begins, but students are asymptomatic or attribute

mild symptoms to hangovers/allergies. By the time the first student seeks a test, the virus has spread to 50 others.

- *Actionable Recommendation: The "Sewage Signal".*
  - Universities should consider implementing wastewater monitoring at the building level (dorms), in line with the national protocols and latest updates on this method. A positive signal in the wastewater of a specific dorm triggers targeted clinical testing (pool testing) of all residents in that building [7, 26]. This method has been successfully used to identify and isolate asymptomatic carriers before widespread community transmission occurs [29].

8.10.2 The Social Network Factor

Transmission in universities is driven not just by location but by social networks. Students cluster by course, sports team, and social groups.

- *The Science:* Contact tracing studies show that transmission is highly clustered (superspreading events). "Hybrid" transmission routes—involving both close contact and shared air—are common in social gatherings [39].
- *Actionable Recommendation: Pods and Bubbles.*
  - Create "social pods" or "bubbles" of students who live and socialize together. If infection occurs, it is contained within the pod. This requires administrative support to align housing assignments with social or academic cohorts [89]. Alternatively, across the board have more cross ventilation and outdoor activities so that even within these pods transmission can decrease.

8.11 Active Transport: The School Run Reimagined

The journey to school or university is often as risky as the destination. Public buses and carpools represent enclosed, high-density environments.

- *The Science:* Studies of particulate matter (PM) and viral transmission in transport suggest that private cars and buses can accumulate high viral loads if windows are closed [93]. Conversely, active transport (walking, cycling) occurs outdoors, where infinite dilution virtually eliminates long-range airborne transmission.
- *Real-World Scenario:* A parent drives three children from different households to school in a car with windows up. One child is infectious. The small volume of the car cabin (~3 m^3) leads to rapid saturation of the air with viral aerosols.
- *Actionable Recommendation: The Walking School Bus.*
  - Promote *Active Transport*. Walking or cycling to school not only reduces infection risk via outdoor dilution but also improves cardiovascular health, reducing comorbidities that worsen COVID-19 outcomes [4, 56].

- *Administrative:* Schools should facilitate "Walking School Buses"—groups of children walking together under adult supervision. This structural intervention simultaneously addresses obesity, pollution, and infection control [79]. If not feasible, naturally ventilated vehicles may be used.

8.12 Specialized Settings: Gyms and Music Rooms

Certain activities inherently carry higher risks due to physiology.

8.12.1 The High-Exertion Risk

Gymnasiums and sports centers involve heavy breathing. During vigorous exercise, pulmonary ventilation rates can increase from ~6 L/min (rest) to >100 L/min. This increases both the *emission* of aerosols by an infected person and the *intake* of aerosols by susceptible persons [20]. Computational and experimental work in indoor sports settings further underscores that ventilation requirements increase sharply during vigorous activity [9].

- *Actionable Recommendation:*
  - *Ventilation:* Gyms require significantly higher ventilation rates than classrooms. If mechanical ventilation cannot be increased, outdoor classes are the safest alternative.
  - *Distancing:* The "2-meter rule" is insufficient for heavy exertion. Aerosol plumes can travel further when expelled with force. Distance should be increased to >3–4 m indoors during high-intensity interval training (HIIT) or cardio classes [9].

8.12.2 The Choir Paradox

Singing and playing wind instruments generate high volumes of aerosols. The Skagit Valley Chorale outbreak is a seminal case study where 53 of 61 attendees were infected during a single rehearsal [50].

- *Actionable Recommendation:*
  - *HEPA Filtration:* In case 100% indoors is the only option, portable HEPA filters should be placed close to the source (the singer/musician) to capture the plume before it disperses. If not, then choir practices may be done in semi open ventilated spaces, as suitable for most Indian school conditions.
  - *Masking:* Use of instrument masks (with slits for mouthpieces) and bell covers for wind instruments can reduce aerosol emission without silencing the music [80].

8.13 The Healthcare Paradox: Visiting the Doctor Without Getting Sick

For the average citizen, the healthcare facility represents a paradox: it is the locus of healing, yet historically, it has also been a primary node of transmission. During the SARS-CoV-1, MERS, and COVID-19 outbreaks, nosocomial (hospital-acquired) transmission played a significant role in amplification events. While Chap. 5 detailed the engineering controls required for isolation wards, this section addresses the *user experience*. How does a patient or visitor navigate a hospital or clinic safely in the post-pandemic era?

8.13.1 The Waiting Room Vulnerability

The waiting area is often the weakest link in the infection control chain of a clinic. Unlike the negative-pressure isolation rooms used for known infectious patients, waiting rooms are often mixed-use spaces where undiagnosed infectious individuals (index cases) share air with susceptible patients (e.g., those with comorbidities or immunocompromised states) [75].

- *The Science:* Research conducted on hospital waiting areas in Delhi highlighted that these spaces often operate at high occupant densities with inadequate ventilation, creating favorable conditions for airborne transmission of pathogens like *Mycobacterium tuberculosis* and SARS-CoV-2. Simulation studies have shown that without specific displacement ventilation or air purification, droplets and aerosols can linger and disperse widely, crossing the "physical distance" barriers typically marked on seats. Furthermore, studies on super-spreading events have demonstrated that a single index case in a poorly ventilated space can infect multiple individuals within a short timeframe, even without direct contact. Air sampling in hospitals has repeatedly detected airborne SARS-CoV-2 RNA, reinforcing the role of shared air in clinical spaces [39].
- *Real-World Scenario:* A patient visits an ophthalmology clinic. The waiting room is small (20 m^2), packed with 15 people, and cooled by a split air conditioner (recirculating air). An asymptomatic carrier is present. The CO_2 level rises to 1500 ppm. After 45 min of waiting, the patient enters the doctor's chamber, but the exposure event has already occurred in the lobby.
- *Actionable Recommendation: The "Wait-Outside" Protocol and PPE Upgrade.*
  - *Behavioural:* If the waiting room appears crowded or stuffy (sensory indicators of poor ventilation), patients should request to wait outdoors or in their vehicle until called via mobile phone. This practice, termed "parking lot waiting rooms," was effectively utilized during the pandemic to de-densify indoor spaces.
  - *Personal Protection:* In healthcare settings, the probability of high viral load is elevated. Therefore, this is the specific environment where upgrading from a cloth or surgical mask to a respirator (N95, FFP2, or P2) provides the most

significant benefit. A systematic review indicated that N95 respirators are significantly more effective than surgical masks in preventing respiratory viral infections in healthcare settings, particularly against aerosolized pathogens. Comparative reviews show N95/FFP2 advantages over surgical masks for aerosolized pathogens, with known tolerability considerations [52].
  - *Administrative:* Patients should embrace *Telemedicine* for non-urgent consultations. The rapid expansion of digital health technologies allows for triage and routine follow-ups without physical presence, thereby breaking the transmission chain entirely for those interactions.

8.13.2 Navigating Shared Medical Equipment

While airborne transmission is dominant, the healthcare environment contains high-touch surfaces. However, the risk from fomites (contaminated surfaces) in these settings is often mitigated by standard cleaning protocols. The greater risk may often lie in "transient" spaces like elevators and public restrooms within the hospital.

- *The Science:* Bioaerosols can be generated from toilet flushing (toilet plume) and can persist in the air of small, enclosed restrooms. Elevators are enclosed volumes where air exchange may be slow; a study of elevator transmission dynamics suggests that infectious aerosols can remain suspended even after the index case has exited.
- *Actionable Recommendation:*
  - *Elevator Etiquette:* Avoid speaking in elevators to minimize aerosol emission. Face the walls rather than other occupants to direct respiratory plumes away from faces. If possible, take the stairs—not only for cardiovascular health but to utilize the typically larger volume of air in stairwells compared to the elevator cab. Switch on the fan, if possible and if not too uncomforting.
  - *Restroom Safety:* Always close the toilet lid before flushing to contain the aerosol plume. Minimize time spent in public hospital restrooms and ensure masks remain on at all times.

8.14 The Retail and Hospitality Sector: Dining and Shopping

The economic necessity of reopening the hospitality sector stands in tension with aerobiological reality. Restaurants and bars pose a unique challenge because the primary infection control measure—masking—must be suspended to eat and drink.

8.14.1 The "Dining out" Dilemma

The outbreak in a Guangzhou restaurant, where families sitting at adjacent tables were infected via the air conditioning airstream, served as a pivotal case study for airborne transmission [40].

- *The Science:* In the Guangzhou case, the air conditioning unit created a recirculation loop that transported viral aerosols from an index case to tables downwind, while those outside this airstream remained uninfected. This demonstrated that in poorly ventilated spaces, "physical distancing" of 1–2 m is insufficient if the airflow pattern carries pathogens further. Furthermore, loud talking in bars can increase aerosol emission rates by an order of magnitude or more, depending on the individual, turning a social gathering into a potential super-spreading event.
- *Real-World Scenario:* A family dines indoors. The restaurant is noisy, forcing diners to speak loudly. Windows are closed for climate control. The ventilation system is mixing air rather than replacing it.
- *Actionable Recommendation: The Acoustic and Airflow Check.*
  - *Acoustics:* Choose venues where music volume is low. High background noise forces occupants to raise their voices (the Lombard effect), exponentially increasing the release of respiratory fluids. A "quiet" restaurant may be biologically safer than a loud one (Context being aerobiology).
  - *Ventilation Awareness:* Prefer "semi-indoor" or outdoor seating (terraces). If indoors, look for open windows or doors. Studies on semi-indoor terraces using CO_2 as a proxy showed significantly better ventilation and lower infection risk compared to fully enclosed spaces. Empirical measurements confirm substantially lower CO_2 (and thus lower rebreathed fraction) on semi-indoor terraces [65].
  - *Strategic Seating:* Avoid sitting directly in the draft of a split air conditioner or wall fan. The air blowing on you has likely passed over other occupants first.

8.14.2 The Shopping Mall Ecosystem

Large modern shopping malls often have centralized HVAC systems with better filtration than small shops, but they also have high occupant density and specific hotspots like food courts and restrooms.

- *The Science:* Large volumes (atria) allow for dilution, but "canyons" or corridors with shops on both sides can trap pollutants. A study on disease transmission in an auditorium (analogous to a cinema or large venue) showed that displacement ventilation (supplying air from the floor) was superior to mixing ventilation in preventing cross-infection, but most malls use mixing ventilation [31].
- *Actionable Recommendation:*
  - *Short Duration:* Risk is a function of *concentration* x *time*. Reduce the duration of shopping trips.

  - *Masking in Transition:* Wear high-quality masks in corridors, elevators, and restrooms.
  - *Avoid Peak Hours:* Shopping at off-peak times reduces occupant density, thereby increasing the effective ventilation rate per person (L/s/person).

8.15 Public Gatherings: Faith, Culture, and Aerosols

Religious and cultural gatherings are essential for societal well-being but are believed to have been the site of numerous super-spreading events (SSEs) [36].

8.15.1 The Aerobiology of Worship

From the Shincheonji Church outbreak in South Korea to the Skagit Valley Chorale in the USA, religious settings often combine high density, long duration, and vocalization (singing/chanting).

- *The Science:* Singing releases aerosols at a rate comparable to coughing. When a choir sings, the viral load in the air increases rapidly. In the Skagit Valley outbreak, an attack rate of >50% was observed despite some physical distancing, proving that shared air in an enclosed room may be the vector. A review of mass gatherings highlighted that such religious events were linked to significant transmission chains globally.
- *Actionable Recommendation: Hybrid Worship and Ventilation.*
  - *Ventilation Protocols:* Religious buildings should implement "purge cycles" (opening all doors/windows) between services. CO_2 monitors should be visible to the congregation; if levels exceed 800 ppm, doors must be opened or occupancy reduced.
  - *Modified Rituals:* Humming or listening to recorded music is safer than communal singing. If singing is essential, it should be done outdoors or while wearing masks.
  - *Shorter Services:* Reducing the duration of the gathering directly reduces the cumulative dose of exposure.

8.16 The "Hygiene Theatre" Trap: Surface vs. Air

Early in the pandemic, the focus was heavily on deep cleaning surfaces (fomites). While hygiene is important, the obsession with surface disinfection at the expense of air quality has been termed "Hygiene Theatre."

8.16.1 The Disinfection-Toxicity Trade-Off

- *The Science:* SARS-CoV-2 transmission is now understood to occur predominantly through inhalation of aerosols. While fomite transmission is theoretically possible, real-world data suggest it is rare compared to inhalation. Conversely, the indiscriminate use of chemical disinfectants (spraying, fogging) introduces volatile organic compounds (VOCs) and secondary pollutants into the indoor air. Exposure to chemicals like quaternary ammonium compounds and bleach can trigger respiratory inflammation and exacerbate conditions like asthma and multiple chemical sensitivity (MCS). Fragranced cleaning products can emit reactive VOC mixtures that aggravate respiratory symptoms [81].
- *Real-World Scenario:* A school "sanitizes" classrooms by fogging them with disinfectant every evening. The windows are kept closed to "let the chemical work." The next morning, students enter a room with residual chemical aerosols. The ventilation is poor. The risk of viral transmission remains high (due to poor ventilation), and a new risk of chemical respiratory irritation is introduced.
- *Actionable Recommendation: Clean Air First.*
  - *Prioritize Ventilation:* Opening a window is more effective against COVID-19 than just wiping down a grocery bag. Resources should be shifted from excessive surface cleaning to HVAC upgrades and air purification (HEPA).
  - *Safer Cleaning:* Use soap and water for surfaces. Reserve strong disinfectants for high-touch healthcare settings. Avoid "fogging" in occupied spaces.
  - *Chemical Awareness:* For individuals with chemical sensitivities, the "new normal" of hyper-hygiene can be exclusionary. Buildings should choose cleaning products with low VOC emissions.

8.17 FAQs: Everyday Infection Control

Q1: Is it safe to wait in a hospital waiting room? A: Hospital waiting rooms can be high-risk areas due to the mix of potentially infectious patients and often inadequate ventilation. To minimize risk, wear a high-quality respirator (N95/FFP2), minimize time spent in the waiting area, and if possible, wait outdoors or in your vehicle until your appointment.

Q2: Are outdoor dining terraces completely safe? A: While safer than indoor dining due to dilution, outdoor terraces are not risk-free. If a terrace is enclosed by plastic sheets or walls (semi-indoor), ventilation can be restricted, allowing viral particles to accumulate. True open-air seating is best.

Q3: Can cleaning surfaces too much be harmful? A: Yes. Excessive use of chemical disinfectants (especially fogging) can release volatile organic compounds (VOCs) that irritate the lungs and may exacerbate asthma or chemical sensitivities. Hygiene should focus on hand washing and targeted cleaning of high-touch surfaces, rather than broadcasting chemicals into the air.

Q4: Why is singing in religious services risky? A: Singing and loud vocalization release significantly more aerosol particles than quiet breathing. In enclosed spaces like churches or temples, this can rapidly increase the viral load in the air, leading to super-spreading events. Outdoor settings for such religious activities should be preferred.

Q5: How can I tell if a room is poorly ventilated? A: Sensory cues include stuffiness, lingering odors (like food or body odor or moist walls or undried carpets) and condensation on windows. A portable CO_2 monitor is a reliable tool; readings consistently above 800–1000 ppm indicate that you are breathing a significant amount of air exhaled by others.

8.18 The Floating Petri Dish: Cruise Ships and Confined Hospitality

Perhaps no built environment captured the public imagination—and dread—during the early phase of the COVID-19 pandemic quite like the cruise ship. These vessels represent a unique intersection of high-density hospitality, complex HVAC engineering, and prolonged exposure durations. From the *Diamond Princess* to the *Grand Princess*, cruise ships served as unintended, "floating laboratories" that provided the world with the first definitive evidence of the transmissibility and severity of SARS-CoV-2. As we move into a post-pandemic era, understanding the aerobiology of these "floating cities" is essential not just for travelers, but for facility managers of any high-density accommodation, including hotels and dormitories.

8.18.1 The *Diamond Princess* Case Study: Ventilation vs. Quarantine

The outbreak on the *Diamond Princess* in February 2020 remains a seminal event in modern epidemiology. Of the 3711 passengers and crew on board, over 700 were infected [66]. Retrospective analyses have revealed that the ship's environment facilitated transmission not merely through fomites or close contact, but through the mechanics of airflow and the failure of onboard quarantine protocols.

- *The Science:* A systematic review of transmission on cruise ships identified that transmission occurred significantly among passengers sharing cabins, but also spread across decks and cabins via crew members and potentially the ventilation system [66]. Genomic sequencing studies of the *Diamond Princess* outbreak showed that linked genomes were found in clusters, but the rapid spread suggested that the ship's HVAC system, which recirculated air to conserve energy (a standard maritime practice to manage humidity and temperature), likely may have contributed, alongside crew movement and close-contact interactions [66, 70].

- *The "Piston Effect" in Corridors:* Cruise ship corridors are often narrow, low-ceilinged, and poorly ventilated compared to open decks. Movement of people and service carts creates turbulent wakes (piston effects) that can transport suspended aerosols from one cabin door to another. Kakimoto et al. [33] noted that food service workers were disproportionately affected, likely acting as super-spreaders or vectors as they moved through these corridors delivering meals during the quarantine period [66].

8.18.2 Recommendations for the Traveler and Operator

For the everyday user considering cruise travel or hotel stays, risk assessment must shift from surface hygiene to air hygiene.

- *Actionable Recommendation: The "Balcony Rule".*
  - *Traveler:* If booking a cruise or hotel room, prioritize cabins/rooms with opening windows or balconies. The ability to induce natural ventilation with marine air (which is generally typically much lower in human-associated pathogens due to high dilution) is the single most effective risk mitigation strategy available to the occupant. Keeping the balcony door ajar may situationally create a positive pressure in the room relative to the corridor, preventing potentially contaminated corridor air from infiltrating the personal living space [66].
  - *Behavioral:* Avoid spending prolonged periods in indoor common areas (casinos, buffets, theatres) where ventilation rates are often variable and occupant density is high. Prefer outdoor decks for dining and socializing.
- *Actionable Recommendation: HVAC Verification*
  - *Operator/Policy:* Operators must upgrade HVAC systems to minimize recirculation. If recirculation is necessary for thermal control, HEPA filtration (H13 or higher) or UV-C disinfection within the ducts is non negotiable. Travelers should explicitly ask operators about their air exchange rates (ACH) and filtration standards before booking. Carbon dioxide levels should be displayed.

8.19 The Forgotten Frontline: Correctional Facilities and Institutional Settings

While cruise ships are voluntary environments, correctional facilities are involuntary, high-density settings where occupants have zero control over their environment. The pandemic exposed the catastrophic vulnerability of prisons, jails, and detention centers, where infection rates often exceeded those of the surrounding communities by orders of magnitude [34, 35]. This crisis highlighted the intersection of architectural neglect, overcrowding, and airborne transmission.

8.19.1 The Aerobiology of Incarceration

Correctional facilities share aerobiological characteristics with cruise ships but lack the ventilation standards. They are characterized by:

1. *Overcrowding:* Occupancy often exceeds design capacity, reducing the effective air volume per person.
2. *Poor Ventilation:* Many facilities rely on outdated HVAC systems or passive ventilation that is often blocked for security or thermal reasons.
3. *Static Population:* Unlike a shop where customers leave, inmates are static receptors, exposed to the same air volume for 24 h a day.

- *The Science:* A systematic review by Kim et al. [34, 35] found that the incidence rate of COVID-19 among people experiencing imprisonment was significantly higher than in the general population. For example, in the United States, the case rate was according to one estimate 5.5 times higher in prisons. The environmental drivers identified included dormitory-style housing (shared air), inability to physical distance, and insufficient ventilation [34, 35]. The review highlighted that outbreaks in these settings are often explosive; once the virus is introduced, the attack rates have been reported to be extremely high in certain outbreaks.

8.19.2 Mitigation Strategies for Institutional Resilience

The solutions for prisons are applicable to other institutional settings like homeless shelters and barracks.

- *Actionable Recommendation: Depopulation and Cohorting.*
  - *Administrative:* The most effective intervention identified was *depopulation*—reducing the number of occupants to increase the effective air volume and physical distance per person [34, 35]. Where this is politically impossible, *cohorting* (grouping individuals by infection status) is essential, but only if the cohorts are aerially segregated.
- *Actionable Recommendation: Engineering Retrofits.*
  - *Upper-Room UVGI:* In crowded spaces where increasing air change rates is infrastructure-prohibitive, upper-room ultraviolet germicidal irradiation (UVGI) may be situationally a highly effective retrofit. As discussed in previous chapters, it creates a "disinfection zone" above occupants' heads, relying on natural convection to clean the air. This is particularly suitable for high-ceilinged cell blocks or dormitories [34, 35, 58].
- *Actionable Recommendation: Universal Masking in Common Areas.*
  - *Behavioral:* Given the inability to distance, high-quality masking (N95/KN95) for both staff and residents is critical during outbreaks. Staff may be the source vectors introducing the virus into the facility; therefore, screening and masking of staff are the primary firewalls [34, 35].

8.20 The Hazards of Renewal: Renovation and Fungal Bioaerosols

As we upgrade buildings for better ventilation, we paradoxically introduce a new risk: the release of dormant pathogens during construction. The renovation of older buildings, particularly to improve energy efficiency (weatherization) or HVAC systems, can disturb microbial ecosystems established over decades.

8.20.1 The Hidden Fungal Reservoir

Buildings are not sterile; they are microbiomes. Moisture damage in walls, ceilings, and HVAC insulation allows fungi like *Stachybotrys chartarum* (toxic black mold), *Aspergillus versicolor*, and *Penicillium* species to colonize building materials [43]. These fungi produce mycotoxins and allergens. When a building is renovated—walls opened, ceilings tiles removed—these spores are aerosolized.

- *The Science:* Mahmoudi and Gershwin [43] detailed how *Stachybotrys* produces trichothecene mycotoxins, which are potent inhibitors of protein synthesis. Inhalation of these toxin-laden spores has been associated in some studies with severe health outcomes, though causality is still under absolute confirmation for pulmonary hemorrhage (in infants), neurotoxicity, and severe immune dysregulation. Studies have shown that the concentration of airborne fungal spores may increase by 1000-fold during demolition or renovation activities if containment measures are not used [15, 43].
- *Real-World Scenario:* An office building undergoes an HVAC retrofit to improve COVID-19 safety. The contractors remove old, water-stained ceiling tiles without containment. Dust containing *Aspergillus* spores rains down onto carpets and desks. When the new high-velocity AC system is turned on, it resuspends this dust. Occupants return to a "safer" building but begin reporting headaches, fatigue, and respiratory irritation—classic sick building syndrome (SBS) triggered by fungal bioaerosols [82].

8.20.2 Construction Hygiene Protocols

To prevent "renovation sickness," strict containment protocols must be followed.

- *Actionable Recommendation: Isolation of Work Zones.*
  - *Engineering:* Construction areas must be negatively pressurized relative to occupied zones to prevent dust escape. HEPA-filtered vacuums or wet mopping must be used for cleanup, never brooms which re-aerosolize dust [43].
- *Actionable Recommendation: Pre-Occupancy Flush Out.*
  - *Operational:* After renovation and before re-occupancy, the building must undergo a "flush out"—running the HVAC system at 100% outdoor air for

several days to dilute VOCs (from new paints/adhesives) and remove suspended particulates [10, 13]. Post-renovation off-gassing can include 2-ethyl-1-hexanol from building materials and floorings [86].

- *Actionable Recommendation: Moisture Management.*
  - *Maintenance:* The root cause of fungal growth is moisture. Any water intrusion must be dried within 24–48 hours to prevent spore germination. Porous materials (drywall, carpet) that have been wet for >48 hours should generally be discarded, not dried [43].

8.21 Future-Proofing Cities: The 15-Minute City and Spatial Resilience

The pandemic has forced urban planners to rethink the fundamental structure of cities. The centralized model—where millions commute to a central business district (CBD) via crowded transport—proved to be a liability. The emerging paradigm is the "15-minute city" or "20-minute neighborhood."

8.21.1 Decentralization as Infection Control

The concept of the 15-minute city is that all essential services (work, school, healthcare, shopping) should be accessible within a 15-minute walk or bike ride from home.

- *The Science:* A systematic review by Zhang et al. [93] and Yang et al. [92] found that population density alone was not the primary driver of transmission; rather, *connectivity* and *mobility* were key. Cities with high mobility flows (long commutes) facilitated rapid viral diffusion. Conversely, decentralized neighborhoods acted as "compartments" that slowed transmission. Faedda et al. [18] highlighted that the 15-minute city model enhances resilience by reducing reliance on crowded public transport and enabling active mobility (walking/cycling), which allows for natural physical distancing.
- *Real-World Implication:* In a future pandemic, a 15-minute city does not need to lock down entirely. If an outbreak occurs in District A, District B can continue functioning because the two are not obligate-linked by a mass daily commute. This is "urban compartmentation."

8.21.2 The Role of Green Infrastructure

Urban design reviews indicate that access to green spaces (parks) is not just a psychological amenity but a physiological necessity during pandemics.

- *The Science:* Gemmell et al. [25] reviewed the impact of the built environment on child health during COVID-19, noting that access to outdoor play spaces was critical for physical activity and mental well-being. Furthermore, outdoor environments provide "infinite dilution" for aerosols.

- *Actionable Recommendation: Reclaiming the Outdoors.*
  - *Policy:* Cities should prioritize the permanent expansion of sidewalks and the creation of "parklets" (converting parking spaces to seating) to allow for outdoor dining and socializing, which is aerobiologically safer than indoor alternatives [18].

8.22 The "New Normal" Checklist for Building Occupants

As we synthesize the lessons from healthcare, transport, hospitality, and the home, a "New Normal" checklist emerges for the everyday user of the built environment. This is a mental heuristic to evaluate any indoor space.

The "S.A.F.E." Protocol for Entering Buildings

1. *S—Smell:* Does the air smell stale, chemically, or musty? (Indicates poor ventilation or mold).
2. *A—Auditory:* Is it quiet enough to speak without shouting? (Loud environments increase aerosol emission; see Section "The Retail and Hospitality Sector: Dining and Shopping").
3. *F—Freshness/Flow:* Can you feel air movement? Is there a supply of fresh air (open windows/doors)?
4. *E—Expanse:* Is there enough volume (high ceilings) and floor area to dilute aerosols and maintain distance?

If a space fails the S.A.F.E. test, the occupant should minimize time spent there or upgrade their PPE (masking).

8.23 Points to Reflect

We have till now extended our journey into the specific, often overlooked environments of ships, prisons, and renovating buildings, and zoomed out to the scale of the city itself.

- *Cruise ships* demonstrated the failure of "recirculation" and the danger of corridors.
- *Prisons* highlighted the lethal cost of overcrowding and static populations.
- *Renovation* reminded us that sealing buildings for energy efficiency must not trap biological hazards like mould.
- *Urban Design* offers a path forward through decentralization—breaking the transmission chains by redesigning how we live and move.

8.24 The Economics of Healthy Buildings: Counting the Cost of "Cheap" Air

For decades, the dominant narrative in facility management and construction has been cost containment. Energy efficiency may have been the primary metric of a building's performance, often achieved by sealing envelopes tighter and reducing the intake of "expensive" outdoor air that required heating or cooling. The COVID-19 pandemic, however, has brutally exposed the false economy of this approach. We have learned that while energy is a line item on a budget, health *is* the budget.

8.24.1 The Price of Pandemic vs. Prevention

The economic devastation wrought by SARS-CoV-2—measured in trillions of dollars in lost GDP, collapsed supply chains, and healthcare expenditures—dwarfs the cost of ventilation upgrades. A report by the Royal Academy of Engineering [67] provides a stark quantification of this reality. Their analysis suggests that in the UK alone, the total societal cost (health, social, and economic) of another severe pandemic could equate to £23 billion per year over a 60-year cycle by one rough estimate. Even in non-pandemic years, the rough approximate cost of seasonal influenza, often driven by indoor transmission, is estimated at £8 billion annually [67].

Contrast this with the cost of intervention. Increasing ventilation rates, upgrading filtration to MERV-13/HEPA, and installing CO_2 monitors represent a fraction of these losses. Fisk [23] estimated that in the United States, improved indoor environments could result in annual savings of roughly $6–$14 billion from reduced respiratory disease, about $1–$4 billion from reduced allergies and asthma, and predictively $20–$160 billion from direct improvements in worker productivity [23]. The post-pandemic economic imperative is clear: investing in "infection-resilient" infrastructure is not a luxury; it is a high-yield insurance policy against future biological and economic shocks.

8.24.2 The Productivity Dividend

Beyond preventing disease, cleaner air makes us smarter and faster. Research has consistently shown a correlation between ventilation rates and cognitive function. Wargocki et al. [87] demonstrated that increasing the outdoor air supply rate in an office significantly improved perceived air quality and the productivity of workers performing text processing and simple addition tasks [87]. Similarly, Seppänen et al. [71] estimated that the potential for productivity gains through improved IAQ is enormous, often exceeding the energy costs required to achieve it by a factor of ten or more [71]. Field data also associate higher outdoor air supply and humidification management with reduced sick leave [51].

In the "new normal," tenants and employees will increasingly view IAQ data as a proxy for safety and management competence. Buildings that can demonstrate verifiable "clean air" via real-time monitoring will command market premiums, while "sick buildings" will face obsolescence and liability risks.

8.25 The Regulatory Horizon: From "Comfort" to "Health"

Historically, older but popular ventilation standards like may have been originally oriented to be designed primarily to control body odours and provide "acceptable" air quality for a majority of occupants [6]. They may not have been explicitly designed for infection control. This paradigm is shifting rapidly.

8.25.1 The Rise of "Guide Values" and Legal Mandates

Courts and tribunals are beginning to recognize the right to breathe clean indoor air. In India, the National Green Tribunal's order (OA 143/2016) mandated the formation of a joint committee to frame standards for indoor air quality in public places, explicitly linking IAQ to the Air (Prevention and Control of Pollution) Act, 1981 [14]. The committee's recommendations move beyond vague assurances to specific, measurable parameters for pollutants/variables like $PM_{2.5}$, CO_2, and total volatile organic compounds (TVOCs) [10, 13]. Case studies of early crisis management highlight how governance agility shapes environmental controls during public health emergencies [12].

Future building codes will likely treat ventilation not just as a mechanical service but as a life-safety system, akin to fire suppression. We can anticipate:

1. *Mandatory CO_2 Monitoring:* Visible displays of CO_2 levels in public spaces (schools, cinemas, offices) to serve as a "traffic light" for occupancy safety [62]. Public places should boast the presence of good air, just like a cinema hall boasts of good sound systems, etc.
2. *Infection-Mode Operations:* Building management systems (BMS) pre-programmed with "pandemic modes" that automatically maximize outdoor air, disable recirculation, and activate UVGI systems when a public health threat is declared [46].
3. *Performance Verification:* A shift from "design-based" compliance (what the blueprints say) to "performance-based" compliance (what the sensors say).

8.26 Final Synthesis: Making the Invisible Visible

This book began with the microbiology of the unseen—the viral capsid, the bacterial spore, the fungal hyphae. It journeyed through the physics of how these entities ride the thermal plumes of our breath and the currents of our air conditioning systems. It explored the engineering of filters, the chemistry of disinfection, and the architecture of airflow.

The overarching lesson is that we are not passive inhabitants of our buildings; we are biological components of a complex, dynamic ecosystem. Every cough, every flush, every turn of a thermostat alters the microbial landscape we share.

8.26.1 The "Building as a Patient"

We must learn to treat our buildings with the same diagnostic rigor we apply to our bodies. Just as we monitor our blood pressure and heart rate, we must monitor our buildings' metaphorical pulse (airflow), pressure (differentials), and metabolism (CO_2 levels). The "sick building" is not a metaphor; it is a diagnosis that requires treatment—sometimes a metaphorical lifestyle change (opening windows), sometimes medication (filtration/UVGI), and sometimes surgery (retrofitting HVAC) [41, 43].

8.26.2 A Call to Action

- *To the Architect:* Design for the unseen. Create spaces that breathe. Prioritize natural ventilation and decoupling of thermal control from air provision.
- *To the Engineer:* Innovate for resilience. Develop systems that can surge ventilation without potentially bankrupting the planet.
- *To the Policymaker:* Regulate for health. Recognize that the air inside a school classroom is as much a public good as the water from a tap.
- *To the Individual:* Be aware. Use your knowledge of transmission pathways to navigate the world safely. Close the toilet lid. Open the window. Wear the mask when the air is stagnant.

8.26.3 Conclusion

Navigating the post-pandemic built environment requires a shift in mindset from just "sterile surfaces" to "clean air." The invisible threat is in the air we breathe. By understanding the physics of aerosols—that they accumulate in stagnant air, disperse with ventilation, and are generated by vocalization—individuals can make informed risk assessments in everyday scenarios. Whether waiting for a doctor, dining out, or attending a place of worship, the principles of *Time, Space, People, and Place* apply: minimize time, maximize space (distancing), reduce people density, and ensure the place is ventilated.

The COVID-19 pandemic was a tragedy, but it was also a teacher. It taught us that the walls we build to shelter us from the elements can, if mismanaged, trap us with our own biological exhaust. But it also proved that we have the tools—scientific, engineering, and behavioral—to make our built environments safer.

We have now seen the invisible. We have mapped the aerosol trajectories and sequenced the viral genomes. The evidence base now is sufficiently strong. The responsibility now lies with us to build a world where the air we share sustains life, rather than threatening it. This is the future of the built environment: resilient, responsive, and radiantly healthy.

Acknowledgments Many thanks to Gaurav Shorey and Abdullah Nisar Siddiqui for their kind support. The authors acknowledge the support provided by the institutions including School of Planning and Architecture, New Delhi, All India Institute of Medical Sciences, New Delhi, and Drexel University. Special thanks to Rajshekhar Pullabhatla and Group Captain P Aanand Naidu of ISAC Centre for Built Environment Policy and Tathatara Foundation. Many thanks to Dr. Arthur L Frank, MD. Many thanks to all the people who supported this work in many ways.

Declarations The authors Raja Singh, Nirupam Madaan, and Anil Dewan declare no conflict of interests or competing interests in this work. There is no involvement of human participants, animals, human or animal tissue. All authors declare that there was no specific financial support received from any organization for the submitted work. All authors declare that they have no financial relationships at present or within the previous 3 years with any organizations that might have an interest in the submitted work. While all care has been taken in ensuring the accuracy of this work, any inadvertent error may be reported at the earliest. The authors acknowledge the use of supervised language learning models/large language models for enhancement of the work, with responsibility lying with the authors. For more information, the corresponding author may be contacted at email rajaresearch@proton.me.

CRediT Statement The following is the CRediT statement which declares the author credits for this chapter:

Raja Singh: Conceptualization, Methodology, Formal Analysis, Investigation, Data Curation, Writing-Original Draft, Writing-Review & Editing, Visualization, Project Administration.
Nirupam Madaan: Conceptualization, Resources, Validation, Supervision, Project Administration.
Anil Dewan: Resources, Validation Supervision.

References

1. Abduljabbar RL, Liyanage S, Dia H. A systematic review of the impacts of the coronavirus crisis on urban transport: key lessons learned and prospects for future cities. Cities. 2022;127:103770.
2. Aithinne KAN, Cooper CW, Lynch RA, Johnson DL. Toilet plume aerosol generation rate and environmental contamination following bowl water inoculation with Clostridium difficile spores. Am J Infect Control. 2019;47(5):515–20.
3. Allen JG, Ibrahim AM. Indoor air changes and potential implications for SARS-CoV-2 transmission. JAMA. 2021;325(20):2112–3.
4. Andersen ZJ, de Nazelle A, Mendez MA, Garcia-Aymerich J, Hertel O, Tjønneland A, et al. A study of the combined effects of physical activity and air pollution on mortality in elderly urban residents: the Danish diet, cancer, and health cohort. Environ Health Perspect. 2017;123(6):557–63.
5. Asadi S, Wexler AS, Cappa CD, Barreda S, Bouvier NM, Ristenpart WD. Aerosol emission and superemission during human speech increase with voice loudness. Sci Rep. 2019;9(1):2348.
6. ASHRAE. Ventilation for acceptable Indoor Air Quality (ANSI/ASHRAE Standard 62.1–2019). American Society of Heating, Refrigerating and Air-Conditioning Engineers; 2019.

7. Betancourt WQ, Schmitz BW, Innes GK, Prasek SM, Brown KMP, Stark ER, et al. COVID-19 containment on a college campus via wastewater-based epidemiology, targeted clinical testing and an intervention. Sci Total Environ. 2021;779:146408.
8. Bhagat RK, Wykes MSD, Dalziel SB, Linden PF. Effects of ventilation on the indoor spread of COVID-19. J Fluid Mech. 2020;903:F1.
9. Blocken B, van Druenen T, van Hooff T, Verstappen PA, Marchal T, Marr LC. Can indoor sports centres be allowed to re-open during the COVID-19 pandemic based on a certificate of equivalence? Build Environ. 2020;180:107022.
10. Central Pollution Control Board (CPCB). (2023a). Minutes of the fifth meeting of the joint committee for Indoor Air Quality (IAQ) management held on March 13, 2023. Government of India.
11. CDC. Guidelines for preventing the transmission of mycobacterium tuberculosis in health-care settings. MMWR. 2005;54(RR-17):1–141.
12. Choi H, Cho W, Kim MH, Hur JY. Public health emergency and crisis management: case study of SARS-CoV-2 outbreak. Int J Environ Res Public Health. 2020;17(11):3984.
13. Central Pollution Control Board (CPCB). Report of the joint committee on indoor air quality management. Ministry of Environment, Forest & Climate Change, Government of India; 2023b.
14. Central Pollution Control Board (CPCB). Report of the joint committee on indoor air quality management (In original application 143/2016 (WZ) with original application 206/2022). Ministry of Environment, Forest & Climate Change, Government of India; 2022.
15. Cooley JD, Wong WC, Jumper CA, Straus DC. Correlation between the prevalence of certain fungi and sick building syndrome. Occup Environ Med. 1998;55(9):579–84.
16. Curtius J, Granzin M, Schrod J. Testing mobile air purifiers in a school classroom: reducing the airborne transmission risk for SARS-CoV-2. Aerosol Sci Technol. 2021;55(5):586–99.
17. Escombe AR, Oeser CC, Gilman RH, Navincopa M, Ticona E, Pan W, et al. Natural ventilation for the prevention of airborne contagion. PLoS Med. 2007;4(2):e68.
18. Faedda S, Plaisant A, Talu V, Tola G. The 15-minute city as a hybrid model for knowledge-based urban development: a systematic review. Int J Environ Res Public Health. 2022;19(13):791656. https://doi.org/10.3389/fpubh.2022.791656.
19. Ferrari S, Blázquez T, Cardelli R, Puglisi G, Suárez R, Mazzarella L. Ventilation strategies to reduce airborne transmission of viruses in classrooms: a systematic review of scientific literature. Build Environ. 2022;222:109366.
20. Fikenzer S, Uhe T, Lavall D, Rudolph U, Falz R, Busse M, et al. Effects of surgical and FFP2/N95 face masks on cardiopulmonary exercise capacity. Clin Res Cardiol. 2020;109(12):1522–30.
21. First MW, Weker RA, Yasui S, Nardell EA. Monitoring human exposures to upper-room germicidal ultraviolet irradiation. J Occup Environ Hyg. 2005;2(5):285–92.
22. Fisk WJ, Black DR, Brunner G. Benefits and costs of improved IEQ in US offices. Indoor Air. 2011;21(5):357–67.
23. Fisk WJ. Health and productivity gains from better indoor environments and their relationship with building energy efficiency. Annu Rev Energy Environ. 2000;25(1):537–66.
24. Fisk WJ, Rosenfeld AH. Estimates of improved productivity and health from better indoor environments. Indoor Air. 1997;7(3):158–72.
25. Gemmell E, Ramsden R, Brussoni M, Brauer M. The impact of the built environment on children's health behaviors during the COVID-19 pandemic: a systematic review. Int J Environ Res Public Health. 2022;19(19):12966. https://doi.org/10.1186/s12966-022-01359-0.
26. Gibas C, Lambirth K, Mittal N, Juel MA, Barua VB, Roark H, et al. Implementing building-level SARS-CoV-2 wastewater surveillance on a university campus. Sci Total Environ. 2021;782:146749.
27. Gormley M, Aspray TJ, Kelly DA, Rodriguez-Gil C. Pathogen cross-transmission via building sanitary plumbing systems in a full scale pilot test-rig. PLoS One. 2017;12(2):e0171556.
28. Gu J, Han B, Wang J. COVID-19: gastrointestinal manifestations and potential faecal-oral transmission. Gastroenterology. 2020;158(6):1518–9.
29. Harris RJ, Hall JA, Zaidi A, Andrews NJ, Dunbar JK, Dabrera G. Effect of vaccination on household transmission of SARS-CoV-2 in England. N Engl J Med. 2021;385(8):759–60.

30. Hodgson M. Indoor environmental exposures and symptoms. Environ Health Perspect. 2002;110(suppl 4):663–7.
31. Huang J, Hao T, Liu X, Jones P, Ou C, Liang W, Liu F. Airborne transmission of the Delta variant of SARS-CoV-2 in an auditorium. Build Environ. 2022;219:109212.
32. Johnson S. The ghost map: the story of London's most terrifying epidemic--and how it changed science, cities, and the modern world. Riverhead Books; 2006.
33. Kakimoto K, Kamiya H, Yamagishi T, Matsui T, Suzuki M, Wakita T. Initial investigation of transmission of COVID-19 among crew members during quarantine of a cruise ship—Yokohama, Japan, February 2020. MMWR Morb Mortal Wkly Rep. 2020;69(11):312–3.
34. Kim MS, Seong D, Li H, Chung SK, Park Y, Lee M, et al. Comparative effectiveness of N95, surgical or medical, and non-medical facemasks in protection against respiratory virus infection: a systematic review and network meta-analysis. Rev Med Virol. 2022a;32(5):e2336.
35. Kim H, Hughes E, Cavanagh A, Norris E, Gao A, Bondy SJ, McLeod KE, Kanagalingam T, Kouyoumdjian FG. The health impacts of the COVID-19 pandemic on adults who experience imprisonment globally: a systematic review. PLoS One. 2022b;17(5):e0268866. https://doi.org/10.1371/journal.pone.0268866.
36. Lee M, You M, Ryoo H. Religious gatherings and COVID-19: a review of the literature. J Relig Health. 2022;61:866–919.
37. Li W, Chong A, Hasama T, Xu L, Lasternas B, Tham KW, Lam KP. Effects of ceiling fans on airborne transmission in an air-conditioned space. Build Environ. 2021;198:107887.
38. Li Y, Leung GM, Tang JW, Yang X, Chao CY, Lin JZ, et al. Role of ventilation in airborne transmission of infectious agents in the built environment-a multidisciplinary systematic review. Indoor Air. 2007;17(1):2–18.
39. Liu Y, Ning Z, Chen Y, Guo M, Liu Y, Gali NK, et al. Aerodynamic analysis of SARS-CoV-2 in two Wuhan hospitals. Nature. 2020;582(7813):557–60.
40. Lu J, Gu J, Li K, Xu C, Su W, Lai Z, et al. COVID-19 outbreak associated with air conditioning in restaurant, Guangzhou, China, 2020. Emerg Infect Dis. 2020;26(7):1628.
41. Lyles WB, Greve KW, Bauer RM, Ware MR, Schramke CJ, Crouch J, Hicks A. Sick building syndrome. South Med J. 1991;84(1):65–75.
42. Madewell ZJ, Yang Y, Longini IM Jr, Halloran ME, Dean NE. Household transmission of SARS-CoV-2: a systematic review and meta-analysis. JAMA Netw Open. 2020;3(12):e2031756.
43. Mahmoudi M, Gershwin ME. Sick building syndrome. III Stachybotrys chartarum. J Asthma. 2000;37(3):191–8.
44. Mao N, An CK, Guo LY, Wang M, Guo L, Guo SR, Long ES. Transmission risk of infectious droplets in physical spreading process at different times: a review. Build Environ. 2020;185:107307.
45. Marr LC, Tang JW, Van Mullekom J, Lakdawala SS. Mechanistic insights into the effect of humidity on airborne influenza virus survival, transmission and incidence. J R Soc Interface. 2019;16(150):20180298.
46. Megahed NA, Ghoneim EM. Indoor air quality: rethinking rules of building design strategies in post-pandemic architecture. Environ Res. 2021;193:110471.
47. Meggs WJ. Neurogenic inflammation and sensitivity to environmental chemicals. Environ Health Perspect. 1993;101(3):234–8.
48. Meggs WJ. Neurogenic switching: a hypothesis for a mechanism for shifting the site of inflammation in allergy and chemical sensitivity. Environ Health Perspect. 1995;103(1):54–6.
49. Menzies D, Popa J, Hanley JA, Rand T, Milton DK. Effect of ultraviolet germicidal lights installed in office ventilation systems on workers' health and wellbeing: double-blind multiple crossover trial. Lancet. 2003;362(9398):1785–91.
50. Miller SL, Nazaroff WW, Jimenez JL, Boerstra A, Buonanno G, Dancer SJ, et al. Transmission of SARS-CoV-2 by inhalation of respiratory aerosol in the Skagit Valley Chorale superspreading event. Indoor Air. 2021;31(2):314–23.
51. Milton DK, Glencross PM, Walters MD. Risk of sick leave associated with outdoor air supply rate, humidification, and occupant complaints. Indoor Air. 2000;10(4):212–21.

52. Mitchell BG, Dempsey K, Stewardson AJ, Friedman D, Cole K, Sim MR, et al. P2/N95 respirators & surgical masks to prevent SARS-CoV-2 infection: effectiveness & adverse effects. Infect Dis Health. 2022;27(2):81–95.
53. Morawska L, Tang JW, Bahnfleth W, Bluyssen PM, Boerstra A, Buonanno G, et al. How can airborne transmission of COVID-19 indoors be minimised? Environ Int. 2020;142:105832.
54. Morawska L, Johnson GR, Ristovski ZD, Hargreaves M, Mengersen K, Corbett S, et al. Size distribution and sites of origin of droplets expelled from the human respiratory tract during expiratory activities. J Aerosol Sci. 2009;40(3):256–69.
55. Moreno T, Rothenberg SJ, Querol X. Tracing surface and airborne SARS-CoV-2 RNA inside public buses and subway trains. Environ Int. 2021;147:106326.
56. Mueller N, Rojas-Rueda D, Salmon M, Martinez D, Ambros A, Brand C, et al. Health impact assessment of cycling network expansions in 7 European cities. Prev Med. 2018;109:62–70.
57. Nair AN, Anand P, George A, Mondal N. A review of strategies and their effectiveness in reducing indoor airborne transmission and improving indoor air quality. Environ Res. 2022;213:113579.
58. Nardell EA. Air disinfection for airborne infection control with a focus on COVID-19: why germicidal UV is essential. Photochem Photobiol. 2021;97(3):493–7.
59. Nardell EA, Keegan J, Cheney SA, Etkind SC. Airborne infection. Theoretical limits of protection achievable by building ventilation. Am Rev Respir Dis. 1991;144(2):302–6.
60. Nazarenko Y. Air filtration and SARS-CoV-2. Epidemiol Health. 2021;42:e2020049.
61. Patterson PD, Mcilvaine QS, Nong L, et al. Masking by health care and public safety workers in non-patient care areas to mitigate SARS-CoV-2 infection: a systematic review. JACEP Open. 2022;3:e12699.
62. Peng Z, Jimenez JL. Exhaled CO_2 as a COVID-19 infection risk proxy for different indoor environments and activities. Environ Sci Technol Lett. 2021;8(5):392–7.
63. Redlich CA, Sparer J, Cullen MR. Sick-building syndrome. Lancet. 1997;349(9057):1013–6.
64. Reed NG. The history of ultraviolet germicidal irradiation for air disinfection. Public Health Rep. 2010;125(1):15–24.
65. Rivas E, Santiago JL, Martín F, Martilli A. Impact of natural ventilation on exposure to SARS-CoV 2 in indoor/semi-indoor terraces using CO_2 concentrations as a proxy. J Build Eng. 2022;46:103725.
66. Rosca EC, Heneghan C, Spencer EA, Brassey J, Plüddemann A, Onakpoya IJ, Evans D, Conly JM, Jefferson T. Transmission of SARS-CoV-2 associated with cruise ship travel: a systematic review. Trop Med Infect Dis. 2022;7(10):290. https://doi.org/10.3390/tropicalmed7100290.
67. Royal Academy of Engineering. Infection resilient environments: time for a major upgrade. London: Royal Academy of Engineering; 2022.
68. Rudnick SN, Milton DK. Risk of indoor airborne infection transmission estimated from carbon dioxide concentration. Indoor Air. 2003;13(3):237–45.
69. Sassi HP, Reynolds KA, Pepper IL, Gerba CP. Evaluation of hospital-grade disinfectants on viral deposition on surfaces after toilet flushing. Am J Infect Control. 2018;46(5):507–11.
70. Sekizuka T, Itokawa K, Kageyama T, Saito S, Takayama I, Asanuma H, Nao N, Tanaka R, Hashino M, Takahashi T, et al. Haplotype networks of SARS-CoV-2 infections in the Diamond Princess cruise ship outbreak. Proc Natl Acad Sci. 2020;117(33):20198–201.
71. Seppänen O, Fisk WJ, Lei QH. Ventilation and performance in office work. Indoor Air. 2006;16(1):28–36.
72. Seppänen O, Fisk WJ. Association of ventilation type with SBS symptoms in office workers. Indoor Air. 2002;12(2):98–112.
73. Seppänen OA, Fisk WJ, Mendell MJ. Association of ventilation rates and CO_2 concentrations with health and other responses in commercial and institutional buildings. Indoor Air. 1999;9(4):226–52.
74. Shen J, Duan H, Zhang B, Wang J, Ji JS, Wang J, et al. Prevention and control of COVID-19 in public transportation: experience from China. Environ Pollut. 2020;266:115291.
75. Singh R. The risk status of waiting areas for airborne infection control in Delhi hospitals. Cureus. 2022;14(3):e23211.

76. Singh R, Dewan A. Bioaerosol spread of COVID-19 and TB in air conditioned spaces: how the court spearheaded the movement in India. J Commun Dis. 2022a;54(1):30–5.
77. Singh R, Dewan A. Air conditioners, airborne infection prevention and air pollution in buildings in New Delhi. Int J Tuberc Lung Dis. 2022b;26(3):288–90.
78. Singh R, Dewan A. Rethinking use of individual room air-conditioners in view of COVID 19. Creat Space. 2020;8(1):15–20.
79. Smith M, Hosking J, Woodward A, Witten K, MacMillan A, Field A, et al. Systematic literature review of built environment effects on physical activity and active transport-an update and new findings on health equity. Int J Behav Nutr Phys Activity. 2015;14(1):158.
80. Stockman T, Zhu S, Kumar A, Wang L, Patel S, Weaver J. Measurements of emission rates of aerosol particles from a wind instrument. Aerosol Sci Technol. 2021;55(3):273–9.
81. Steinemann A. Fragranced consumer products: exposures and effects from emissions. Air Qual Atmos Health. 2016;9:861–6.
82. Straus DC. Fungal contamination in sick building syndrome. Front Biosci. 2011;E3(2):562–80.
83. Sundell J, Levin H, Nazaroff WW, Cain WS, Fisk WJ, Grimsrud DT, et al. Ventilation rates and health: multidisciplinary review of the scientific literature. Indoor Air. 2011;21(3):191–204.
84. Thornton GM, Fleck BA, Fleck N, Kroeker E, Dandnayak D, Zhong L, Hartling L. The impact of heating, ventilation, and air conditioning design features on the transmission of viruses, including the 2019 novel coronavirus: a systematic review of ultraviolet radiation. PLoS One. 2022;17(4):e0266487.
85. Vardoulakis S, Espinoza Oyarce DA, Donner E. Transmission of COVID-19 and other infectious diseases in public washrooms: a systematic review. Sci Total Environ. 2022;803:149932.
86. Wakayama T, Ito Y, Sakai K, et al. Comprehensive review of 2-ethyl-1-hexanol as an indoor air pollutant. J Occup Health. 2019;61:19–35.
87. Wargocki P, Wyon DP, Sundell J, Clausen G, Fanger PO. The effects of outdoor air supply rate in an office on perceived air quality, sick building syndrome (SBS) symptoms and productivity. Indoor Air. 2000;10(4):222–36.
88. Wells WF, Wilder TS. The environmental control of epidemic contagion: I. An epidemiologic study of radiant disinfection of air in day schools. Am J Hyg. 1942;35(1):97–121.
89. World Health Organization. Considerations for school-related public health measures in the context of COVID-19. World Health Organization; 2020.
90. Wu Y, Guo C, Tang L, Hong Z, Zhou J, Dong X, et al. Prolonged presence of SARS-CoV-2 viral RNA in faecal samples. Lancet Gastroenterol Hepatol. 2020;5(5):434–5.
91. Wu S, Harber P, Yun D, et al. Respirator physiological effects under simulated work conditions. J Occup Environ Hyg. 2011;6(4):221–7.
92. Yang L, Iwami M, Chen Y, Wu M, van Dam KH. Computational decision-support tools for urban design to improve resilience against COVID-19 and other infectious diseases: a systematic review. Prog Plan. 2022:100657. https://doi.org/10.1016/j.progress.2022.100657.
93. Zhang X, Sun Z, Ashcroft T, Dozier M, McAllister DA. Neighbourhood design and the transmission of COVID-19 and other respiratory viruses: a systematic review. Health Place. 2022;76:102827. https://doi.org/10.1016/j.healthplace.2022.102827.
94. Zhang Q, Jenkins PL. Evaluation of ozone emissions and exposures from consumer products and home appliances. Indoor Air. 2017;27(2):386–97.

Index

R. Singh et al., *Infection Control in the Everyday Built Environment*,
https://doi.org/10.1007/978-981-95-8624-0

GPSR Compliance

The European Union's (EU) General Product Safety Regulation (GPSR) is a set of rules that requires consumer products to be safe and our obligations to ensure this.

If you have any concerns about our products, you can contact us on ProductSafety@springernature.com

In case Publisher is established outside the EU, the EU authorized representative is:

Springer Nature Customer Service Center GmbH
Europaplatz 3
69115 Heidelberg, Germany

Batch number: 10732090

Printed by Printforce, the Netherlands